D0787582

Arthur S. Elstein, Ph. D.

Professor, Office of Medical Education
Research and Development,
Michigan State University

Howard S. Frazier, M.D.

Professor of Medicine, Harvard Medical School;
Director, Center for the Analysis of Health Practices,
Harvard School of Public Health

Duncan Neuhauser, Ph. D.

Professor of Community Health,
Case Western Reserve Medical School

Raymond R. Neutra, M.D., Dr. P.H.

Associate Professor, School of Public Health,
University of California, Los Angeles

Barbara J. McNeil, M.D., Ph. D.

Associate Professor of Radiology,
Harvard Medical School

Clinical Decision Analysis

Milton C. Weinstein, Ph.D.

Professor of Policy and Decision Sciences,
Harvard School of Public Health,
Harvard University

Harvey V. Fineberg, M.D., Ph.D.

Associate Professor of Health Services,
Harvard School of Public Health,
Harvard University

W. B. Saunders Company
Philadelphia   London   Toronto   Mexico City   Rio de Janeiro   Sydney   Tokyo

W.B. SAUNDERS COMPANY
A Division of
Harcourt Brace & Company

The Curtis Center
Independence Square West
Philadelphia, Pennsylvania 19106

Library of Congress Cataloging in Publication Data

Weinstein, Milton C
  Clinical decision analysis.

  1. Medicine, Clinical—Decision making.
2. Probabilities. I. Fineberg, Harvey V., joint
author. II. Title. [DNLM: 1. Decision making.
2. Diagnosis. WB141 W424c]
RC48.W44 610.69'52 79-66719
ISBN 0-7216-9166-8

Clinical Decision Analysis   ISBN 0-7216-9166-8

Last digit is the print number: 9

To Howard H. Hiatt, M.D.,
who brought us together

A Physician's Foreword

In 1956 a young theoretical nuclear physicist named Freeman Dyson was spending the summer in San Diego, California. He writes in his autobiography as follows:

> In September, the summer's work in San Diego was coming to an end, and I took a bus ride to Tijuana, in Mexico, to buy presents for my family. As I was walking through Tijuana after dark, a small dog ran up to me from behind and bit me in the leg. Tijuana was so overrun with sickly and mangy dogs that there was no chance whatever of identifying and catching the animal that bit me. So I went to a clinic in La Jolla every day for fourteen days to take the Pasteur treatment against rabies. Before giving me the first injections, the doctor there impressed on me forcefully the fact that the treatment itself was risky, causing in one case out of six hundred an allergic encephalitis that was almost as often fatal as rabies. He told me to figure the odds carefully in coming to a decision about the treatment. Consequently having decided to take the shots, I was under some emotional strain for the last two weeks of the summer.

Dyson and his doctor are confronted with a choice; treat or do not treat. Treating runs a risk of harm which the doctor assumes is one in six hundred. The probability that the dog had rabies can only be guessed at. Dyson faces fourteen days of disruption and some financial cost if he chooses the Pasteur treatment. Unlike many patients Dyson is thoroughly familiar with probabilistic reasoning, and the doctor was justified in allowing this patient to choose. Even Dyson, like someone who has placed a large bet at the gambling table, is under strain while he awaits the outcome.

This is but one example of the kinds of decisions that are made in clinical medicine every day. They range from such seemingly minor actions as determining what laboratory procedures to order or what interpretation to place on the results obtained, to the decisions whether or not to perform major surgery that may, in itself, present a substantial risk to the patient. Traditionally, the physician makes decisions on the basis of accumulated knowledge and judgment, with a dash of intuition. There has been a tendency to emphasize "completeness" in the selection of diagnostic tests and procedures so as to avoid criticism from superiors or peers. Consideration of cost has been regarded as irrelevant or close to immoral, and concepts such as cost-effectiveness, cost-benefit, or even probability are not often considered by the clinician in reaching a decision.

We are coming to realize that a more systematic approach to clinical decision making can improve the effectiveness of the physician, and that an appropriate concern for the fiscal health of the patient and society must be considered along with physical and mental well-being.

The analytic tools of decision analysis—incorporating statistics, epidemiology, and economics along with clinical knowledge and humanistic concerns—can greatly enhance the capacity of the physician using them to provide the best of medical care from the resources available. It is such an organized approach that is outlined in this book. It should be recognized that clinical decision analysis does not provide automatic answers, but rather serves as a framework around which to organize one's thinking about a problem. It should assist those with less experience to deal with clinical problems more effectively. It does not replace experience; however, it can be a framework in which added experience can improve clinical decisions. One hopes that these ideas will be a solid foundation for developing that unclearly defined, but highly desired attribute, "good clinical judgment."

FREDERICK C. ROBBINS, M.D.

Dean
Case Western Reserve School of Medicine

President-Elect
Institute of Medicine

A Decision Analyst's Foreword

All entering 800 Master of Business Administration (MBA) candidates at the Harvard Business School, the School where I profess, are exposed to the full array of conceptual topics covered in this book—but, of course, in that course the cases and examples reflect the problems faced by the managerial decision maker. Practically every prestigious MBA program in the country now requires a heavy dose of decision analysis in its core curriculum. If this course were now to be dropped from this core curriculum, there would be a howl of anguish from students, from other faculty, and from our younger alumni. Fifteen years ago, when decision analysis was first introduced into the core curriculum, there was a howl of a different kind: What are those guys trying to do? Decision making is an art, not a science, and you can't automate the mysterious, creative, indescribable insights of the experienced practitioner. Sound familiar? Well, the task of decision analysis is not to displace but to help; and even though it takes time to help and time is precious, I think the effort will be worth it in clinical medicine. Decision analysis may falter not because it will displace the man or woman of experience but because it might demand too much from these experts.

This book is ripe for publication. It could have been written fifteen years ago but it would have fallen flat. Now I sense a change of mood. Fifteen years ago when one of my doctoral students (at the Business School!) wrote a dissertation on the clinical treatment of sore throat, there were only a handful of doctors in the Boston area interested in clinical decision analysis; now in Boston there are two handfuls of proselytizers, scores of interested and receptive practitioners, and still more intrigued, but somewhat skeptical, agnostics. This masterful book will state the case for the introduction of decision-analytical thinking in clinical medicine. To me decision analysis is just the systematic articulation of common sense: any decent doctor reflects on alternatives, is aware of uncertainties, modifies judgments on the basis of accumulated evidence, balances risks of various kinds, considers the potential consequences of his or her diagnoses and treatments, and synthesizes all of this in making a reasoned decision that he or she decrees right for the patient. All that decision analysis is asking the doctor to do is to do this a lot more systematically and in such a way that others can see what is going on and can contribute to the decision process.

Granted that there are dangers in premature formalizations. The mind of the expert is a miraculous synthesizer, and the quality of the decisions made by just gut-feel may be far better than the decision maker's ability to articulate the reasons for his or her decisions. There is a tendency in any formalization to structure the problem by leaving out subtleties because the formalization may not be able to cope with these subtleties. But medical decisions are important enough and repetitive enough for us to try painstakingly to dissect the decision process. In doing this, there are some obvious pluses: we can systematically incorporate objective statistical data; we can elicit and combine the judgments of several experts; we can adaptively and systematically combine the experiences of others; we can calibrate the experts; we can correct for dysfunctional biases; we can elicit the preferences of patients for different medical outcomes. Admittedly, all this can also be done in an informal unstructured process, but then cumulative learning is not as easily communicated to others. Some might look on this change as a sad development: science pushing aside art. Ill-developed scientific reasoning may be worse than accumulated artistic wisdom, but scientific (formalized) reasoning, if documented and constructively criticized, can eventually become a more preferred option—for some medical practitioners and for some medical problems.

In this book you will learn how to structure clinical decision problems, how to systematically formulate the intertwining roles of diagnosis and treatment, how to incorporate hard data and soft intuition in probabilistic calculations, how to formalize the combined objectives of doctor, patient, and society, and how to use analyses to help (not to dictate!) the choice of a final decision. Practically all of you who complete this program of study will learn a new way of thought, together with a new vocabulary that will help you to articulate to yourself and to others important features of clinical decision problems. Even though most of you will not actually personally employ the full quantitative armamentarium of decision analysis, you will be able to synergistically interact with those few specialists who will think and analyze problems in terms of a decision analytic paradigm, and also you will feel more comfortable reading the medical research literature, which, I predict, will increasingly feature decision analysis. Why? Because those doctors who have already taken the time to learn this theory are, for the most part, convinced of its relevance and importance.

This book, written by experts who both know the intricacies of decision analysis and understand clinical practice, should launch a major new development in medical education and practice.

HOWARD RAIFFA, Ph. D.

Frank P. Ramsey Professor of Managerial Economics

Harvard University

Preface

This text was conceived and developed in the Center for the Analysis of Health Practices at the Harvard School of Public Health, an environment that has fostered interdisciplinary research in health care as well as the development of teaching material of which this book is an example. The book had its origins in a set of classroom materials that we developed during the academic year 1974–75. All seven of us participated that year in formulating and teaching an elective course at Harvard Medical School on medical decision making. We were rewarded by several visits to Harvard by Lee Lusted, one of the pioneers in the application of decision theory to medical decision making. It was a unique opportunity to pursue this project which, more than five years later, has reached fruition in the form of this text. The book is truly a multidisciplinary product, representing our collective backgrounds in medicine, statistical decision theory, epidemiology, health services administration, economics, and psychology.

Since offering that first elective course, we have used the contents of this book to help teach decision-analytic concepts to students at many levels of medical education, including second-year medical students, residents, fellows, and practicing physicians participating in continuing medical education. We have also made use of these materials at schools of public health, in courses that stress the cost-effectiveness of medical practices from the societal perspective.

Many colleagues read through the manuscript and offered us much needed criticism and advice. Howard Raiffa and Frederick Mosteller, especially, deserve our thanks for their extraordinarily close reading of an earlier draft and for giving us the benefit of their experience as authors of major texts. Other colleagues who read and commented on drafts include John Bailar, Benjamin Barnes, Peter Braun, Charles Fried, Charles Hatem, Anthony Komaroff, Leighton Read, Herbert Sherman, Robert Stern, William Taylor, and David Young. We also benefited from the reactions and comments of many students, especially Peter Barkin and Deborah Zarin.

The product you see would not have been possible without the contributions of our fellow staff members at the Center for the Analysis of Health Practices. The production of the manuscript proceeded smoothly, thanks to the managerial talents of Eleanor Druckman. Various drafts were typed most capably and energetically by Linda Fasciano, Sue Kaufman, Penny Kefalas, Laurie Pearlman, Najla Salhaney, Carol Weisberg, and Paula Zimlicki. Their careful work made it possible to use interim drafts in our teaching. The arduous bibliographic work for this book was coordinated by Dawn Renear, without whose help we could not have attempted to produce the cross-indexed Bibliography that accompanies the text.

To each of these colleagues and associates, and to the others whom we have almost surely (but unintentionally) overlooked, we offer our sincere thanks. We are also grateful to the Robert Wood Johnson Foundation for the support it has provided to the Center for the Analysis of Health Practices.

MILTON C. WEINSTEIN, Ph.D.

HARVEY V. FINEBERG, M.D., Ph. D.

Boston

June, 1980

Contents

Chapter One

The Elements of Clinical Decision Making

1.1 THE PHYSICIAN AS DECISION MAKER

You are a physician in the practice of internal medicine. One of your patients, a 34-year-old mother of two, comes to your office complaining of urinary frequency and dysuria for the past three days. You immediately suspect a bacterial infection of the urinary tract, although she has had no fever, chills, or flank pain. Findings from her physical examination are normal, and a microscopic analysis of her urine shows only one to two white blood cells per high-power field. You consider taking a culture of the urine for bacterial growth, the results of which will not be ready for two days. Meanwhile, you have to decide whether to start treatment with an antibiotic and, if so, which drug to prescribe. You are aware of the risk of adverse reactions to the drug, but the patient seems anxious to be relieved of her symptoms, and if she does have an infection it could become worse without treatment. If you do not prescribe an antibiotic at this time, you may schedule a return office visit in two days when the results of the urine culture are available and assess the status of the symptoms before you decide whether to prescribe an antibiotic. By waiting, you would be in a position to base your choice of drugs on the results of testing the cultured bacteria for their sensitivity to various antibiotics. Or you may simply schedule a return visit without ordering a culture or prescribing medication to see whether the symptoms resolve. What should you do now? What will you do in two days?

The physician caring for patients is repeatedly faced with decisions, some routine and some complicated. Should I admit the patient to the hospital? Should I order an electrocardiogram, or a barium enema, or a test to determine the bilirubin level, or a radionuclide scan, or another diagnostic test? Shall I operate now or wait to see if the symptoms change? Should I perform an open or a closed biopsy? Should I prescribe an antibiotic before the culture results

1

are back or only afterward? Whatever else they may be doing for patients — examining, reassuring, or curing them — physicians are continually making decisions about the care of their patients. In some clinical situations the decisions seem fairly straightforward, and any well-trained clinician might reach the same conclusions and act the same way. Other situations are more ambiguous, and the decisions are much less clear-cut. The patient's signs and symptoms may not fall into any well-defined diagnostic category, or experts may disagree about the correct diagnosis or the most appropriate therapy. Regardless of whether the clinical circumstances are obvious or exceedingly complex, some decisions, and often many decisions, have to be made. Even in choosing not to intervene — not to order any tests or undertake any special treatment — the physician still makes a decision that carries its own consequences.

UNCERTAINTY IN CLINICAL DECISIONS

Clinical decisions are not only unavoidable but also must be made under conditions of uncertainty. This uncertainty arises from several sources, including the following:

Errors in Clinical Data.   Data gathered from patient histories, physical examinations, or laboratory tests are subject to error. For example, the patient may state one complaint, but the physician hears another. Or a blood sugar level is reported to be 120 mg/100 ml, but the chemistry-analyzer was miscalibrated and the true figure is 105 mg/100 ml. Errors may be due to inaccurate recordings by the observer, faulty observation, or misrepresentation of the data by an instrument or by the patient. The implication is that there is uncertainty surrounding every piece of data, no matter how precisely stated it may be.

Ambiguity of Clinical Data and Variations in Interpretation.   Information obtained by physical examination or a diagnostic procedure may be intrinsically ambiguous and may thus be interpreted differently by different observers. Virtually every visual, auditory, and tactile bit of information from the physical examination varies to some degree in its prominence from patient to patient. Observers may differ in their ability to detect these signs and in their propensity to record them. Furthermore, even physicians who can agree that they feel, hear, or see the same thing or technicians who can assure the accuracy of an observation may apply different perceptual thresholds in determining the presence or absence of some clinical sign.

Uncertainty About Relations Between Clinical Information and the Presence of Disease.   The relations among clinical signs, symptoms, and disease are not the same in every patient. Even if one could accurately and unambiguously determine the patient's clinical signs and symptoms, uncertainty would often remain about the presence or absence of disease. Pathognomonic signs, that is, signs whose presence indicates that a particular condition is undoubtedly present, have been recognized for only a few diseases. Even then, these signs are not typically manifest in very many cases of those diseases and are, therefore, rarely helpful. In a typical situation a symptom or sign often occurs in the presence of the disease in question but may be absent, and that same sign is sometimes present even in the absence of the disease.

Uncertainty About the Effects of Treatment.   Finally, the effects of any treatment are uncertain in any given patient. Even in cases in which a diagnosis can be made with certainty and a preferred treatment is well established, the treatment will still fail in some patients who may be indistinguishable a priori from those in whom the treatment will be successful. The natural history of the disease, that is, what would happen in the absence of intervention, is itself usually uncertain in any particular case.

VALUES AND TRADE-OFFS IN CLINICAL DECISIONS

A characteristic of clinical decisions in addition to uncertainty is the need to make value judgments about which risks are worth taking. Is the risk of mortality from cardiac surgery justified by the possibility of a longer life or an improved quality of life? Are the side effects of antihypertensive drugs justified by the possible prevention of stroke or myocardial infarction? Value judgments and trade-offs concerning the possible outcomes of treatment are made continually, if implicitly. Somehow these value judgments are combined with all of the other information at the physician's disposal in reaching a clinical decision.

THE ART AND SCIENCE OF CLINICAL DECISION MAKING

Making good decisions in the face of uncertainty may be the "art" of medicine, but, like art, it has its own rules and standards and can be studied systematically, learned, and perfected by the application of rational principles.

Medical students and physicians master the "science" of medicine by learning innumerable facts and some theory about normal and diseased biologic processes. Later, they gain experience in the "art" of evaluating and treating patients in a clinical setting, but typically they receive little or no training in systematic methods for making decisions regarding patient care. Clinical decision analysis is intended to complement and enhance, not replace, the clinical judgment that comes only with experience.

1.2   THE LOGIC OF DECISION ANALYSIS

Decision analysis is a systematic approach to decision making under conditions of uncertainty.[114,204] Although decision analysis was not developed specifically to solve problems of patient care, it has been applied to numerous clinical problems, and some have advocated its much wider application in the clinical setting.[190,225] Since decision analysis is designed to deal with "choice under uncertainty," it is naturally suited to the clinical setting.

We believe that decision analysis is a valuable tool for physicians and others concerned with clinical decision making, both for decisions affecting individual patients and for social policy decisions affecting populations of patients. The ability of physicians collectively to command a vast array of powerful and expensive diagnostic and therapeutic interventions carries with it a social responsibility to use these resources wisely.

WHAT IS DECISION ANALYSIS?

Decision analysis is an approach that is (1) explicit, (2) quantitative, and (3) prescriptive. It is explicit in that it forces the decision maker to separate the logical structure of the decision problem into its component parts so that they can be analyzed individually and then recombined in a systematic way to suggest a decision. The analytic process forces the decision maker to consider explicitly the timing of choices that must be made and the data that will need to be acquired to make informed decisions and to identify explicitly the uncertainties involved and the relative values of possible outcomes.

The approach is quantitative in that the decision maker is compelled to marshal evidence and beliefs about the key uncertainties (using the language of probability) and to be precise about the values placed on possible outcomes.

Most important, decision analysis is meant to be prescriptive, not descriptive. It is intended to aid physicians in deciding what they *should* do under a given set of circumstances, so that their decisions will be consistent with their underlying assessments of the structure of the decision problem, of the uncertainties, and of the valued outcomes. Decision analysis, as we apply it, is not meant to describe or model the intuitive thought process of the physician unaided by formal analysis. Psychologic studies of the ways in which physicians think through clinical decisions[61] do provide many instructive lessons, some of which suggest both advantages and limitations of the analytic (as contrasted with the intuitive) approach to clinical decision making.

THE ELEMENTS OF THE DECISION-ANALYTIC APPROACH

The starting point in clinical decision analysis is a decision that must be made on behalf of a patient or a population of patients. In the example that opened this chapter, the decision was twofold: whether to order a urine culture and whether to begin antibiotic treatment immediately. Often, additional diagnostic or therapeutic decisions will follow, and these, too, need to be anticipated at the time of the initial decision. In the example, another round of decisions will be faced when the urine culture results are known and the patient's symptoms have been followed for two days.

The decision-analytic approach entails four basic steps, which are summarized by the flow diagram in Figure 1–1. These four steps are to

I. Identify and bound the decision problem.
II. Structure the decision problem over time.
III. Characterize the information needed to fill in the structure.
IV. Choose a preferred course of action.

We shall consider these one at a time, keeping in mind the clinical decision problem described at the outset of this chapter. That scenario was routine, but its elements will serve to illustrate the approach, which is also applicable to more complicated clinical situations.

Step I: Identify and Bound the Decision Problem

The first step is to define what specifically is the decision problem at hand and what considerations the decision maker wants to take into account in reaching that decision. This step entails breaking the clinical problem down into its component parts, which are of four types:

Alternative Actions.   The decision maker identifies the choices among alternative actions that may be taken with regard to the patient at different

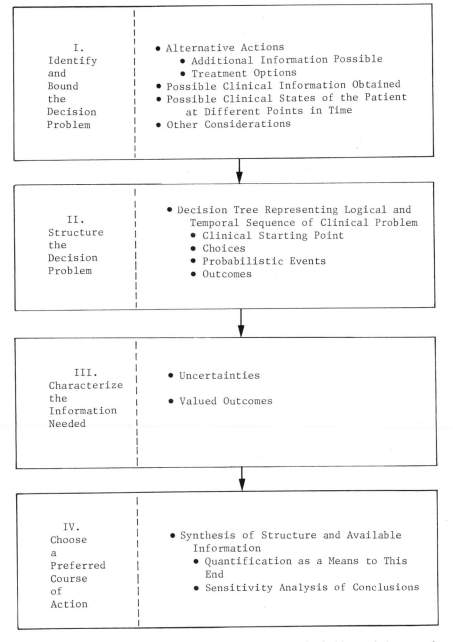

Figure 1–1 The decision-analytic approach.

points in time. One important type of choice is whether to seek additional clinical information (e.g., repeat the urinalysis, obtain a more detailed patient history, do a more extensive physical examination, consult experts on urinary tract infection, do a urine culture). If additional data are necessary, the physician must decide what information is to be acquired and what tests are to be run. Another important type of choice concerns whether to undertake treatment (e.g., treat with antibiotics) and, if it is undertaken, what type of treatment is to be administered (e.g., ampicillin or another antibiotic) and when it is to be altered or discontinued.

Clinical Information Obtained. The decision maker identifies the bits of clinical information that will be available in making the various decisions. This information may include the results of laboratory or other tests (e.g., urinalysis or urine culture), the evolution of a patient's symptoms (e.g., whether the dysuria persists), or the patient's response to treatment (e.g., adverse drug reactions). After considering the information that might bear upon one or more of the choices among alternative actions, the decision maker may go back and amend the list of alternative actions. The changes may take the form of additional options to acquire clinical information or alterations in the timing of their acquisition.

Clinical States of the Patient. The decision maker next specifies the aspects of the patient's health that are of particular concern in this decision context. The clinical states of concern may be the patient's presentation at the outset of a clinical problem (e.g., dysuria); possible worsening or improvement at intermediate stages before, during, and after treatment; and possible final outcomes, such as the relief of symptoms, chronic impairment, or death.

Other Considerations. There may be other considerations that bear upon the decision but do not relate directly to the patient's health. One consideration might be financial costs. Another concern might be the possible effects on future generations of a mutagenic treatment such as radiation.

In practice, the product of this first step of analysis might be simply a list of each of these types of considerations. The structuring of these component parts is the task of the second step.

Step II: Structure the Decision Problem Over Time

The second basic step in the four-step process (Figure 1–1) is to structure the decision problem. After identifying the components of the clinical problem, the decision maker or analyst must structure them in a logical and temporal sequence that clearly displays points at which choices must be made among alternative actions and points at which information is obtained or outcomes are revealed. We emphasize the importance of incorporating time in this structure to highlight the events and information that precede each decision point. The outcomes associated with each possible scenario of actions and events are also specified in this framework.

The product of this second step of analysis is a decision tree, which is a kind of flow diagram that is especially helpful in highlighting the sequential nature of events and decisions over time. The decision tree is introduced in Chapter Two and will be one of the principal tools in our development of decision analysis in subsequent chapters.

Step III: Characterize the Information Needed to Fill in the Structure

The third step of analysis involves identifying the nature of the uncertainties and the valued outcomes associated with the structure of step II.

Uncertainties. The uncertainties in a clinical situation — errors and ambiguity in clinical data and uncertainty in diagnosis and in the effects of treatment — will have been identified in step I and built into a temporally logical structure in step II. It remains to further characterize each uncertain element. The ability to consider these one at a time is a by-product of the process of separating the problem into its elemental units and then restructuring them in a logical way.

For each uncertain element, the decision maker might first seek to understand the factors underlying the uncertainty. For example, what are the chances that the urine culture will be positive? This depends on the chances that a patient who has these symptoms and signs actually has a bacterial infection, on the chances that the culture will detect it if it is present, and on the chances that the culture will be positive in the absence of infection because of contamination of the specimen and limitations of the technique. Focusing on this particular uncertainty, the decision maker will then bring to bear upon this problem the sources of data that might clarify the nature of the uncertainty. The medical literature, consultation with colleagues, and personal experience are all appropriately considered.

We advocate that the decision maker go further and seek quantitative information, using the language of probability, to be more precise about the magnitudes of these uncertainties. Quantitative assessments of probability (e.g., "There is a 10 per cent chance that...") are more specific and less ambiguous than semiquantitative language (e.g., "It is unlikely that..."). Another advantage is that by using the quantitative language of probability it is possible to base decisions upon the most complete use of the information available.

In Chapter Three we introduce the concept of probability as a way of quantifying uncertainties and demonstrate the powerful approaches to decision making that the language of probability makes possible.

Valued Outcomes. The personal values of the patient and the physician regarding possible outcomes come clearly into play in reaching clinical decisions. For example, how does the patient feel about risking an adverse antibiotic reaction in order to improve the chances of an early cure? It is important to identify such values and trade-offs early in the decision-making process so that the attitudes of the patient and the physician can be probed. Trade-offs between various levels of health status and between the quality of life and mortality often come into play. Formal approaches to utility, or value, assessment can be very helpful in probing one's own values about trade-offs involving survival, death, and the eventual quality of life. One important nonhealth outcome, economic resource cost, might also be identified at this step of the analysis if it is relevant to the particular decision.

Step IV: Choose a Preferred Course of Action

The final step — choosing the action to be taken — requires a synthesis of the information generated in step III using the structure of step II. We shall develop two aspects of this synthesis.

Quantification of Uncertainties and Valued Outcomes. In our development of the decision-analytic approach, we shall demonstrate how quantification of uncertainties and also of valued outcomes can be a most satisfactory and appealing aid to synthesizing information. But while we advocate the use of numbers, we do not believe it necessary to express every uncertainty as a numerical probability and every outcome as a numerical utility. Indeed, for many decisions, carrying the formal approach through the first three steps will suggest a preferred course of action even without quantification. When no obvious preferred action emerges, quantification can help clarify one's beliefs and preferences and lead to a logical decision.

Sensitivity Analysis. When a formal structure and quantitative assessments are used, it is usually advisable to do what is called sensitivity analysis.

This is accomplished by systematically varying the different structural assumptions that are built into the decision tree (i.e., factors included or excluded) and the numerical assessments (i.e., probabilities and utilities) to see if the conclusions change.

If the conclusions do not change appreciably when the numbers are varied over the plausible range, this is reassuring. In many cases a decision does not depend on precise estimates of probability or utility. In such circumstances one need not agonize over estimates based on "soft" data. If conclusions do vary with varying assessments, then one should think harder about the probability estimate or utility valuation in question and possibly consider factors previously kept outside the analysis that may sway the issue. Since a decision cannot be avoided, the best estimates will ultimately have to be used, with the salient factors considered, and the decision will have to be based accordingly.

When the decision applies to a population or to a future stream of individual patients, a sensitivity analysis has the additional merit of suggesting areas in which clinical research would be most valuable in resolving the uncertainties that are found to make the most difference in the clinical decision.

WHY DECISION ANALYSIS?

Many physicians think decision-analytically without realizing that they are doing so. Some formalization, especially in complex decisions, may help them to do even better. As you learn about the decision-analytic approach, you will undoubtedly form your own opinion about its merits. Nevertheless, we would like to suggest the following advantages to consider while working through the book. At this point, you may view these as working hypotheses to be evaluated in light of your own experiences in medicine, both with and without clinical decision analysis. We shall return with a more expansive discussion of its advantages and shortcomings at the conclusion of the book in Chapter Ten.

The Importance of Vocabulary.   Decision analysis provides the clinician with a vocabulary and a language that can be used to articulate concerns about a clinical situation. The language of probability and utility can aid communication. Quantification helps to avoid the ambiguities of "semiquantitative" terms such as *rarely, sometimes,* and *almost always.*

The Value of Structuring a Clinical Decision Problem.   Thinking through the structure of a problem may be most profitable to the clinician, even without quantification. Being systematic about the sequence of decisions and observed events, identifying the key uncertainties and the sources of evidence concerning them, and focusing on the key value trade-offs and considering them separately from the uncertainties all may be of value. The key is the breaking-down-and-putting-back-together feature of decision analysis that allows one to focus on one aspect of a complex decision at a time.

Clarifying Medical Controversies.   If controversies were structured in a decision-analytic framework, the nature of the disagreement might become clearer. What do we agree about? (Do we accept the same structure of the problem?) Can we agree about what it is that we disagree about? (Is it a probability assessment or a value judgment?) Can we agree on what further information might bring us closer together? (What clinical studies would we agree to accept as a basis for the currently contested probability assessment?)

1.3 THE ORGANIZATION OF THE BOOK

This book begins with a basic framework that permits the user of decision analysis to work through all four steps of the analytic approach. In Chapter Two the decision tree is introduced as a way of structuring a decision problem over time. Chapter Three presents the language of probability and demonstrates that a decision tree can be used to help make the best clinical decision in situations in which the object is to maximize the probability of some desirable outcome (e.g., cure) or to minimize the probability of some adverse outcome (e.g., death).

While the material presented in Chapters Two and Three represents a complete pass through the four analytic steps, the framework to that point is incomplete and not fully applicable to many clinical situations. The rest of the book unfolds several additional layers of the framework so that it becomes applicable to a wider range of clinical decisions.

Chapters Four through Six are devoted to various aspects of probability in clinical decision making. For example, interpretation of diagnostic tests using probabilities is an extremely important subject, since almost all clinical decisions involve the use of diagnostic information. Chapter Four addresses the use of test information to revise probability estimates for alternative diagnoses. Also included in Chapter Four is an approach to the ubiquitous question of how to draw the line between "positive" and "negative" test results for tests that have no natural dividing line. For example, what level of blood sugar is high enough to warrant treatment for diabetes? The decision-analytic approach leads to an answer that depends on the specific decision context.

Chapter Five goes beyond Chapter Four in addressing the question, What is the value of a clinical test? Decision analysis is used to help assess the value of information obtained from a single test that may be subject to error, the value of multiple tests (e.g., two imaging studies of the renal arteries and not just one, three cardiac enzyme studies and not just one or two), and the value of repeated tests (e.g., repeated blood electrolyte determinations during a hospital stay, repeated blood pressure readings at successive office visits).

Chapter Six raises the difficult issue of the sources of probability estimates. How can a numerical probability be assigned to an event, such as long-term survival from a new surgical procedure, when there is not enough objective evidence upon which to base such an assessment? We will examine the ways in which a clinician can combine both objective and subjective information to derive probability assessments to use in decision analysis.

Through Chapter Six little attention is paid to the difficult problem of assigning values to outcomes, including the values associated with risk taking and with trade-offs among chances at different kinds of health outcome. Chapter Seven addresses the issues of outcome valuation directly and provides both qualitative and quantitative aids to decision making. Using the quantitative approach that is developed in that chapter, we demonstrate how it is possible to generalize the decision-analytic model of Chapters Two and Three to situations in which the outcomes are not only uncertain but also have many attributes.

Through Chapter Seven we will have addressed primarily the problems of the physician who is confronted with a decision for an individual patient. Decisions on the societal level differ in one major respect: Because of insurance, it is uncommon for the individual to pay directly the full cost of medical care, and cost considerations that do not enter into individual doctor-patient decisions are of concern at the level of collective decision making. We reserve for Chapter Eight the introduction of cost and limited resources into the decision-analytic framework. At that point we will extend the method to deal with decision makers at levels beyond that of the individual provider of care who seeks to do the best for each patient.

Having developed the analytic framework as far as is our intent in this introductory text, we devote Chapter Nine to a synthesis of the material by presenting several formal applications of clinical decision analysis.

As you work through this book you will undoubtedly realize some limitations of clinical decision analysis. Indeed, we will address many of them ourselves. We will also point out its strengths relative to more intuitive approaches to medical judgment. We urge you to suspend judgment until the arguments have been fully laid out. Chapter Ten summarizes some of the major strengths and shortcomings of clinical decision analysis, and you may want to refer to that chapter from time to time. The final chapter also discusses some of the ethical implications of clinical decision analysis for medical decisions that involve individual patients as well as decisions that affect society as a whole.

An extensive bibliography of applications, methods, and foundations of clinical decision analysis is provided.

Finally, a word about the clinical examples used in the text. Although most of them have been chosen to be reasonably close to an actual clinical problem, it is often necessary for pedagogic reasons to simplify reality. In each case we shall specify the simplifying assumptions we are making. It is, of course, not our intent to teach the substance of medicine in this book, but we have done our best not to violate it unduly.

1.4 THE OBJECTIVES AND SCOPE OF THE BOOK

We have several objectives in mind as we introduce various techniques and concepts in this book. At one level we expect that the practicing physician reader will have mastered, in an operational sense, the fundamentals of clinical decision analysis. Basic skills, such as sketching a decision tree, revising probabilities, or assessing simple outcome measures, will be presented and reinforced by numerous examples and exercises. At a second level we have tried to introduce the reader to a variety of techniques and ideas that have become a growing part of the medical research literature, but without the intention that these will be mastered by all readers in an operational way. The intent with respect to such topics as multiattribute utility analysis and cost-effectiveness analysis is to give the reader an intellectual appreciation of these ideas as well as the ability to comprehend research papers that make use of them. Some readers, of course, will want to pursue these topics further and may even want to undertake research along these lines; for them, we include in the bibliography several references to intermediate and advanced works on these topics.

At a third level we hope that an understanding of the principles of decision analysis will seep into the subconscious cognitive processes of decision makers at all levels of the health care system and that this may lead to more consistent, and maybe even better, decisions. The theory and methods we develop here offer a systematic approach to the use of information to help make decisions. We believe that the physician will be able to apply the principles presented in practice, without necessarily writing much down on paper, and that with practice the approach will become automatic and natural. While we cannot hope to prove here that the approach and the thought process it fosters will lead to better clinical decisions, it is that objective rather than the dissemination of the mechanics or theory that motivates our pedagogic interest in this area.

Before getting into the substance of clinical decision analysis, we should clarify what this text is *not* intended to offer its readers. First, although a wide range of statistical and analytic techniques have been suggested for application to medical decision making, we concentrate on just one: decision analysis. Although we barely introduce the topic, modern computer technology permits one to use sophisticated machinery in decision analysis, thus allowing more complexity to be introduced into an analysis. In the course of our discussion we shall also introduce some terms and methods that were developed in epidemiology, psychologic theories of perception and cognition, information theory, operations research, and economics, but this text is not intended to be an introduction to any of these important areas.

While many decision-making aids have been advanced, we believe that none offers the medical decision maker a more flexible, practical, and yet rigorously logical approach than does decision analysis. We focus primarily on the essentials of that approach, which, we believe, can be enlightening and useful to the medical decision maker.

Chapter Two

Structuring Clinical Decisions Under Uncertainty

2.1 CLINICAL DECISION TREES

The structure of a clinical decision problem over time involves an often complex interaction of decisions made by the clinician and the unfolding of events, such as test results or changes in the patient's condition. The example of a patient with possible urinary tract infection, which introduced Chapter One and to which we shall return in this chapter, is a case in point. As in virtually all clinical decision problems, some events that occur are within the control of the physician (e.g., ordering a culture, prescribing an antibiotic), and others are beyond the physician's control (e.g., the result of the culture, the patient's response to the antibiotic). The former are what were referred to in Chapter One as actions; the latter are events that, from the viewpoint of the physician at least, are subject to uncertainty.

The **decision tree**, the fundamental analytic tool for decision analysis, is a way of displaying the proper temporal and logical sequence of a clinical decision problem. Its form highlights the three structural components that were described briefly in the first chapter: the alternative actions that are available to the decision maker; the events that follow from and affect these actions, such as the clinical information obtained or the clinical consequences revealed; and the outcomes for the patient that are associated with each possible scenario of actions and consequences.

Our purpose in this chapter is to enable you to build decision trees as a means of systematically modeling the structure of a clinical decision problem. We will also define the concept of a **strategy** as a sequence of contingent clinical decisions over time, and we will use the decision tree as an aid in identifying alternative clinical strategies. In Chapter Three, after introducing the quantitative notion of probability, we will demonstrate how the structure of a decision tree can be used to determine the best strategy for patient care. In this chapter, however, we do nothing quantitative; we concentrate on the structuring of clinical decision problems using decision trees.

As will be our approach throughout the book, we develop the basic concepts in the light of clinical examples, which in this chapter include the management of a patient with possible appendicitis and the management of a patient with suspected urinary tract infection.

OBSERVATION OF A PATIENT WITH POSSIBLE APPENDICITIS

Let us begin by building a decision tree for the management of a patient with acute abdominal pain. As we construct the decision tree for this problem, we will define the structural elements in such a way that it will become evident how virtually any clinical decision may be so modeled.

The appendix, for reasons that are still incompletely understood, may become infected and inflamed and as a result may perforate. The treatment of choice for appendicitis is surgery to remove the appendix. Unfortunately, but not unusually, the signs and symptoms that suggest appendicitis may also occur in other pathologic conditions and are often produced by nonspecific abdominal pain (NSAP), by which we mean a self-limited condition without any notable consequences for the patient. For purposes of discussing this problem we shall consider only the diagnostic possibilities of appendicitis and NSAP. Whether a patient has appendicitis or NSAP becomes more evident from the evolution of symptoms over time, but if surgery is delayed for patients with appendicitis, there is the added risk of perforation and possible death even in otherwise healthy patients. On the other hand, operating on patients with NSAP exposes them needlessly to the risks of general anesthesia and surgery.

A patient comes to the emergency room of a community hospital with signs and symptoms that the chief resident calls equivocal for appendicitis. He decides to consult with the chief of surgery, who agrees that the symptoms and signs are equivocal. She knows that patients with such symptoms and signs often have NSAP and, if an operation is performed, will have had unnecessary surgery. Some such patients, however, have an inflamed appendix which may perforate by the time of surgery. She wonders if it might be beneficial to hold this patient for six hours in the emergency room to see whether the symptoms improve or worsen (or remain the same) before deciding whether to operate. The prime concern of the chief is to give this patient the greatest possible chance of survival. How might she go about structuring and analyzing this problem?

Decision Nodes and Chance Nodes

The approach that we suggest for the chief of surgery begins with sketching a decision tree. Since the decision tree is intended to take particular cognizance of the timing of actions and consequences over time, let us begin at the beginning. By convention, a decision tree is built from left to right. First, the chief of surgery must make a decision: Do I decide now whether to operate, or do I wait six hours to see how the signs and symptoms evolve? This choice becomes the first branching point of the decision tree and is denoted in Figure 2–1. We call such a branching point a **choice node** or a **decision node.** It is represented as a small square with alternative actions branching out to the right.

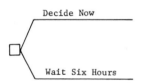

Figure 2–1   The initial choice node in the decision tree for possible acute appendicitis.

Definition. A **choice node** (also called a **decision node**) denotes a point in time at which the decision maker can elect one of several alternative courses of action. It is represented in a decision tree as a small square (□).

Note that the path followed from a choice node is controlled by the decision maker.

Let us follow the upper branch in Figure 2–1 to see where it may lead. Suppose that the chief of surgery were to decide not to wait but to make her choice immediately. The next decision of importance is whether to operate or to send the patient home. This is another choice node, and this further branching is indicated on our expanding decision tree in Figure 2–2.

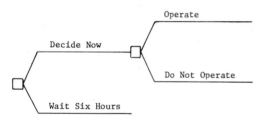

Figure 2–2   The initial sequence of decisions in the management of a patient with possible acute appendicitis.

Again, following the upper branch for the time being, suppose that the chief of surgery decides to operate right away. During surgery it will become known whether the patient actually has appendicitis or NSAP and, if it is appendicitis, whether the appendix has perforated or is just inflamed. This result is uncertain and beyond the physician's control. We call such a branching point a **chance node.** It is represented as a small circle with several possible events branching out to the right.

Definition. A **chance node** denotes a point in time at which one of several possible events beyond the control of the decision maker may take place. It is represented in a decision tree as a small circle (○).

The chance node following the decision to operate is shown in Figure 2–3. Since the same possibilities exist following the alternative decision not to operate, a similar structure is shown for that main branch in Figure 2–3.

The last event of importance is the ultimate outcome to the patient — survival or death. One way to portray this final result is shown in Figure 2–4; another set of chance nodes is appended to each branch to denote the possibilities of survival and death. The outcome to the patient depends then on the result at the last chance node.

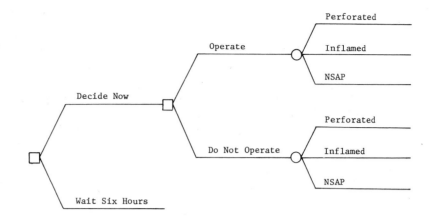

Figure 2–3 *The branching of the decision tree for appendicitis following a decision to decide now.*

Generally, we will associate with each **path** in a decision tree (e.g., decide now → operate → inflamed → survive) an outcome (e.g., survival or death).

Definition. A **path** (also called a **scenario**) in a decision tree is a particular sequence of actions and events beginning with a particular choice at the initial choice node and following a particular event or choice at each subsequent chance or choice node from left to right.

In Figure 2–4, 12 complete paths beginning with "decide now" are represented; of these, 6 lead to the outcome "survival," and 6 lead to the outcome "death." By convention, we denote an outcome at the end of a path by enclosing its description in a box, as shown in Figure 2–4.

Another way to define the outcomes of the decision tree in Figure 2–3 is to assign to each path a probability of death. We will define more fully what we mean by "probability" in Chapter Three. For now, think of the probability of

Figure 2–4 *The complete branching of the decision tree for appendicitis following a decision to decide now.*

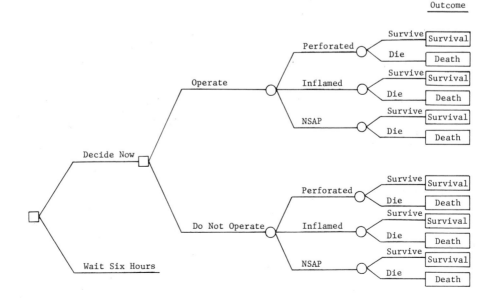

death as the percentage of patients following a given path who die. For example, if the decision is to operate and the patient's appendix is inflamed, the probability of death might be 1 per cent. To simplify the presentation of the decision trees in this example, we will display the branching up to the point shown in Figure 2–3 (rather than the complete branching of Figure 2–4). Implicitly associated with the outcome at the end of each path (e.g., decide now → operate → NSAP) is a probability of death.

Now let us return to the task of structuring this decision problem by following the "wait six hours" branch. The chief of surgery will observe the evolution of the patient's signs and symptoms at the end of six hours. To simplify, consider three possibilities: The patient's condition may worsen, it may remain about the same, or it may improve. What the chief observes is not within her control but is subject to chance, and this branch point is a chance node, as shown in Figure 2–5. This type of chance node is very common in clinical decision problems; it represents the result of obtaining clinical information. Sometimes clinical information comes from a laboratory test, a roentgenogram, or another diagnostic study; often, as in this example, the clinical information comes simply from observation of the patient.

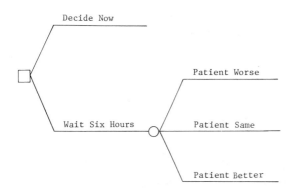

Figure 2–5   The result of the information obtained by waiting six hours.

For each of the three possibilities — worse, same, or improved — what follows next is a decision: to operate or not to operate. These alternatives are represented by choice nodes, as shown in Figure 2–6.

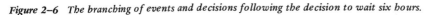

Figure 2–6   The branching of events and decisions following the decision to wait six hours.

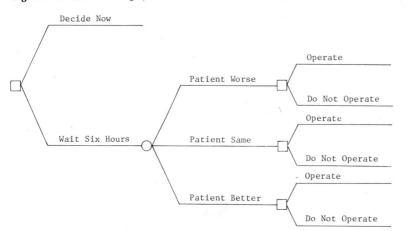

If the decision is to wait six hours and the patient's condition improves, why would the chief of surgery consider operating as a possible action? The answer, of course, is that she would not. If she were going to operate after six hours even if the patient were better, what would the reason for the six-hour delay be? Similar questions could be raised about the option of not operating even if the patient's condition worsens; what would the reason be for not sending the patient home in the first place if the surgeon were not going to operate regardless of the patient's condition? We include these decision nodes in Figure 2–6 for the sake of completeness. In this case, however, it would be perfectly permissible to "prune" the decision tree by eliminating the branches that would never be followed, as shown in Figure 2–7. We will see in Chapter Three how the analysis of this decision tree reinforces the appropriateness of this pruning. In general, if you are considering acquiring clinical information at some risk to the patient or at some cost, then it makes sense to do so only if some subsequent decision might be affected by the information. We shall see another example of this point later in this chapter.

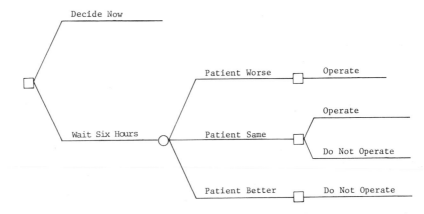

Figure 2–7 *The "pruned" branches at the decision nodes following observation for six hours.*

The complete decision tree for this problem is shown in Figure 2–8. Study it carefully to be sure you understand its logic.

Identifying Key Uncertainties

Each chance node in a decision tree suggests an uncertainty, including in this example the risk of mortality associated with each path. Specifically, in order to evaluate whether it is worthwhile to observe patients for six hours, we need to assess the following:

1. The chances of a patient with an inflamed appendix, a perforated appendix, or NSAP dying (or surviving) with or without surgery.
2. The chances of a patient with equivocal symptoms improving, worsening, or staying the same after six hours.
3. The chances of a patient whose status was originally equivocal having a perforated, inflamed, or normal appendix both at the outset and after six hours of observation.

Information bearing on these issues might be derived from clinical or epidemiologic studies or from informed guesses. We believe that it is appropriate, and

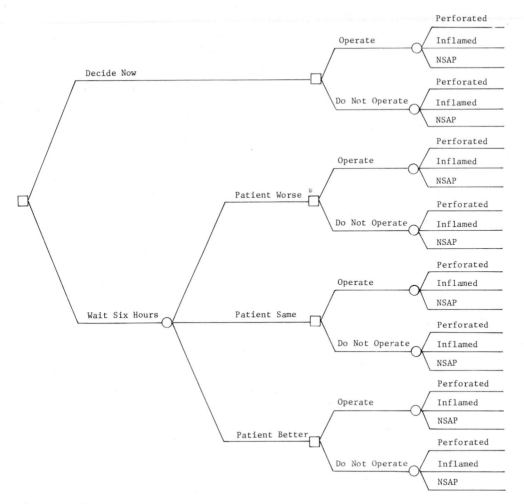

Figure 2–8 *The completed decision tree for a patient with possible appendicitis.*

quite helpful, to use the language of probability to quantify these uncertainties. In the next chapter we shall continue the analysis of this example and assign probabilities to each of the key uncertainties.

Specifying Valued Outcomes

In this example the chief of surgery has specified that she is concerned mainly with the chances of survival. This is the outcome we associate with each path of the decision tree in Figure 2–8. However, other attributes of the outcome may be of concern, such as the length of hospitalization, the nonfatal consequences of possible surgical complications, and even the fear and anxiety of the patient. At this stage, the chief of surgery may wish to make note of these other attributes of outcome, while limiting the formal analysis to her main concern for survival. In Chapter Seven, we introduce methods for incorporating multiple attributes into the analysis.

Foliating the Decision Tree

There is no limit as to how complex a decision tree can become. It is important, however, to simplify in order to get your thinking straight and to permit you to proceed with the tree. Most clinicians make similar kinds of simplifications in their daily practices. Part of the art of clinical decision analysis, as in actual clinical decision making, is to know when to simplify a problem.

It is often valuable, after having made a simplifying assumption, to go back and "unsimplify" a bit to see if the more detailed structure adds any qualitative (or, as we shall develop in Chapter Three, quantitative) insights. We might call this process "foliation," the opposite of "pruning."

In our example one simplification was that the condition of the patient after six hours would be one of three possibilities: worse, the same, or better. A clinician might wish to make finer distinctions among the possible patient presentations; thus, the decision maker might expand the possibilities to seven (e.g., much worse, worse, slightly worse, the same, slightly better, better, much better) or even more. These possibilities would appear as new branches in the decision tree (and we include an exercise to build a more detailed tree in the problem set at the end of the chapter).

The caveat is that, while part of being a good clinician is thinking of all the possibilities, an equally important part is knowing what to think about and what to set aside for the time being. The simpler the decision tree that captures the essence of the clinical problem, the more likely is decision analysis to yield valuable insights.

MANAGEMENT OF URINARY TRACT INFECTION

Let us return to the clinical decision problem presented at the beginning of Chapter One, the 34-year-old mother of two in whom you, her internist, suspect a bacterial infection of the urinary tract. You have to decide whether to begin treatment now with an antibiotic and whether to culture the urine for bacterial growth and test any cultured bacteria for sensitivity to different antibiotics. There is a chance that, even if it is a bacterial infection, the organism may not grow in culture, and if present, it may not be sensitive to your first-choice antibiotic. It is also possible that bacterial growth in the culture will be attributable to a contaminant rather than to infection and that the antibiotic sensitivity test will fail to reflect the true sensitivity of the organism in the urinary tract. The results of the urine culture and the antibiotic sensitivity test will not be available for two days. For purposes of this exercise, we will ignore the risk of side effects from medication. You may also assume that a history has been taken and that a physical examination, a urinalysis, and a Gram stain have already been performed and that none of the findings is contributory to a diagnosis.

To get started on the structure of this decision problem, we take as our interim stopping point a follow-up visit three days after the patient's initial visit, at which time she may or may not feel better.

If you wish, you may spend a few minutes drawing a decision tree for this problem on your own.

The Timing of Decisions and Test Results

Figure 2–9 shows one possible decision tree for the clinical problem just outlined. Study the sequence of chance and decision nodes to see if you agree with the order in which they occur. Notice that two possible antibiotics — A and B — have been introduced. Of course, the decision tree can be expanded to

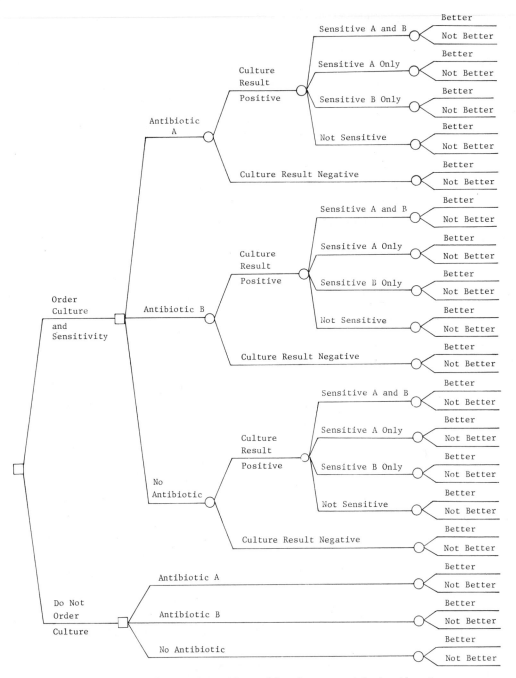

Figure 2–9 *A decision tree for a patient with possible urinary tract infection (days 1 through 3).*

allow for other drugs. In addition, the possible drug reactions in the cases in which antibiotics are prescribed may be included; this can be done by means of another column of chance nodes following the "better" and "not better" branches.

Would it be correct in this problem to list the chance node denoting the culture results *before* the node denoting the choice of antibiotics, as shown in Figure 2-10?

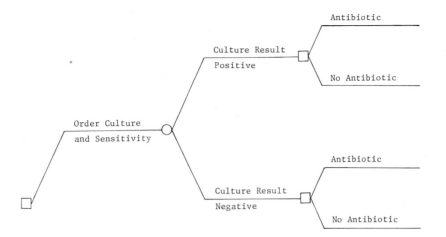

Figure 2–10 An incorrect sequence of chance and decision nodes.

Figure 2–10 would not be an appropriate way to diagram the problem because it implies that the culture results would be known before the first decision of whether to prescribe an antibiotic is made. In an actual situation, culture results would be available only after the first decision about antibiotics has been made. In general, the position of decision nodes in relation to the information available and the relationship between chance events and actions in the tree diagram must reflect the logic and timing of the clinical situation.

Would it be correct in this problem to add a chance node to indicate the presence or absence of bacterial infection following the "culture result positive" branch? The answer, again, is no, because the "true" disease of the patient is not known to the physician at that time. On day 3 the doctor must decide whether to continue the antibiotic or substitute another and whether to reorder the culture, without knowing whether the positive culture is the result of a bacterial infection or a contaminant. In most clinical decision problems, the underlying disease is not known with certainty until after many of the treatment decisions have already been made, even though test results may strongly suggest a particular diagnosis. It is often appropriate to place chance nodes describing test results (e.g., "culture result positive" or "culture result negative") before the next treatment decision (e.g., "continue antibiotic" or "switch antibiotic"), because the test result is known before the decision must be made. However, it would be wrong to draw the decision tree as if perfect knowledge of the diagnosis (e.g., "bacterial infection" or "no bacterial infection") preceded treatment decisions when, in fact, such knowledge is not available prior to the decision.

Sequences of Decision Nodes and Chance Nodes

Notice in Figure 2–9 that the last three branches following the "order culture and sensitivity" strategy are sequential chance nodes. The description of a particular path does not depend in any way on the order in which *adjacent* chance nodes are listed, so that it would have been equally correct to list the "better" or "not better" node before the "culture result" node.

Sequences of *adjacent* decision nodes can be collapsed into a single node without disrupting the logic of the analysis. In the appendicitis example it would be perfectly logical if, instead of portraying the "decide now" or "wait six hours" node and the immediately adjacent "operate" or "do not operate" node sequentially (Figure 2–2), you chose to consolidate them into a single choice node with three branches: "decide now; operate," "decide now; do not operate," and "wait six hours" (Figure 2–11). Note that the structure of the tree to the right of that point would be the same under both variants.

It would not be correct, however, to invert the order of chance and choice nodes (e.g., to put the chance node denoting whether the patient is better, the same, or worse before the choice node concerning whether to wait six hours), since that would change the timing of decisions and the information upon which they must be based.

THE POTENTIAL VALUE OF CLINICAL INFORMATION

Urinary Tract Infection

Before we generalize from these examples, reflect a moment about the potential value of a urine culture in a patient whose signs and symptoms are suggestive of a urinary tract infection. We know that the culture results cannot influence our first decision. If you look back at Figure 2–9, you will notice that as far as the problem is diagramed no decision follows the "culture result" chance node. If this diagram were a complete description of the clinical problem, then taking a culture would be entirely superfluous. (A urine culture presents no risk at all to the patient and so has no direct impact on patient outcome. Also, we are ignoring financial costs until Chapter Eight.)

In fact, the clinical problem extends beyond the diagram of Figure 2–9, and, if the patient is not better, the results of the culture on day 1 can be very helpful to our next decision. For example, the subsequent decision to continue or initiate an antibiotic would depend on the culture results, and the choice of antibiotic would be affected by knowledge of the type and sensitivity of the organism causing the infection.

The lesson here is that, for the purposes of the clinical situation at hand, information can be useful only if it might affect a subsequent clinical decision. The quantitative formulation using probabilities in the next chapter will reinforce this point. This point may not be valid, of course, if the information has research value or if it is obtained for medicolegal reasons.

Figure 2–11 An equivalent formulation of the initial decision nodes of the decision tree for a patient with possible appendicitis.

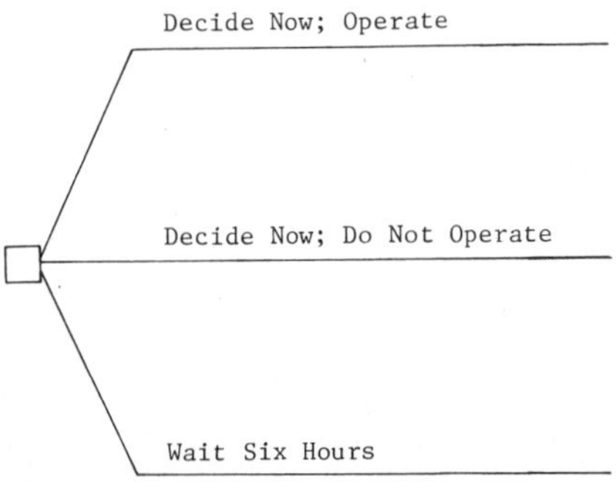

Decide Now; Operate

Decide Now; Do Not Operate

Wait Six Hours

A Culture for Gonorrhea

Consider another example that deals with a possible infection and the question of bacteriologic culture. A 28-year-old woman comes to you because of sexual exposure three days previously to a man who is known to have gonorrhea. She denies sexual contact with anyone else, and your knowledge of her as a patient leads you to believe her. Therefore, you rule out the possibility that she might have exposed anyone else to the infection. After establishing that she has no allergy to penicillin, you decide to treat her with that antibiotic according to the regimen recommended by the Center for Disease Control.

Should you also take a culture for gonococci? In this case, if your only concern is for the physical health of the patient, the answer is no, because you will have administered the definitive treatment before the results of the culture are known. In order for a test to affect a clinical decision, the results must become known prior to the time the decision is made. On the other hand, you may choose to perform such a test in order to satisfy the patient's curiosity. The value of such a test would be measured in terms of peace of mind rather than any tangible health benefit.

In Chapter Three we will consider a clinical problem in which we can assess the value of additional information, specifically, that obtained from a diagnostic biopsy. We will also develop the concept of *expected value of clinical information* and relate this concept to the appendicitis and urinary tract infection examples.

A GENERALIZED FORMULATION OF CLINICAL DECISION PROBLEMS

A typical clinical situation involves a patient who may have a disease and a physician who must make decisions on behalf of the patient. As we indicated in Chapter One, most clinical decisions fall into one of two categories, namely, (1) decisions regarding whether to seek additional diagnostic information (and, if so, how), and (2) decisions concerning which treatments, if any, are to be employed. Additional information can come from inquiry into the patient's history, from physical examination, and from imaging and laboratory or other diagnostic tests. Possible treatments include the full gamut of physical, pharmacologic, surgical, radiologic, and other modalities.

The prototypical clinical situation may be modeled in a generalized form of a decision tree, as shown in Figure 2–12. As shown on the left, a patient has a certain set of signs and symptoms. The first choice point, decision node $\boxed{1}$, is whether to seek additional information and, if so, what diagnostic tests or other means to use. The possible actions are represented by a "fan" of branches that denote a spectrum of possibilities.

If the physician decides to seek more information, there follows an array of possible results or pieces of information, which are shown by the fan of branches emanating from chance node $\textcircled{A}$.

The next decision, at node $\boxed{2}$ or $\boxed{3}$, is whether to prescribe treatment and, if so, what type. At this point the physician may have reached an inference of disease or made a presumptive diagnosis, as indicated in Figure 2–12. In fact, psychologic studies of clinical cognition suggest that physicians form initial diagnostic hypotheses very early in their evaluation of patients (see Section 2.3), and some inference of disease might have been represented as early as node $\boxed{1}$. In decision-analytic terms, however, the physician's hypotheses or beliefs about

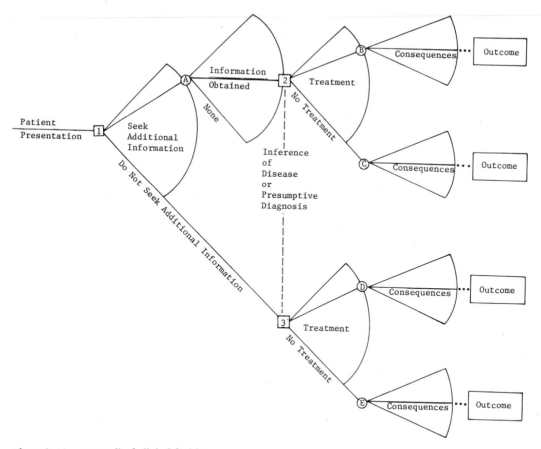

Figure 2–12 A generalized clinical decision tree.

disease are not decisions; that is, they are not choices among alternative actions. In general, the probabilities of disease enter the decision tree at chance nodes Ⓑ, Ⓒ, Ⓓ, and Ⓔ, and they affect the probabilities of reaching different outcomes. Since the probabilities of each possible disease affect the probabilities of each response to treatment at these chance nodes, the method of analysis that we will present in Chapter Three will automatically incorporate the physician's diagnostic judgments. However, the diagnosis itself is not a decision; the treatment is the decision, and the responses to treatment reflect the probabilities of various diseases.

The consequences of treatment ultimately lead to final outcomes, which are valued in their own right, such as the quality of life and survival. Obviously, each clinical situation contains its own specifics, and the art of building useful decision trees involves gauging their appropriate depth and pruning their width to keep them within manageable but still meaningful proportions.

2.2 CLINICAL STRATEGIES

The term **strategy** in common usage connotes a sequence of decisions that are made over time, with each decision based on the information available at the time the decision must be made. It suggests the feature of planning ahead, that is, contingency planning. All of these aspects are embodied in the formal, decision-analytic definition of a strategy, which we present in this section.

EXAMPLES OF CLINICAL STRATEGIES

In the appendicitis example presented at the beginning of this chapter, there are really four competing strategies. They are as follows:

Strategy 1. Decide now and operate.
Strategy 2. Decide now and do not operate.
Strategy 3. Wait six hours. If the patient gets better, do not operate; if the patient stays the same or gets worse, operate.
Strategy 4. Wait six hours. If the patient gets better or stays the same, do not operate; if the patient gets worse, operate.

Notice the presence of the "if...then" construction in strategies 3 and 4; the future decision (six hours later) of whether to operate is made contingent upon the intervening information (i.e., the course of the patient's condition). In strategies 1 and 2, however, all decisions are made prior to the availability of new information.

Strictly speaking, we might have listed still other strategies, such as the following:

Strategy 5. Wait six hours. If the patient gets worse, do not operate; if the patient stays the same or gets better, operate.
Strategy 6. Wait six hours. Operate regardless of the patient's condition.

We rule these out, however, for reasons given in the section on decision nodes and chance nodes (p. 17).

In the urinary tract infection example, which we laid out only partially, several strategies are possible, including the following:

Strategy 1. Prescribe antibiotic A; order a culture and a sensitivity test. If the culture is negative, have the patient discontinue the antibiotic. If the culture is positive and the bacteria are sensitive to antibiotic A, have the patient continue antibiotic A. If the culture is positive and the bacteria are sensitive to antibiotic B but not to antibiotic A, prescribe antibiotic B.
Strategy 2. Prescribe antibiotic A; order a culture and a sensitivity test. If the symptoms cease, have the patient continue antibiotic A for a full course of treatment. If the symptoms continue, the culture is positive, and the bacteria are sensitive to antibiotic A, have the patient continue antibiotic A. If the symptoms continue, culture is positive, and the bacteria are sensitive to antibiotic B but not to antibiotic A, prescribe antibiotic B. If the symptoms continue and the culture is negative, have the patient discontinue the antibiotic and reevaluate the patient (e.g., seek additional history, reexamine the patient, and take additional urine cultures).
Strategy 3. Order a culture and a sensitivity test, but prescribe no antibiotic. If the culture is negative and the symptoms continue, reevaluate the patient. If the culture is negative and the symptoms cease, undertake no treatment. If the culture is positive, prescribe an antibiotic to which the bacteria are sensitive.

The possibilities expand as the amount of information obtained and the number of action alternatives increase. You might wish to generate additional strategies for this example.

THE FORMAL CONCEPT OF A STRATEGY

Once you have a decision tree, it is a straightforward matter to generate an exhaustive list of possible strategies. The following definition indicates why this is so.

Definition. A **strategy** is a specification of the action to be taken at each decision node in a decision tree.

Let us apply this definition to the appendicitis example, the decision tree for which is shown in Figure 2–8, to see if it agrees with the intuitive concept of a strategy.

In Figure 2–8 there are five decision nodes. However, if the first decision is to decide now, there is only one subsequent choice; if the first decision is to wait six hours, there are three subsequent choices to specify, even though only one will actually have to be faced. The number of theoretically possible strategies in this problem is ten; two are associated with the "decide now" branch and eight with the "wait six hours" branch. These include such noncontenders as hypothetical strategies 5 and 6 of the previous section, however. If we prune the tree according to Figure 2–7, we are left with only four alternative strategies. These are the four we listed in the previous section.

Specifying an action at each decision node is, in effect, specifying a contingency plan. Having worked out your preferred strategy, you could leave it in the hands of an associate to carry out if the associate is capable of initiating the treatments and securing the diagnostic information required.

In reality, a difficulty in doing so is that unexpected events often occur, events that you did not build into your decision tree. For example, the patient with acute abdominal pain may be diabetic. This can affect your subsequent decision making in ways you had not anticipated and may lead you to generate several new strategies along the way. If you had thought that the unforeseen event was a real possibility and that it might affect your immediate actions, you could have built it into your tree in the first place.

DECISION TREES IN REDUCED FORM*

Having defined the concept of a strategy, we are in a position to describe another form of decision tree that highlights the choices among strategies. We construct this form of decision tree by indicating at the first decision node the choice among all possible strategies rather than just the choice among possible actions at the initial point in time. In effect, all decisions are specified in contingent form at the first decision node. Then the chance nodes follow, and outcomes are assigned to each path as before.

An example for the appendicitis problem is shown in Figure 2–13. This

---

*This section is not essential to the material that follows and may be skipped without loss of continuity.

tree is derived directly from the decision tree of Figure 2–8, but with the pruning suggested by Figure 2–7. Four branches emanate from the first decision node; these correspond to the four strategies that were previously identified. The remainder of the decision tree involves only chance nodes, the decision nodes in Figure 2–8 having been collapsed into the four alternative strategies. We shall say that the clinical decision tree in Figure 2–13 is in **reduced form.**

Definition. A decision tree is in **reduced form** if its decision nodes all precede its chance nodes.* Ordinarily, the initial decision node specifies the choice among the possible alternative strategies.

---

*Some writers[204] refer to this form as **normal form.** We feel, however, that the word *normal* carries more than enough meanings and connotations as it is, so we adopt this alternative terminology.

Figure 2–13   *The reduced form of a decision tree for a patient with possible appendicitis.*

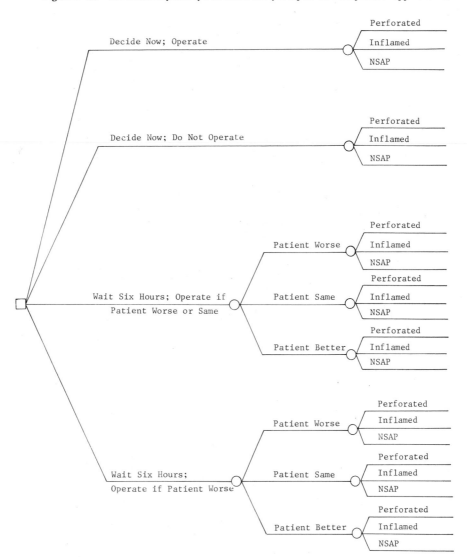

In contrast, we shall use the term **extensive form** to refer to the ordinary, time-sequenced decision tree that we will be using most of the time.

It may seem that by expressing the decision tree in reduced form, we are violating one of our basic principles: that a decision tree should be true to the timing of decisions and the acquisition of information. In fact, the reduced form does not violate this principle. It simply takes advantage of the fact that a strategy (that is, a sequence of decisions made contingent on subsequent events) may be specified in advance, even though the actual decisions may not. Thus, it is perfectly appropriate to decide now to wait six hours and to operate if the patient gets worse or stays the same. It would be inappropriate, however, to decide now to wait six hours and then operate, because that would be prejudging the currently uncertain course of the patient's condition during the six hours.

The reduced form can simplify the calculation of the best strategy in a complicated decision problem. The reduced form highlights the dependencies of the optimal course of action on the underlying probabilities assigned at chance nodes, which, in effect, facilitates sensitivity analysis with respect to probability assessments.

2.3 DECISION ANALYSIS, PSYCHOLOGY, AND THE "ART" OF CLINICAL DECISION MAKING

Making clinical decisions is a complex skill that is learned gradually as the physician deals with patients, observes more experienced clinicians, and discusses with them the rationale underlying their decisions. Clinical training provides an opportunity for learners — medical students, interns, residents, postdoctoral fellows, and practitioners — to make their own decisions and to review them with others.

The rules or principles underlying decision making are ordinarily not formalized. Indeed, clinicians are often reluctant to state such principles formally for fear that they might be applied in situations for which they were not intended. This is one reason why clinicians view judgment as more art than science and why it is so often characterized as an informal, intuitive process.

Decision analysis as a prescriptive formalization of the process of clinical decision making is an alternative to the intuitive approach. Throughout our development of the principles of clinical decision analysis, the process of intuitive clinical reasoning will be compared and contrasted with the procedures of decision analysis. We offer the following brief dramatization of a clinical decision-making episode to illustrate the importance of uncertainty and value judgment and the need to structure and simplify complex decision problems. It also strongly suggests the value of clinical decision analysis.

A CLINICAL EPISODE

As the scene opens, an intern is discussing a patient recently admitted to the hospital with the senior medical resident and a consulting surgeon.

Actors: *Intern (I); Senior Medical Resident (R); and Surgeon (S)*

   I: That's a great case you just admitted. My first patient with amebic dysentery involving the cecum.

R: Oh? Well, I've asked a surgical consultant to go over the patient with us. Why don't you go ahead and present her problem?

I: She's a 20-year-old single woman of Jamaican extraction who came to the emergency ward two hours ago with abdominal pain. She's been well in the past. She had her normal breakfast of grapefruit, coffee, toast, and butter six hours ago, and then about an hour after eating noticed the gradual onset of steady abdominal pain that she can't describe very precisely, but it seems to have been in the upper part of her abdomen. The pain has steadily worsened, and she says it's now most prominent in the right lower quadrant of her belly. It doesn't radiate to her shoulder or back, and she has had no other episodes like this. She's eaten nothing since breakfast because of loss of appetite and had three loose brown stools prior to coming to the emergency ward. She had a fourth stool while here.

Two weeks ago she returned from a month's vacation in Jamaica, where she visited her family. She traveled with a friend who developed a diarrheal disease late in the month. After returning, her friend was worked up for the diarrhea and was told that she had amebic dysentery.

Physical examination showed an oral temperature of 99 degrees, a pulse of 72, a blood pressure of 115 over 65, and respirations of 20. She has no rash or jaundice, and there are no abnormal findings of her head, neck, and chest. She has no surgical scars on her abdomen; her liver and spleen are not palpable, and I felt no masses. There is no rebound tenderness, but she complained on palpation of the right lower quadrant of her abdomen, and I think she may have a little guarding there.

The only other problem found on physical examination is tenderness in her right knee without detectable joint fluid or any other signs of inflammation in the joint.

Her laboratory studies show a white blood cell count of 10,000, with 70 per cent polys and 4 per cent young forms. A urinalysis shows no protein or sugar, but the sediment shows 5 red blood cells per high-power field. Findings from routine blood chemistries are normal. We looked at that stool she passed in the emergency ward. It was brown and soft and didn't contain any mucus, blood, or white blood cells but did show active amebae.

She'll be going to x-ray shortly for a barium enema to see if she has amebic ulcers of the colon.

R: How do you put that all together?

I: Well, with the recent travel history and amebae in the stools, it seems sure to be amebic dysentery. Because of the pain in the right lower quadrant, she must have involvement of the cecum.

S: I'm impressed that you took the trouble to do the smear of the stool. I saw a lot of amebiasis when I was serving in Vietnam, and the likelihood of it presenting as localized pain in the right lower quadrant is very slim. Also, there's a good chance that anyone who has spent time in Jamaica would show amebae in the stool. The important thing is to distinguish between *Entamoeba histolytica* and *Entamoeba coli*, because the *coli* aren't pathogens. Hospital labs in this part of the country simply don't see enough of the two to make the distinction with any reliability. It's even possible she does have amebic dysentery, but another more common problem may be causing most of her symptoms now and threatening her life.

I think we ought to back up a little and consider some other diagnoses. What about her sexual history? Did you see any discharge from the cervix?

I: She denied ever having had intercourse, and she didn't have any discharge from the cervix. A smear didn't show any evidence for gonorrhea.

S: Did she complain of pain when you moved her cervix?

I: No. I thought we had a diagnosis; what are you driving at?

S: Then it's very unlikely that pelvic inflammatory disease is the cause of her pain.

R: What about her periods? Have they been regular?

I: She started having periods at age 12, and they've varied from three weeks to two months in between. Her last one was six weeks ago.

R: What about an ectopic pregnancy?

I: I mentioned before that she denies intercourse!

R: Maybe we shouldn't rely so much on the history. If she has an ectopic pregnancy, she could bleed to death into her peritoneal cavity right under our noses. Did you feel a mass in her fallopian tubes on pelvic examination?

I: No.

S: I think we'd do better to focus on her abdominal pain rather than on the diarrhea. Acute appendicitis seems to me the best way to put her story together. If she really has guarding on her abdominal exam, we should operate promptly before her appendix perforates.

R: We both should feel her abdomen, but before we get to that, I'm disturbed by those red blood cells in the urine. Was it a catheterized specimen?

I: Yes, but there were only five red blood cells per high-power field. According to the books, that may be normal.

R: Well, I'd put my cutoff point lower than five and be worried about the possibility that the cells are evidence of a renal stone on the right. The trouble is that the catheterization itself could have caused this number of red blood cells, and I don't think we can use this evidence one way or the other. But I do think we should get a plain abdominal x-ray film rather than the barium enema to look for a stone. Unless her belly feels much worse now, I think we should sit tight and reevaluate her in several hours.

I: Right. There isn't any rebound tenderness. Besides, Rovsing's sign* is just about diagnostic for appendicitis, and she doesn't have it.

S: You may be interested to know that in 20 years of general surgery I've seen Rovsing's sign only a couple of times. Also, in this situation, rebound tenderness is not as important as guarding.

R: If this were a man, it would be easy: We should operate right away. But it isn't and we could just as well be dealing with pelvic inflammatory disease, a twisted ovarian cyst, an ectopic pregnancy, or plain old mesenteric lymphadenitis as with acute appendicitis. With that much uncertainty, I think we should wait and see how her condition changes over the next few hours.

S: Treatment for a twisted ovarian cyst, ectopic pregnancy, or acute appendicitis is all the same: It's surgical and we don't have to decide precisely what the diagnosis is.

---

*Rovsing's sign is present when pressure on the left side of the abdomen (over the descending colon at a point symmetrically opposite to McBurney's point) elicits pain on the right side (at McBurney's point).

R: Even apparently obvious surgical cases may not be what they seem; remember the patient we had last week who died on the operating table? We can't accept the risk of death from anesthesia unless we're sure she has a surgical problem.

S: The odds against death caused by anesthesia are very high, but if her appendix perforates, her chances of dying increase. How would you feel about presenting her case at Mortality Conference if we just watch her while her appendix perforates?

Why don't we go feel her abdomen and repeat the pelvic and rectal examinations to see what the situation is now? Then we can add things up and decide whether she's got a surgical belly or not.

CHARACTERISTICS OF THE INTUITIVE APPROACH TO CLINICAL REASONING

This vignette illustrates several characteristics of both good and poor intuitive clinical reasoning. The problem, like nearly all clinical problems, begins with a complaint. Something is wrong, but the underlying cause of the complaint is unclear. The clinician's task is to collect relevant data and clarify the problem so that appropriate actions can be taken.

Sequential data acquisition is a basic feature of nearly all clinical problem solving, and decisions are made regularly about which data are needed in a particular case and which are irrelevant and superfluous. The meaning of any particular finding is not self-evident. Many findings (e.g., fever, pain in the right lower quadrant of the abdomen, abdominal tenderness, sore throat, headache) are common to more than one disease, and some interpretation of the data by the clinician is required.

All three clinicians in the vignette are trying to simplify the problem by finding some way of combining a variety of data into a smaller number of categories for further reflection. The intern puts forth a single diagnosis (amebic dysentery with involvement of the cecum) and tries to reconcile as many data as he can with that conclusion. The resident suggests a number of alternatives and finds some evidence for each. The surgeon focuses mainly on two categories according to whether surgical treatment is appropriate or not.

To help make decisions about data collection and to aid in the process of interpreting the data, clinical reasoning commonly employs the strategy of generating and testing hypotheses about the diagnosis. Typically, a small set of hypotheses is generated very early in the clinical encounter and is based on very limited data compared with that which will eventually be collected.[61] Often the chief complaint or the data obtained in the first few minutes of interaction with the patient are sufficient to establish this small set of working hypotheses. The clinician can then ask, What findings would be observed if a particular hypothesis were true?, and the approach to data collection follows from the answer to this question.

This type of strategy transforms the ill-defined, open-ended question, What is wrong with the patient?, into a series of more closed, better defined problems. Could it be acute appendicitis? a twisted ovarian cyst? pelvic inflammatory disease? ectopic pregnancy? This set of alternatives can be tested and is much more manageable for the problem solver. By constructing a set of hypothesized end points, the clinician can work backward from the diagnostic criteria of each hypothesis to the work-up to be conducted. This simplifies the data search considerably.

If a clinician proceeded purely by generating and testing hypotheses, each work-up might differ substantially from its predecessors, since the set of problem formulations that are evaluated would be different for each patient. But we know that this is not the case. There are routine components to most, if not all, diagnostic work-ups. Routines are established partly as labor-saving devices. They simplify clinical work by making it unnecessary to figure out what will be done each time de novo. But they have other purposes as well. A problem may be so common or so important that a clinician may indeed wish to consider it for each patient, and clinical evaluation for such problems becomes routine.

Routine data collection also helps to protect clinical reasoning from prematurely narrowing the search to a few possibilities. Hypotheses can be powerful blinders. By helping decision makers to structure information, they may also prevent them from seeing that alternative interpretations are plausible. One purpose of routine data collection is to search for information that might, in turn, suggest hypotheses that the clinician would not otherwise consider.

This reasoning process can be summarized in four major stages:

1. *Data acquisition,* in which information is obtained by the clinician using a variety of methods.
2. *Hypothesis generation,* in which alternative problem formulations are retrieved from memory.
3. *Data interpretation,* in which the data are interpreted in light of the alternative hypotheses under consideration.
4. *Hypothesis evaluation,* in which the data are used to determine if one of the diagnostic hypotheses already generated can be confirmed. If not, the problem must be recycled: New hypotheses are generated, and additional data are collected until one of the hypotheses is verified.

Two modes of clinical inference may be observed in the vignette; one is diagnostically oriented, and the other is more concerned with therapeutics. Both are concerned with alleviating the patient's problem by rational action, but this goal can be approached in different ways.

HOW DECISION TREES CAN LEAD TO BETTER DECISION MAKING

A major advantage of informal or intuitive clinical reasoning, as observed in the vignette, is its flexibility. The method imposes few restrictions upon the decision maker and leaves much to discretion and ingenuity. Moreover, the process of hypothesis generation is one for which the decision-analytic approach offers little help.

On the other hand, constructing a decision tree diagram has many advantages over trying to assess a clinical situation intuitively. Designing the tree requires that you note the relevant uncertainties and possible actions, some of which might otherwise be overlooked. The tree helps to identify the pieces of clinical information that will be available before each decision must be faced, so that information that cannot affect a decision need not be collected. Also, the tree allows you to concentrate on one part of the problem at a time without losing the total picture, and it enables you to integrate in a meaningful way your thinking concerning all parts of the problem.

Clearly, a practicing physician cannot produce a full decision tree for each patient. Indeed, the structuring of the problem into a manageable decision tree may occasionally lead to undue simplification of the problem and the forfeiture of open-mindedness. However, experience in sketching decision trees for typical cases can yield insights that the clinician will keep in mind when treating similar cases. Decision trees are also particularly helpful in dealing with typical situations for which routines have not been established by the clinician.

The process of structuring a clinical decision problem with the aid of a decision tree can be the most valuable part of decision analysis. In subsequent chapters we will demonstrate how the judicious use of numbers (i.e., probabilities) can help even more. In Chapter Four, for example, we will refer to the vignette to show how intuitive reasoning can lead to clearly erroneous inferences and how decision analysis can help to avoid those pitfalls. By the time you reach Chapter Ten, we hope that you will have a good sense of the specific advantages as well as the limitations of clinical decision analysis.

2.4 SUMMARY OF CHAPTER TWO

A clinical **decision tree** is a schematic display of the temporal and logical structure of a clinical situation in which one or more decisions must be made. The decision tree requires the decision maker to identify alternative actions that might be taken at different points in time, information that may be obtained at different points in time, and the possible consequences of the actions. The decision tree highlights uncertainties about the patient and the clinical problem. The primary aim of the decision tree is to help the clinician separate the problem into manageable parts and think clearly about the actions that are available and their timing in relation to the information available. Further, by using quantitative measures of uncertainty (i.e., probabilities), the clinician can use a decision tree as an aid to selecting an optimal course of action by the methods that will be developed in Chapter Three.

Three basic building blocks of the decision tree are

1. **Choice nodes** (or **decision nodes**), at which one of two or more alternative actions may be selected.
2. **Chance nodes,** at which the status of the patient is revealed, test information becomes available, or other events beyond the control of the clinician occur.
3. **Outcomes,** which describe what happens to a patient along each **path** of events in the decision tree in terms of attributes held to be of value (e.g., mortality, health status).

By convention, a decision tree is built from left to right, with choice nodes represented by squares and chance nodes by circles and with outcomes specified at the right-hand "tips" of the tree.

The timing of decisions and the relation of choice nodes to chance nodes must accurately reflect the clinical reality. If a decision must be made before an item of clinical information becomes available, then the choice node corresponding to that decision must precede the chance node corresponding to the point at which the information becomes known. If a decision must be made without perfect knowledge of a patient's disease, then the corresponding choice node must precede the chance node at which the "true" disease is revealed. For decision-analytic purposes, however, the exact sequence of adjacent chance nodes and the grouping of adjacent choice nodes do not matter.

Clinical information is useful only if it has the potential to affect some subsequent clinical decision. Inspection of the decision tree can help identify what, if any, decisions are to be made contingent upon the information obtained.

A clinical **strategy** is a complete specification of the actions to be taken at each decision node under each contingency. It is possible to redraw a decision tree in **reduced form,** in which the initial decision node represents a choice among strategies and all subsequent nodes are chance nodes.

Decision-analytic structuring has many advantages over the intuitive approach to clinical decision making. Among these advantages is the ability to focus on one aspect of the decision problem at a time without losing sight of the whole. Another advantage is that decision analysis compels the decision maker to consider the relation between the information acquired and subsequent decisions that might be affected; for example, clinical data that would become available too late to affect a decision need not be acquired. Realization of the full value of clinical decision analysis, as for all tools of clinical decision making, comes only with experience.

EXERCISES FOR CHAPTER TWO

EXERCISES FOR SECTION 2.1

1. *Vascular Insufficiency in a Diabetic Patient*
   A 68-year-old patient has suffered for years from peripheral vascular disease. Now, after a penetrating foot injury, the patient has developed an infection and appears to have developed gangrene in the left foot. One possible response would be prompt amputation, but at this stage there is the possibility that the patient's foot might heal under more conservative, nonsurgical care. If surgical amputation is delayed, however, there is a risk that the gangrene could spread, necessitating amputation above the knee or even resulting in death. If surgery is performed now, the amputation can be done below the knee, with less resultant disability and deformity than that associated with amputation above the knee. Limb amputation is a relatively safe procedure, but there is always some risk of operative mortality.

   a. Draw a decision tree for this problem.
   b. Identify the outcomes of concern and indicate the outcome at the tip of each path.

2. *Appendicitis*
   a. In the appendicitis example in this chapter (p. 13) there were only three possibilities for progression of the patient's condition during the six-hour observation period: better, the same, or worse. Draw a modified decision tree in which you consider a more refined array of possibilities (e.g., much worse, worse, slightly worse).
   b. To what extent would it be permissible to prune the tree drawn in part a in view of the fact that waiting six hours has value only if it might affect the subsequent decision to operate?
   c The period of six hours was selected arbitrarily. You may want to observe the patient at the end of perhaps three hours and then reassess the situation to determine whether you want to observe the patient for another three hours or whether you want to decide then about surgery. Modify the decision

tree of Figure 2–8 to include the possibility of an assessment after the first three hours and a reassessment after six hours.

3. *Renovascular Disease*

For a small percentage of individuals with high blood pressure, the cause is an obstruction of one or both of the renal arteries, which is known generally as renovascular disease (RVD). For such patients the disease can often be corrected surgically, and this usually results in lowered blood pressure.

One test for RVD is the intravenous pyelogram (IVP), an x-ray procedure designed to measure kidney function. The IVP is not a perfect indicator of RVD, however; a patient with an abnormal IVP may not have RVD, and a patient with a normal IVP may have RVD.

The only way to confirm the presence or absence of RVD after an IVP has been done is by renal arteriography, a procedure that involves some risk of death. Arteriography will reveal with certainty whether the patient has RVD and, if so, whether it is operable. No surgeon would operate unless renal arteriography were performed and revealed an operable lesion.

Surgery itself poses a risk of death and sometimes does not even result in lowered blood pressure in a patient with RVD. The alternative to surgery for a patient with or without RVD is medical management with antihypertensive drugs, which may or may not be successful in lowering the blood pressure.

Draw a decision tree for the management of possible RVD in a patient with high blood pressure. Begin with the decision of whether to order an IVP and consider the subsequent decisions of whether to perform renal arteriography and surgery. Consider as possible end points mortality or survival and success or failure in lowering the blood pressure. Ignore all other complications.

4. *The Management of Sore Throat* [206]

A 23-year-old man comes to you, his physician, with a severe sore throat. Excluding unusual cases, the sore throat may be caused either by streptococcal bacteria (strep) or by a virus. If the sore throat is, in fact, caused by strep, the best treatment is penicillin, whereas if it is caused by a virus, rest and symptomatic relief are all that should be prescribed.

Failure to treat a strep throat may result in glomerulonephritis or rheumatic heart disease. Treatment with penicillin (whether correct or incorrect) may cause an adverse reaction, which usually consists of two to seven days of extreme discomfort with a rash and itching and, in very rare cases, death. You intend to ask the patient about his history of penicillin reactions, but you know that he may not be aware if he is susceptible.

If the patient has a strep throat and penicillin treatment is delayed by one day, assume that the patient will remain ill for one extra day; if penicillin is not given, assume that he will remain ill for about two extra days. In any case, assume that a patient with strep throat that is treated promptly will be ill for about five days.

The physician may take a throat culture, which will indicate the presence or absence of strep; the results of this culture will be known one day later. This culture may not give perfect information, however, because (1) the bacteria may die before they are "planted," (2) a positive result may be caused by contamination, and (3) the presence of streptococci in the throat does not necessarily indicate that the sore throat is caused by the bacteria.

Your immediate problem is to decide whether to take a culture or to prescribe penicillin or both on the first day.

Draw a decision tree for this clinical problem. Continue only as far as the information presented here allows.

EXERCISES FOR SECTION 2.2

5. *Strategies for Renovascular Disease*
a. Using the solution to Exercise 3 for Section 2.1, list the strategies that are being considered.

b. Explain why the following is not a viable strategy: Perform an IVP. Perform arteriography. Operate if arteriography indicated RVD that is operable; treat medically if arteriography indicates that the condition is not RVD or is not operable.

Chapter Three

Probabilities and Clinical Decisions

3.1 PROBABILITIES IN MEDICINE

In this chapter we introduce the most basic quantitative tool in clinical decision analysis: probability. Using a decision tree to structure a clinical decision problem enables one to focus on those events that are uncertain from the viewpoint of the decision maker. By going a step further and assigning probabilities to those events, the decision maker is able to make judgments as to which of several strategies is more likely to lead to a favorable outcome. In this chapter we shall develop a process for analyzing a decision tree once probabilities have been assigned at chance nodes. This process — averaging out and folding back — enables the decision maker to compare in quantitative terms the efficacy of alternative courses of action.

The fundamentals of probability that we shall use in this book are covered in Section 3.2 using medical examples. Those of you who are familiar with the basic concepts of probability theory and probability notation may skip that section or skim the section as a review. Others are urged to study that section carefully, since we shall build upon the material presented therein.

To introduce the use of probability in clinical decision analysis, we begin with a historical example of the use of probability in clinical decision making.

BENJAMIN FRANKLIN AND SMALLPOX

Benjamin Franklin argued implicitly in favor of the application to individual patients of probabilities based on previous experience with similar groups of patients. Before the discovery of cowpox vaccination for smallpox, it was known that immunity from smallpox could be achieved by a live smallpox inoculation, but the procedure entailed a risk of death. When a smallpox epidemic broke out in Boston in 1721, the physician Zabdiel Boylston consented, at the urging of the clergyman Cotton Mather, to inoculate several hundred citizens. Mather and Boylston reported their results:

Out of about ten thousand Bostonians, five thousand seven hundred fifty-nine took smallpox the natural way. Of these, eight hundred eighty-five died, or one in seven. Two hundred eighty-six took smallpox by inoculation. Of these, six died, or one in forty-seven.*

Though at first skeptical, Franklin eventually saw the advantages of inoculation and advocated the practice. After presenting statistics such as those just given, Franklin said:

In 1736, I lost one of my sons, a fine boy of 4 years old, by the smallpox taken in the common way. I bitterly regretted that I had not given it to him by inoculation. This I mention for the sake of parents who omit that operation, on the supposition that they should never forgive themselves if a child died under it. My example shows that the regret may be the same either way, and that therefore the safer should be chosen.[221]

Franklin here urges the strategy with the lower probability of death, having derived the probability for an individual patient from observed frequencies in other patients.

PROBABILITIES AS PROPORTIONS IN A POPULATION

At first we shall think of the **probability** of an event as the frequency with which the event occurs in a population. For example, since 6 of the 286 Bostonians who took smallpox by inoculation died, we may take this proportion, 6/286, or about 0.021, as an estimate of the probability that an individual will die if inoculated. Similarly, the proportion 885/5,759, or about 0.154, is an estimate of the probability of death from natural infection.

Some physicians may question the use of probabilities for an individual patient and wonder whether any probability estimates, such as the probability that the patient has a particular disease or the likelihood that the patient will survive an illness, can possibly be valid and meaningful for an individual patient. After all, one might argue that this individual patient either has the disease or does not and either will recover or will not. There is no probability involved. Furthermore, the argument continues, since each patient is unique, probability estimates derived from experience with previous patients cannot possibly apply to any individual case.

In regard to probability it is important to bear in mind the distinction between the truth about an individual patient and the state of our knowledge at the time we must make a decision. After a horse race we can state with certainty that a particular horse won and with equal certainty that every other horse did not win. But at the time the horses enter the starting gate, we can and

---

*From Schmidt.[221] Although the quotation may be historically accurate, the proportions cited overstate the advantages of inoculation. The appropriate death rate to compare with that of those patients who were inoculated would be computed using the entire uninoculated population at risk in the denominator.

do assign probabilities in the form of odds* that each will emerge the winner. It is true that as horses enter the starting gate, the race is yet to be run, but when an ill person enters the clinic, the patient already has or does not have a disease. Yet, from a decision-making point of view, the situations are completely analogous. What is important for a decision maker is the state of his or her beliefs and knowledge at the time a decision must be made and not what may then be — and perhaps may later emerge as — the truth.

At some level of specificity each individual is surely unique, but observations of patients who were seen in the past are still instructive for the care of patients who will be seen in the future. Medical practice is based on the transferability of information from past cases to current and future cases. Indeed, all of science concerns the prediction of future events according to theories derived from past observations. The key to the successful use of information derived from previous cases lies in identifying pertinent similarities between past and present cases.

Probability assessments in medicine, as in other areas, are often based on the observed frequency of similar circumstances in the past. When the weather forecaster says that there is a 20 per cent chance of rain tomorrow, this prediction is based on the frequency of rain on previous days when there were similar meteorologic conditions. However, every day is special, and it either will rain or will not rain tomorrow. But the estimated probability of rain is still quite useful for making many decisions. In the smallpox example, Benjamin Franklin based his judgment on the assumption that the 10,000 Bostonians constituted a population that he was willing to use as a basis for estimating the probabilities of death for his own patients.

The assignment of probabilities to the case of an individual patient may be viewed as a measure of the decision maker's ignorance about all of the special characteristics of that unique individual. We must be cognizant of what we know and do not know about each patient, but a refusal to quantify our ignorance will not lessen it. We argue that a physician should use probabilities to help decide on a strategy for an individual patient.

PROBABILITIES AS MEASURES OF STRENGTH OF BELIEF

It is possible to generalize the notion of probability from frequencies in a population to measures of *strength of belief* that an event will occur or that a state of the world is true, even when objective, frequency-based estimates are not available. We will argue that a physician should prefer quantitative language, such as "85 per cent likely," to semiquantitative language, such as "usually" or "rarely." One trouble with semiquantitative terms is that they can be interpreted differently by different people.[174] We advocate the use of probabilities, not because the numerical assessment in any way adds legitimacy to the opinion of the decision maker, but because it facilitates communication among decision makers and permits the decision maker to derive maximum use from the available information. We will return to this subject in Chapter Six. For the next several chapters, however, we will limit ourselves to the concept of probabilities as frequencies in a population. This will permit us to develop most of the fundamentals of clinical decision analysis without introducing the controversies raised by the use of so-called subjective probability.

---

*The relation between probability and odds is introduced in Chapter Four.

3.2 THE FUNDAMENTALS OF PROBABILITY*

EVENTS, PROPORTIONS, AND PROBABILITIES

Probabilities of Equally Likely Events

Early mathematicians and philosophers writing about probability based their discussions on events that occur equally often. It is useful to begin by thinking about similar events, such as the flip of a coin (in which situation the equally likely outcomes are heads or tails) or the roll of a die (in which case the outcomes are a die face with one, two, three, four, five, or six dots). If an event can occur in only one way, we shall say that the probability of this event is 1. If an event can occur in N equally likely, exclusive ways, then the probability of any one outcome is defined as $1/N$. For example, since a flipped coin is equally likely to show heads or tails, the probability that it will show heads is 1/2, and the probability that it will show tails is 1/2. Similarly, the probability that any one face of a tossed die will show up is 1/6, because a tossed die is equally likely to show each of its six faces. Note that this definition of probability ensures that the sum of probabilities of all of the possible events is 1.0.

The probability that any one of a number of mutually exclusive events will occur is the sum of the probabilities for each of the events. The probability that the die will show an odd-numbered face (i.e., one, three, or five dots) is therefore 1/6 (for one dot) plus 1/6 (for three dots) plus 1/6 (for five dots), or 1/2. An equivalent computation would be the number of ways an odd-numbered face can show up (i.e., three) multiplied by the probability of each odd-numbered face (i.e., 1/6). This may be expressed as

$$3(1/6) = 1/2.$$

Example: *Blood Types of Newborns.* It is known that of 1,000 infants born in Smalltown in 1975, 400 had blood type A. A child who is known to have been born in Smalltown in 1975 requires an immediate transfusion. What is the probability that this child has blood type A?

Since it is equally likely that this child is any one of the 1,000 who were born in 1975, and 400 of these have type A, the probability that this child has type A is

$$400(1/1,000) = 0.4.$$

Probabilities, Proportions, Percentages, Frequencies, and Rates

By definition, probabilities range in value from 0.00 to 1.00.[†] If an event has a probability of 0.00, this means that its occurrence is impossible. A probability of 1.00 means that the event's occurrence is a certainty. A probability of 0.50 means that the event is equally as likely to occur as not to occur.

---

*This section covers elementary material and may be skipped or skimmed by readers who are familiar with introductory probability theory.

[†]Sometimes we will write probabilities to two decimal places (e.g., 0.00, 0.70, 1.00), sometimes to one decimal place (e.g., 0.0, 0.7, 1.0), and sometimes to three or more places, depending on the context.

The example of the blood types in the preceding section illustrates a probability derived from the **proportion** of the members of a population who have a certain characteristic. The proportion of children with blood type A in that population is 400/1,000, or 0.4. Therefore, the probability that the child in need of the transfusion has blood type A (assuming that any of the 1,000 children is equally likely to have come to our attention in need of a transfusion) is 0.4. Until Chapter Six we will use the terms *probability* and *proportion* interchangeably. The terms *rate* and *frequency* will also be used occasionally as synonyms for *proportion*. Thus, we may say that the proportion of children with blood type A is 0.4 or, equivalently, that the rate of blood type A is 0.4, that the frequency of blood type A is 0.4, or that the probability that a child has blood type A is 0.4.

Probabilities and proportions are sometimes expressed in **percentages,** where 0 per cent corresponds to a probability of 0.00 and 100 per cent corresponds to a probability of 1.00. An event with a probability of 0.66 is 66 per cent likely to occur; an event that is 34 per cent likely to occur has a probability of 0.34. In our example we would say that a child born in Smalltown in 1975 is 40 per cent likely to be of blood type A.

Probability Shorthand

We will find it convenient in discussing probabilities to employ some shorthand notation. Suppose that E is an event in whose probability we are interested. For example, E might mean that a patient with acute abdominal pain actually has appendicitis or that a patient with duodenal ulcer will survive a vagotomy.

The probability of event E is denoted by $P[E]$ and read "P of E." Thus, if the probability of E is 0.47, we write

$$P[E] = 0.47.$$

In the blood type example, if A indicates that a child has blood type A, we write

$$P[A] = 0.4$$

because the probability of event A is 0.4.

The Summation Principle

The sum of the probabilities of all possible outcomes of a chance event is always equal to 1.0. This principle must hold even when the possible outcomes have different probabilities. It is taken as a basic axiom. We will use the term **complement** in regard to probability to mean 1.0 minus that probability.

> *Example: The Probability of Blood Types.* The only blood types present in a given population are O, A, B, and AB. If the probability of type O is 0.46, we write
>
> $$P[O] = 0.46.$$
>
> Suppose in addition that
>
> $$P[A] = 0.40$$

and

$$P[B] = 0.10,$$

where $P[A]$ and $P[B]$ refer to the probabilities of types A and B. What is the probability of type AB? Since the sum of the probabilities of all four types must equal 1.0,

$$P[O] + P[A] + P[B] + P[AB] = 1.0,$$

and we can solve for $P[AB]$ as

$$P[AB] = 1.0 - (P[O] + P[A] + P[B])$$
$$= 1.0 - (0.46 + 0.40 + 0.10)$$
$$= 0.04.$$

Hence, the probability of type AB in this population is 4 per cent.

Example: The Sex of Fraternal Triplets. What is the probability that a set of fraternal triplets will include at least one boy and one girl? There are three mutually exclusive and exhaustive possibilities: all boys, all girls, or two of one sex and one of the other sex. There will be at least one girl and one boy as long as the offspring are neither all boys nor all girls. Assume that the birth of a girl is as likely as the birth of a boy. Then, as we shall demonstrate in the section on independence (p. 46), the probability of all girls is (1/2) (1/2) (1/2) = 1/8, and the probability of all boys is the same. Hence, by the summation principle the probability that among the three children there will be at least one of each sex is the complement of the probability that all three will be of the same sex:

$$1 - (1/8 + 1/8) = 3/4.$$

JOINT PROBABILITIES AND CONDITIONAL PROBABILITIES

Joint Probability

What is the probability that the next child born at the community hospital will be a blue-eyed girl? Let us say that the event G denotes the birth of a girl, that the event BL denotes the birth of a blue-eyed child, and that the composite event G and BL denotes the birth of a blue-eyed girl. The probability of this event is written as $P[G \text{ and } BL]$ or equivalently as $P[G, BL]$ and is read "P of G and BL." This is called a **joint probability.**

Definition. The probability of the concomitant occurrence of any number of events is called the **joint probability** of those events. The joint probability of two events, E and F, is written in probability notation as $P[E \text{ and } F]$ or as $P[E, F]$.

Observe that since the event E and F is the same as the event F and E, it is always true that

$$P[E, F] = P[F, E].$$

Example: Hypertension and Obesity. Suppose that hypertension and obesity in a particular population of 10,000 males are distributed as shown in Table 3–1. What is the probability that an individual selected at random from this population is both hypertensive and obese? The answer may be found by expressing the number who are both hypertensive and obese, which is 1,500, as a proportion of the total population of 10,000. Hence,

$$P[\text{Hypertensive and Obese}] = 0.15.$$

This is the joint probability of these two characteristics.

Note that we can also infer from the table the probabilities of hypertension and obesity taken separately. Since 2,000 of the 10,000 men are hypertensive, we have

$$P[\text{Hypertensive}] = 0.20.$$

Similarly,

$$P[\text{Obese}] = 0.30.$$

TABLE 3–1   HYPERTENSION AND OBESITY IN A HYPOTHETICAL
POPULATION OF 10,000 MEN

MALE POPULATION	HYPERTENSIVE	NOT HYPERTENSIVE	TOTALS
Obese	1,500	1,500	3,000
Not obese	500	6,500	7,000
Totals	2,000	8,000	10,000

Example: Rolling a Pair of Dice. Suppose that you roll two dice. What is the probability of rolling two sixes? Notationally, we can express this probability as $P[\text{Six Dots on Second Die } and \text{ Six Dots on First Die}]$. This is the joint probability of this composite event. In this example

$$P[\text{Six Dots on Both Dice}] = 1/36.$$

This answer is derived by multiplying the probability of rolling six dots on one die, which is 1/6, by the probability of rolling six dots on the other die, which is also 1/6:

$$P[\text{Six Dots on Both Dice}] = P[\text{Six Dots on First Die}] \cdot$$
$$P[\text{Six Dots on Second Die}]$$
$$= (1/6)(1/6)$$
$$= 1/36.$$

Now, suppose that we had taken this same approach to the calculation of the joint probability of hypertension and obesity in the previous example. By this method we would have calculated that

$$P[\text{Hypertensive and Obese}] = (0.20)(0.30)$$
$$= 0.06,$$

which conflicts with what we know to be the correct answer, namely, 0.15. Therefore, this multiplication rule for joint probabilities, which seems to work for the dice example, does not always work. When it does work, we shall say that the component events are **independent,** a concept to which we will return (p. 46).

Conditional Probabilities

Consider again the example of hypertension and obesity. Suppose we are told that an individual selected at random from the population indicated in Table 3–1 is hypertensive. What is the probability that this person is also obese? We know that there are 2,000 men with hypertension in the population and that of these, 1,500 are obese. Therefore, we may correctly conclude that the rate of obesity among hypertensive males is 1,500/2,000, or 0.75. This may be interpreted as the probability that a member of the population is obese, given that he is hypertensive.

The probability that a man is obese, given that he is hypertensive, is an example of a **conditional probability.** It is called conditional because it refers to the event that the individual is obese under the condition that he is known to be hypertensive. This conditional probability is denoted by P[Obese|Hypertensive], where the vertical bar is read "conditional upon" or simply "given." Thus, the expression P[Obese|Hypertensive] is read "the probability that the man is obese, given that he is hypertensive."

Definition. The probability that event E occurs, given that event F is known to occur, is called the **conditional probability** of event E given event F. It is denoted by P[E|F].

The relation between joint probability and conditional probability is straightforward and is given in the following formula:

$$P[\text{E and F}] = P[\text{E|F}] \cdot P[\text{F}]. \qquad (3\text{–}1)$$

Equation 3–1 may, in fact, be considered a formal definition of joint probability.

In our example, if E denotes obese and F denotes hypertensive, we have, according to Equation 3–1,

$$P[\text{Obese and Hypertensive}] = P[\text{Obese|Hypertensive}] \cdot P[\text{Hypertensive}].$$

We calculated before that P[Obese|Hypertensive] equals 0.75. Moreover, from Table 3–1 we can calculate that P[Hypertensive] equals 2,000/10,000, or 0.2. Therefore,

$$P[\text{Obese and Hypertensive}] = (0.75)(0.2)$$

$$= 0.15,$$

which agrees with the direct calculation we made in the section on joint probability (pp. 42–43).

Starting with Equation 3–1, we can relate a conditional probability (P[E|F]) to the corresponding joint probability (P[E and F]) and the probability of the underlying event (P[F]). If we divide both sides of Equation 3–1 by P[F], we find that

$$P[E|F] = \frac{P[E \text{ and } F]}{P[F].} \qquad (3\text{--}2)$$

In the hypertension and obesity example, we can derive the conditional probability as follows:

$$P[\text{Obese}|\text{Hypertensive}] = 0.15/0.2$$

$$= 0.75.$$

Pursuing this same example, suppose that we were interested in the probability that an individual is obese, given that he is *not* hypertensive. We can see from Table 3–1 that

$$P[\text{Not Hypertensive}] = 0.8,$$

and that

$$P[\text{Obese and Not Hypertensive}] = 0.15.$$

Thus, we can calculate that

$$P[\text{Obese}|\text{Not Hypertensive}] = 0.15/0.8$$

$$= 0.1875.$$

Hence, in this population the probability that a man who is not hypertensive is obese is 18.75 per cent.

Such statements of conditional probability are based on observed associations and do not necessarily represent a causal relation. We can specify the probability that a hypertensive person will be obese ($P[\text{Obese}|\text{Hypertensive}]$) or the probability that an obese person will be hypertensive ($P[\text{Hypertensive}|\text{Obese}]$) without implying either that hypertension *causes* obesity or that obesity *causes* hypertension.

Example: The Sex of Fraternal Twins. Let us consider the probability that both fraternal twins will be girls. We denote this joint probability by $P[G_1, G_2]$, where G_1 refers to the event that the first child is a girl and G_2 refers to the event that the second child is a girl. Thus, according to Equation 3–1, we have

$$P[G_1, G_2] = P[G_2, G_1]$$

$$= P[G_2|G_1] \cdot P[G_1].$$

We know that $P[G_1]$ equals $1/2$. What is $P[G_2|G_1]$, that is, the probability that the second fraternal twin will be a girl given that the first is a girl? This probability is also $1/2$, because the sex of each twin is determined by an independent genetic process, and the probability that the second twin is a girl does not depend on whether the first is a girl or a boy. Hence,

$$P[G_2|G_1] = P[G_2] = 1/2.$$

Therefore, returning to our initial question,

$$P[G_1, G_2] = P[G_2|G_1] \cdot P[G_1]$$
$$= P[G_2] \cdot P[G_1]$$
$$= (1/2)(1/2)$$
$$= 1/4.$$

As with successive flips of a coin or rolls of a die, the sex determination of fraternal twins is an example of **independent** events, a concept we shall define shortly.

Example: *Rolling a Die.* Suppose that we are told that a die has been rolled and that the result was a face with an odd number of dots. What is the probability that three dots showed up? We denote this probability by $P[\text{Three Dots}|\text{Odd}]$, and we apply Equation 3–2 as follows. Let E represent three dots and let F represent an odd number of dots. Then using Equation 3–2, we obtain

$$P[\text{Three Dots}|\text{Odd}] = P[\text{Three Dots and Odd}]/P[\text{Odd}].$$

Now, $P[\text{Three Dots and Odd}]$ is the same as $P[\text{Three Dots}]$, or 1/6, because if three dots comes up it is automatically odd. And $P[\text{Odd}]$ equals 1/2, since of the six possibilities, three are odd. Hence,

$$P[\text{Three Dots}|\text{Odd}] = (1/6)/(1/2) = 1/3.$$

Independence

In the example of the sex of fraternal twins, the conditional probability of the sex of one twin does not depend on the sex of the other. Using our notation,

$$P[G_2|G_1] = P[G_2].$$

Definition. When the conditional probability of event E, given event F, is the same as the unconditional probability of event E, we say that events E and F are probabilistically **independent.**

When events are independent, Equation 3–1 reduces to a particularly simple form. If E and F are independent,

$$P[E|F] = P[E].$$

Therefore Equation 3–1 reduces to the **product rule for independent events:**

$$P[E \text{ and } F] = P[E] \cdot P[F] \tag{3-3}$$

where E and F are independent.

Example: *The Sex of Fraternal Triplets.* If we recognize that the sex determination of fraternal triplets represents independent events, we can easily see that the probability that all three will be girls is equal to

$$P[G_1, G_2, G_3] = P[G_1] \cdot P[G_2] \cdot P[G_3]$$
$$= (1/2)(1/2)(1/2)$$
$$= 1/8,$$

as claimed in the example in the section on the summation principle (p. 42).

Example: A Coin and a Die. If you roll a die and flip a coin, what is the probability that the die will show five dots and the coin will show a head? Since the chance of the die showing five dots is 1/6 and the chance of the coin showing a head is 1/2, the probability of both occurring is

$$(1/6)(1/2) = 1/12,$$

because the two events are independent.

Recall our example in which events were *not* independent, that is, the hypertension and obesity example. In that case, knowing whether an individual is hypertensive affects the probability that he is obese, and

$$P[\text{Obese}|\text{Hypertensive}] \neq P[\text{Obese}].$$

In this case, the product rule (Equation 3–3) does not hold.

The Summation Principle for Joint Probabilities

A modified version of the summation rule holds for joint probabilities. Referring to the example of hypertension and obesity (Table 3–1), we observe that an individual who is hypertensive may be either obese or not obese. Since these are the only possibilities, we would expect that

$$P[\text{Hypertensive}] = P[\text{Hypertensive and Obese}] + P[\text{Hypertensive and Not Obese}].$$

In the example we have

$$P[\text{Hypertensive}] = 0.15 + 0.05$$
$$= 0.20.$$

This is an example of the **summation principle for joint probabilities.**

Generally, if F_1, F_2, and F_3 are exhaustive and mutually exclusive events (i.e., one, but only one, of these must occur) and E is any other event, it is true that

$$P[E] = P[E, F_1] + P[E, F_2] + P[E, F_3]. \qquad (3-4)$$

If E is an event that has a probability of 1.0 (e.g., that the sun will rise tomorrow), then the terms on the right-hand side of Equation 3–4 must also add up to 1.0; thus, the equation reduces to the summation principle.

We can apply the summation principle for joint probabilities to the example of the coin and the die given in the preceding section on independence (p. 46):

$$P[\text{Five Dots}] = P[\text{Five Dots and Heads}] + P[\text{Five Dots and Tails}]$$
$$= (1/12) + (1/12)$$
$$= 1/6.$$

Remember that the summation principle for joint probabilities applies as well when the events are not independent, as the hypertension and obesity example illustrates.

Example: Operative Mortality With Appendectomy. Let us reintroduce a clinical example that we began to consider in Chapter Two and shall develop in more detail later in this chapter. The example concerns a patient who is seen in the emergency room with symptoms equivocal for acute appendicitis.

The chief of surgery wants to calculate the overall probability that the patient will die in surgery. First, she knows that operative mortality will depend on whether the patient has a perforated appendix (Perf), an inflamed but intact appendix (Inf), or nonspecific abdominal pain (NSAP). (We continue to assume that these three, Perf, Inf, and NSAP, exhaust the possible diagnoses for this patient.) The chief cites evidence from the literature* suggesting that if she were to operate on 1,000 patients whose appendices had perforated, 27 would die in surgery. We may write this as a conditional probability as follows:

$$P[\text{Die}|\text{Perf}] = 0.027.$$

She further states that the surgical risk is much lower if the appendix, although it may be infected, has not perforated:

$$P[\text{Die}|\text{Inf}] = 0.001;$$

that is, there would be one surgical death per 1,000 patients whose appendices are inflamed but not perforated. The risk of death is lowest if the patient has a nondiseased appendix; in that case it is only seven deaths per 10,000 patients:

$$P[\text{Die}|\text{NSAP}] = 0.0007.$$

Second, the chief of surgery assesses that 84 per cent of patients with equivocal symptoms have nonspecific abdominal pain (NSAP), and 16 per cent have appendicitis. Three of the 16 per cent already have perforated appendices, and the remaining 13 have inflamed appendices. Hence, using our shorthand,

$$P[\text{NSAP}] = 0.84,$$
$$P[\text{Inf}] \quad = 0.13,$$
$$P[\text{Perf}] \quad = 0.03.$$

Next, she applies the summation principle for joint probabilities:

$$P[\text{Die}] = P[\text{Die and Perf}] + P[\text{Die and Inf}] + P[\text{Die and NSAP}].$$

Then she uses Equation 3–1 three times to calculate the required joint probabilities:

$$
\begin{aligned}
P[\text{Die and Perf}] \quad &= P[\text{Die}|\text{Perf}] \cdot P[\text{Perf}] \\
&= (0.027)(0.03) \\
&= 0.00081; \\
P[\text{Die and Inf}] \quad &= P[\text{Die}|\text{Inf}] \cdot P[\text{Inf}] \\
&= (0.001)(0.13) \\
&= 0.00013;
\end{aligned}
$$

---

*These data were taken from Neutra.[181]

$$P[\text{Die and NSAP}] = P[\text{Die}|\text{NSAP}] \cdot P[\text{NSAP}]$$
$$= (0.0007)(0.84)$$
$$= 0.00059.$$

Finally, she inserts these joint probabilities into the summation formula to derive the desired answer:

$$P[\text{Die}] = 0.00081 + 0.00013 + 0.00059$$
$$= 0.00153.$$

Therefore, the chief can expect about 1.53 deaths per 1,000 operations performed on patients with equivocal signs of appendicitis.

In the next section we offer a diagrammatic approach to this kind of calculation that does not require the use of algebra and is especially helpful in the analysis of decision trees. This is the process to which we will refer later as **averaging out**.

3.3   ANALYSIS OF PROBABILITY TREES

DIAGRAMING PROBABILITIES

In a decision tree, chance events are diagramed as lines or branches leading from a small circle that represents a chance node. Each branch represents one possible event. Now we add to the label on each branch the numerical probability of the event that corresponds to the branch. Because of the summation principle, the sum of the probabilities of all possible events at a chance node must equal 1.0.

> *Example: Blood Types of Newborns.* The blood type example introduced in Section 3.2 may be diagramed as shown in Figure 3–1. We write the probabilities in parentheses on each branch beside the description of the corresponding event. Thus, the event Type A is accompanied by its probability, 0.40. The sum of the probabilities at this chance node equals 1.00, as it always must.

Figure 3–1   *A probability tree for blood types of newborns in Smalltown.*

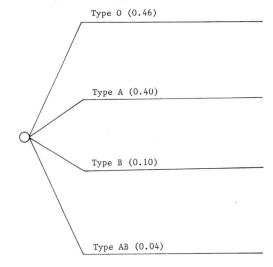

Type 0 (0.46)

Type A (0.40)

Type B (0.10)

Type AB (0.04)

The diagram in Figure 3–1 is not really a decision tree, because it has no decision nodes. We shall call such a diagram a **probability tree.**

Example: The Sex of Fraternal Triplets. The possible sex composition of a set of triplets may be diagramed as shown in Figure 3–2. Notice that the probabilities at every chance node sum to 1.0.

Example: Hypertension and Obesity. The example of hypertension and obesity may be diagramed as shown in Figure 3–3. This example illustrates an important point about probability trees and, by extension, decision trees. The probabilities at chance node Ⓐ are straightforward. However, once we get to chance node Ⓑ, the appropriate probabilities are the *conditional probabilities* for obesity, given that the patient has hypertension. (These were calculated in the section dealing with conditional probabilities [p. 45].) In general, the probability of an event at any stage in the sequence is the conditional probability of that event, given all events preceding it in the sequence. In this example, probabilities at chance nodes to the right of the upper branch following chance node Ⓐ must be conditional probabilities, given that the patient has hypertension. The additional chance node Ⓒ to the right of chance node Ⓑ represents the possibility of having a stroke or of not having a stroke. Probabilities on branches to the right of node Ⓑ would have to be the conditional probabilities of a stroke or no stroke, given that the patient is hypertensive *and* obese. In this way the probability tree keeps track of all the information available at the point at which a particular uncertainty is resolved, and all probabilities are conditional upon all prior information.

PATH PROBABILITIES

In the hypertension and obesity example, the joint probability that the patient is both hypertensive and obese may be calculated by using the probability tree in Figure 3–3. It is simply the product of all the probabilities along

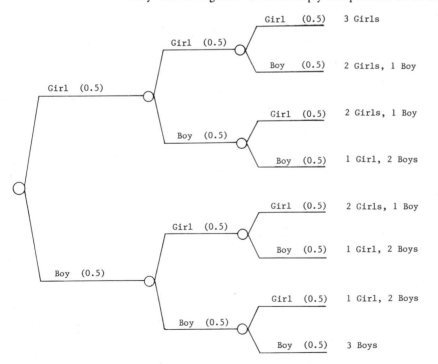

Figure 3–2 A probability tree for the sex of fraternal triplets.

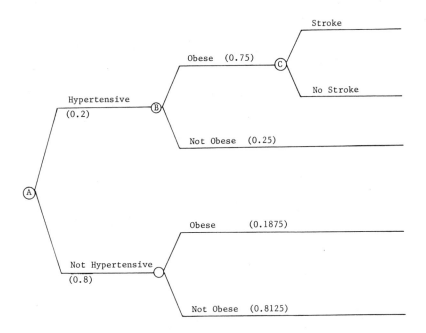

Figure 3–3 A probability tree for the hypertension and obesity example.

the **path** corresponding to the "hypertensive" and "obese" branches, that is, (0.2) (0.75), or 0.15. This is an application of Equation 3–1:

$$P[\text{Hypertensive and Obese}] = P[\text{Hypertensive}] \cdot P[\text{Obese} | \text{Hypertensive}].$$

In the context of a probability tree or a decision tree, we call such a joint probability a **path probability.**

Definition. The **path probability** of a sequence of chance events is the product of all probabilities along that sequence.

AVERAGING OUT PROBABILITIES

A probability tree can facilitate the averaging-out procedure we used in the appendicitis example as shown in Figure 3–4. The probabilities provided by the chief of surgery have been used. We are interested in calculating the overall probability of death.

We average out the overall probability of death by moving from right to left through the sequence of chance nodes as follows. At node Ⓑ the probability of death is 0.027. We indicate this by drawing a "balloon" enclosing the probability and connecting it to the chance node. We interpret this to mean that once we have arrived at chance node Ⓑ, the probability of the outcome in which we are interested, death, is 0.027. We do the same at chance nodes Ⓒ and Ⓓ, as shown in Figure 3–4.

Now we proceed farther to the left, to chance node Ⓐ. We are ready to do so because all nodes at the tips of the branches emanating from Ⓐ have been assigned probabilities for the outcome, death. The probability of death at Ⓐ is calculated by simply multiplying the probability at the tip of each branch by the

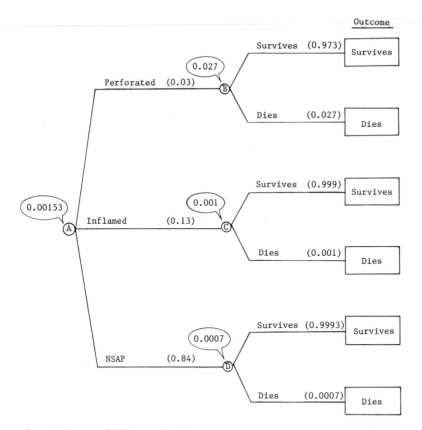

Figure 3–4 *A probability tree for the appendicitis example.*

corresponding probability on the branch and then summing up. According to this procedure, the probability of death at Ⓐ is

$$(0.03)(0.027) + (0.13)(0.001) + (0.84)(0.0007),$$

or 0.00153. We denote this by inserting a balloon containing this number at node Ⓐ. Notice that this is the same answer we derived algebraically in the section on the summation principle for joint probabilities (pp. 48–49).

The procedure we have just used is called **averaging out**, because the calculation involves taking a weighted average of the numbers at the tips of the branches at each chance node. The weights are the probabilities of those branches. The procedure is identical to the algebraic procedure used in the section on the summation principle for joint probabilities.

With this process of averaging out mastered, we are now ready to analyze decision trees in their entirety.

EXPECTED VALUE: A PREVIEW

Later on we shall introduce the concept of **expected value**, which is applied to an "averaged-out" number, such as the 1.53 deaths per 1,000 patients in the appendicitis example. The concept of expected value is important when we want to average out numbers that are not probabilities, such as the number of years of life or the number of days in the hospital. Life expectancy is an example of an expected value. For now, though, we do not need to introduce this concept, since the laws of probability are sufficient to permit us to conduct the averaging-out process for the kinds of examples we shall be using. When we introduce in Chapter Seven examples with outcomes that are more complicated than survival versus death or cure versus no cure, we shall need to develop the concept of expected value more carefully.

3.4 ANALYSIS OF DECISION TREES: OBSERVATION OF PATIENTS WITH POSSIBLE APPENDICITIS

Here we shall develop fully the example of the patient with equivocal symptoms of appendicitis that was introduced in Chapter Two. The problem is whether to observe the patient for six hours or to operate immediately. A decision tree for the problem is shown in Figure 2–8 (p. 18). Using probabilities for each of the chance events, we will use the method of **averaging out** combined with a complementary process called **folding back** to derive an optimal strategy for the management of this patient's condition.

PUTTING PROBABILITIES ON A DECISION TREE

In order to decide whether to wait six hours, probabilities are needed for each chance node in the decision tree. Among these must be probabilities corresponding to the ultimate outcome at the end of each path, the probability of death. In Chapter Two these probabilities were identified as follows:

1. The probability of death (or survival) with and without surgery for patients with perforated appendices, with inflamed appendices, and with NSAP.
2. The probability that patients with equivocal symptoms would improve, stay the same, or worsen after six hours.
3. The probability of a perforated, inflamed, or nondiseased appendix in patients whose status was originally equivocal both at the outset and after six hours of observation.

These probabilities may be derived from clinical or epidemiologic studies or from informed guesses. We shall have much to say about the sources and uses of probability assessments in Chapter Six, but for now let us just assume that the chief of surgery has provided the chief resident with the probabilities he requests.

In our previous discussion of this example the chief cited evidence from the literature suggesting that the mortality from abdominal surgery on a patient with a nondiseased appendix is 0.7/1,000, on a patient with an inflamed appendix is 1/1,000, and on a patient with a perforated appendix is 27/1,000. The chief also stated that of patients whose signs and symptoms are equivocal, 84 per cent have NSAP, 13 per cent have inflamed appendices, and 3 per cent have perforated appendices. Although the chief is not sure, she wants the resident to assume that if he does not remove an inflamed appendix, it will always go on to perforate and if that happens without surgery, the patient has a 50 per cent chance of dying. The chief estimates that after six hours the conditions of patients with equivocal presentations will evolve in the following way:

1. Thirteen per cent of the patients will show worsening symptoms. Of these, 25 per cent will have perforated appendices; 75 per cent will have inflamed appendices; and 0 per cent will have NSAP.
2. Thirty-six per cent will remain unchanged. Of these, 1.7 per cent will have perforated appendices; 6.6 per cent will have inflamed appendices; and 91.7 per cent will have NSAP.
3. Fifty-one per cent will improve, and none of these patients will have appendicitis.

You now have enough data to determine whether waiting six hours or operating immediately will result in the lower probability of death. If you like, you may want to pause for a few minutes and try to solve this problem *without* the aid of a decision tree. It is possible to do so, but using the decision tree makes it much easier.

Now let us insert these probabilities into the decision tree for this problem (Figure 2–8). You may want to do this yourself before looking at the decision tree in Figure 3–5 in which the probabilities are correctly placed. Note that the probabilities of death along each path are shown in terms of deaths per 1,000 patients. These are the numbers in the boxes at the far right of the figure. Of course, these may be converted to probabilities by moving the decimal point three places to the left. However, we will work with deaths per 1,000 patients rather than probabilities to avoid numbers with many zeros.

SPECIFYING VALUED OUTCOMES

From what the chief of surgery has told us, we know that death or survival is the outcome about which we care. At the end of each path in our tree we can substitute a single number, which could be either the mortality or the complementary survival rate if the path is followed to that point. We shall choose here to use mortality as the probability of interest, and our aim (just as with Franklin's choice of inoculation) will be to choose the decision strategy with the lowest mortality. Thus, if in following a given path there is a 2.7 per cent chance of death and a 97.3 per cent chance of survival, this would be indicated in a box at the far right of the path, as shown in Figure 3–5. A more elaborate representation would be to append to the end of each path an additional chance node of the following type:

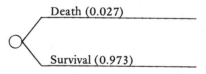

Since the two approaches are equivalent and the former requires less notation, we express the probabilities of death in the boxes simply as 27 deaths per 1,000 patients, or as 0.027.

AVERAGING OUT

With all this information we can now use the decision tree to answer the initial problem faced by the chief resident and generalized by the chief of surgery

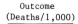

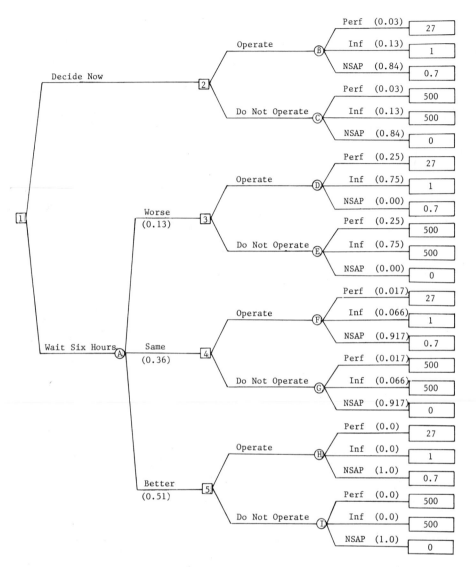

Figure 3–5 *A decision tree for the appendicitis example with probabilities and outcomes inserted.*

in the form of the question, Should patients with equivocal presentations of appendicitis be observed for six hours?

As a first step let us evaluate the mortality for the present policy of operating immediately on all patients with equivocal signs and symptoms. Incidentally, we will be able to double-check whether the benefit of performing surgery in these patients exceeds the benefit of sending them home. We follow the decide now → operate (upper) branch of the tree in Figure 3–5. What is the probability of death at chance node Ⓑ, which is situated just before the final outcomes? At point Ⓑ there is a 0.03 chance of 27 deaths per 1,000 patients, a 0.13 chance of 1 death per 1,000 patients, and a 0.84 chance of 0.7 deaths per 1,000 patients. Hence, the number of deaths per thousand patients at that node is

$$(0.03) (27) + (0.13) (1) + (0.84) (0.7),$$

or approximately 1.53 deaths per 1,000 patients. This is identical to the number we calculated in the section on averaging out probabilities (p. 52); recall that this process of collapsing the probabilities at a chance node is called **averaging out.** Now let us average out at chance node Ⓒ, which follows the decide now → do not operate branch. The death rate at node Ⓒ would be

$$(0.03) (500) + (0.13) (500) + (0.84) (0) = 80 \text{ deaths}/1,000 \text{ patients.}$$

FOLDING BACK

Quite clearly, if one must decide now, the thing to do is to operate, which results in a lower mortality than releasing patients with equivocal signs for appendicitis. Figure 3–6 illustrates the "decide now" branch of our decision tree with the averaged-out death rates shown at chance nodes Ⓑ and Ⓒ.

What is the death rate associated with *decision* node ②? At a decision node remember that you have a choice, so you may select the single most preferred decision branch leading from the node. In this case 1.53 deaths per 1,000 patients is preferred to 80 deaths per 1,000 patients because you want to minimize the probability of death. Therefore, once you have arrived at node ②, you can ensure yourself a death rate of 1.53/1,000 by choosing to operate. We indicate our selection of the "operate" branch at decision node ② by putting two slashes across the "do not operate" branch in Figure 3–7.

In this same figure we indicate the death rate per 1,000 patients associated with decision node ②. This rate, 1.53 deaths per 1,000 patients, is also the probability of death for the entire "decide now" branch.

This process of pruning all but the most preferred branch at a decision node and assigning to it the most advantageous probability is called **folding back** to the decision node. When the outcome with which we are concerned is an unfavorable event, such as death or illness, we fold back by selecting the branch with the *lowest* probability of its occurrence. When the outcome is a favorable

Figure 3–6   The "decide now" branch of the appendicitis decision tree with averaged-out values at chance nodes (deaths per 1,000 patients).

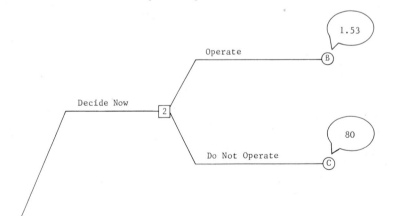

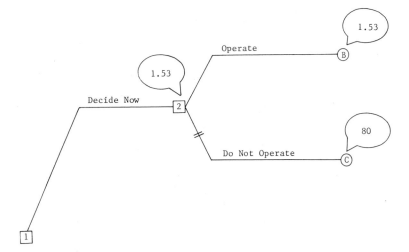

Figure 3-7 *The probability of death (expressed as the death rate per 1,000 patients) for the "decide now" branch.*

event, such as survival or cure, we fold back by selecting the branch with the *highest* probability.

Bear in mind that at a decision node we **fold back** along the *single* best choice, whereas at a chance node we **average out** the probabilities on *all* the branches emanating from that node. We always work backward, from right to left.

FINDING AN OPTIMAL STRATEGY BY AVERAGING OUT AND FOLDING BACK

You can do the same kind of averaging out for chance nodes Ⓓ, Ⓔ, Ⓕ, Ⓖ, Ⓗ, and Ⓘ in Figure 3–5 and then fold back these values to choice nodes ③, ④, and ⑤ along the "wait six hours" branch. The results should look like Figure 3–8.

The probability of death at chance node Ⓐ is obtained by averaging out the probabilities on the three branches that emanate from it. Here, each of the rates at nodes ③, ④, and ⑤ is first weighted by the probability of its respective branch, and then these values are summed. The death rate at node Ⓐ is equal, therefore, to

$$(7.5) (0.13) + (1.17) (0.36) + (0) (0.51) = 1.40 \text{ deaths}/1,000 \text{ patients.}$$

The death rate for the "wait six hours" branch is thus also 1.40 deaths per 1,000 patients, and a much condensed version of the decision problem can be rendered as in Figure 3–9. We obtain this result by starting at the final outcomes, averaging out all the values at each chance node, and folding back along the single best decision to each decision node. The complete decision tree showing each step of the averaging-out-and-folding-back process is portrayed in Figure 3–10.

Finally, we are able to say which of our initial choices is best and to offer a complete statement of the preferred strategy:

1. If your alternatives are to wait six hours or to decide now in patients with equivocal signs and symptoms, you should wait six hours.

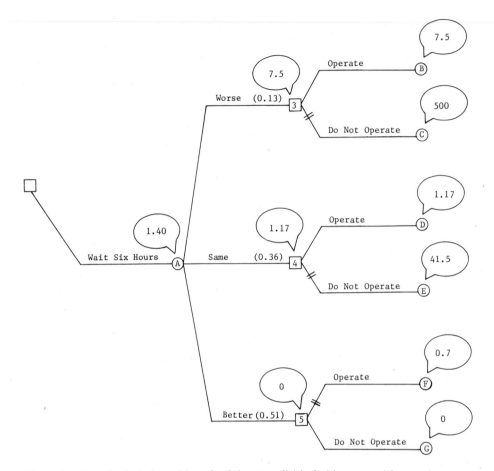

Figure 3-8 The "wait six hours" branch of the appendicitis decision tree, with averaging out at the final chance nodes and folding back to the preceding decision nodes. (The probabilities of death are expressed as rates per 1,000 patients.)

2. If the patient gets worse or remains the same in that period, then you should operate.
3. If the patient improves, then you should not operate.
4. If you were forced to decide now, the preferred strategy would be to operate.

Figure 3-9 A collapsed decision tree to decide now or wait six hours for patients with equivocal presentations of appendicitis.

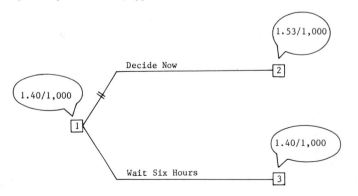

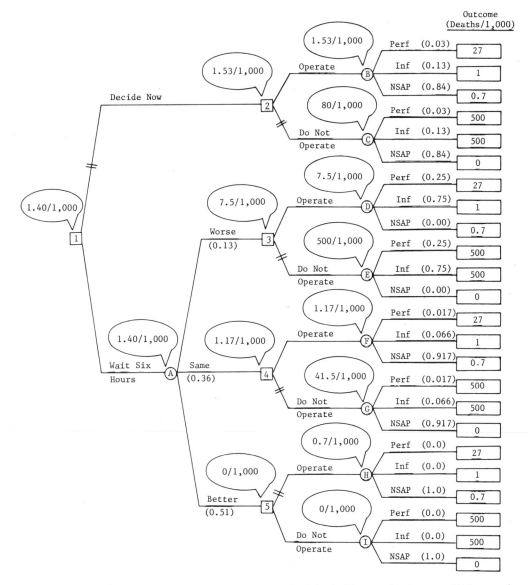

Figure 3–10 *A complete analysis of the decision tree for the appendicitis example.*

Notice that the complete statement of a strategy contains contingent statements, "if . . ., then . . . ." Note as well that the choice "wait six hours" is unrealistically restrictive in that the patient would be available for examination at intervals of much less than six hours. This realization makes us even more confident that waiting is the best strategy.

A difference of 0.13 deaths per 1,000 patients seems small, and one might wonder whether it is wise to be guided by such a slight distinction. When we see results of a scientific experiment, we expect to find a confidence interval indicating the validity of the findings. Should we not have something similar for probabilities in decision trees? The answer is yes and no. We will return to this issue in Section 3–5.

ANALYSIS IN REDUCED FORM*

In Chapter Two we introduced the concept of decision trees in reduced form, in which case all decision nodes are brought up to the front end of the tree in the form of strategies. We now illustrate the use of decision trees in reduced form for this example.

A decision tree in reduced form for the appendicitis problem was shown in Figure 2–13. The analysis of this decision tree is shown in Figure 3–11. Note that the result is identical to that obtained by analysis of the extensive form: The optimal strategy is to wait six hours and then to operate if the patient's

---

*This section is not essential to the material that follows and may be skipped without loss of continuity.

Figure 3–11 *The reduced form of the analysis of strategies for patients with equivocal presentations of appendicitis.*

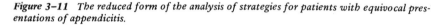

condition remains the same or worsens. The result is the same because the two approaches — the reduced form and the extensive form — are exactly equivalent.

3.5 INTERPRETING THE RESULTS OF A DECISION ANALYSIS

THE MEANING OF SMALL DIFFERENCES

We have raised the question of whether one needs some concept akin to the confidence intervals or significance levels of classical statistics to interpret the uncertainty surrounding the expected values of competing strategies. In the appendicitis example, the strategy to wait six hours had a mortality of 1.40 deaths per 1,000, compared with 1.53 deaths per 1,000 patients with the strategy to operate now. This narrow margin may make one feel uneasy about accepting the results of the analysis.

Part of our response to this unease rests upon the nature of decision analysis. Unlike a scientific experiment, decision analysis is not intended to reveal a scientific truth or a true state of nature. It is intended to help a decision maker choose from among alternative strategies of action. Decision analysis itself does not reduce our uncertainty about the true state of nature, but as long as we must make some choice it does enable us to make rational decisions in light of our uncertainty. If we have adequately specified the situation and represented our beliefs and values as best we can, than any finite difference among alternatives, no matter how minute, should tilt us in favor of the apparently better strategy. We may not be very confident that our selection is best, but according to the available data the chosen strategy is better, even if ever so slightly, than any of its competitors.

SENSITIVITY ANALYSIS

We may justifiably doubt the validity of such an analysis, however, for at least three reasons. First, we may be unsure that one or more of the probabilities that have been used are accurate. In such cases we might compute the analysis again, substituting a range of estimates for the probabilities in question to see whether this alters the conclusion of the analysis. This is an example of **sensitivity analysis**. If the conclusion is stable over a range of estimates around our initial best guess, this should reassure us. If, on the other hand, the conclusion is sensitive to small alterations in a key probability, this may lead us back to the literature or to experts in search of a more refined estimate. However, in the end the decision must still be made.

Consider the analysis of our appendicitis example once again. The analysis says that it is better to wait six hours than to operate now, although the results of this strategy are not much better than the results of the alternative. What would happen if one or more of the probabilities were altered in a direction unfavorable to the conclusion of the analysis? Would the recommended strategy change?

In this case suppose that the probability of the patient's condition worsening in six hours were 0.14 instead of 0.13 and that the probability of the patient's condition improving were 0.50 instead of 0.51. Using Figure 3–10, a straight-forward calculation determines that this change would increase the death rate for the strategy to wait six hours from 1.40 per 1,000 to 1.48 per 1,000 patients. It would still be optimal to wait six hours, but the decision would be less clear-cut. We reemphasize that you still have to make a decision; if 13 per cent or 14 per cent is your best estimate of the probability that the patient will get worse, then the analysis favors waiting six hours.

A second cause of unease over the analysis may be concern that the initial clinical situation was inadequately specified, for example, that an important consideration was omitted from the structure of the problem in the interest of simplicity. In some cases it may be possible to discern in which direction the additional consideration would shift the analysis; if the present conclusion is strengthened, the concern is not serious. In other cases it may be feasible to re-analyze the problem and formally incorporate the additional considerations. In yet other instances the additional considerations will serve as a warning that the analysis should not be accepted unthinkingly. This is another form of sensitivity analysis.

A final source of potential unease relates to the specification of the valued outcomes. Perhaps mortality is not the only real concern for the appendicitis case. Morbidity, including pain and suffering, and anxiety may be involved. If so, an outcome measure that is more complex than mortality would be needed. We describe some approaches to outcome assessment in Chapter Seven. For the time being we note that yet another form of sensitivity analysis involves varying the values attached to outcomes to see how much difference they make in the result of the analysis.

Definition. A **sensitivity analysis** is any test of the stability of the conclusions of an analysis over a range of structural assumptions, probability estimates, or value judgments.

It is useful to perform sensitivity analyses not only to reassure yourself about your own conclusions but also to convince others of the validity of your analysis. We also employ sensitivity analysis in the example to be introduced concerning patients with liver disease (p. 63). In this example we observe how a change in the rate of disease in the population can affect the preferred treatment strategy.

THRESHOLD ANALYSIS

In the sensitivity analysis with respect to the probability that a patient with equivocal symptoms of appendicitis will get worse in six hours, we might have asked how high the probability of the patient getting worse would have to be in order for the optimal strategy to become "operate now." The answer is about 15 per cent. This variant of sensitivity analysis is called **threshold analysis**; it tells us at what level of each of the probabilities, taken one at a time, the decision maker would consider the currently favored strategy no better than its nearest competitor. We shall soon see another example of threshold analysis.

3.6 THE EXPECTED VALUE OF CLINICAL INFORMATION

Recall the urinary tract infection example of Chapter Two (Section 2.1).

We observed that if no further decisions had to be made, the urine culture would have no value to the decision maker. No subsequent decision depends in any way on the result of the test.

In the appendicitis example, by contrast, the decisions following the strategy to wait six hours do depend on the results of this "test," or observation period. The preferred decision for at least one group following the six-hour observation period — the decision not to operate on patients who get better — is *different* from the best decision in the absence of the "wait" strategy, namely, the decision to operate on everyone with equivocal presentations. This difference means that the strategy to wait six hours could at least *conceivably* be the preferred strategy. Our further computations, which are summarized in Figure 3–10, show that the benefits of this change in decision for the patients who do get better indeed more than offset the drawbacks of delaying the decision to operate on those who get worse. Hence, the decision to wait six hours is, in fact, the preferred strategy.

In general, performing a test to gain additional information is worthwhile only if (1) at least one decision would change given some test results and (2) the risk to the patient associated with the test is less than the expected benefit that would be gained from the subsequent change in decision. In this section we use a simple example to demonstrate how one can estimate the **expected value of clinical information.**

CHRONIC PROGRESSIVE LIVER FAILURE

Patients displaying the signs of chronic progressive liver failure may have one of at least two conditions requiring different treatments: chronic progressive hepatitis or cirrhosis. Assume that if a patient has chronic progressive hepatitis, treatment with steroids may increase the probability of two-year survival from 67 per cent to 85 per cent. If the patient has cirrhosis, which may be clinically indistinguishable from chronic hepatitis, treatment with steroids will do no good at all. All steroid treatment carries a risk of complications, which may include gastrointestinal bleeding and thromboembolic accidents. Assume that this risk of complication would lower the two-year survival rate of a patient with cirrhosis from 50 per cent to 48 per cent. Also assume that a liver biopsy would allow a perfect diagnosis in all cases and would lead to the institution of appropriate treatment. However, there is a 1/1,000 chance of these sick patients dying from the biopsy itself.* Should a biopsy be performed?

If you consider only the alternative diagnoses of hepatitis and cirrhosis and take survival for two years as the outcome about which you are concerned, how would you structure a decision tree for this clinical situation? What additional probabilities would you need in order to decide whether to perform a biopsy? You may wish to take a few minutes to draw a decision tree; when you have finished, look at Figure 3–12.

The key difference between the "biopsy" and "no biopsy" branches lies in the order of the chance node denoting hepatitis or cirrhosis and the decision node denoting steroids or no steroids. With a biopsy we can determine the diagnosis *before* we choose the type of therapy; hence, the chance node precedes

---

*In this, as in all the clinical examples used in this book, you are reminded that the problem structure and the probabilities used are illustrative and intended for pedagogic purposes only.

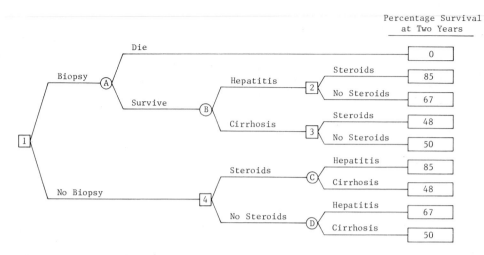

Figure 3–12 *A decision tree for patients with chronic progressive liver failure.*

the choice node. Without a biopsy, the choice of therapy comes first, and the probabilities of alternative diagnoses follow. You are correct if you surmised that the important probabilities that were omitted are the probabilities of a patient's having hepatitis or cirrhosis, that is, the rates of these diseases among patients with similar presentations. Assume that you are at General Hospital, where 80 per cent of chronic progressive liver failure is caused by cirrhosis and 20 per cent by chronic progressive hepatitis. If there were no opportunity to perform a biopsy, would a patient with chronic progressive liver failure be better off treated with steroids or without?

In this case the preferred treatment in the absence of information supplied by a biopsy would be steroids. This is shown in Figure 3–13, which is an analysis of the "no biopsy" branch of Figure 3–12. Notice that we average out at chance nodes Ⓒ and Ⓓ and that we fold back to decision node ⁴ . In so doing we have chosen the branch with the higher probability of survival (55.4 per cent).

A Threshold Analysis

In the absence of the information provided by a biopsy, would the preferred treatment be steroids regardless of the probabilities of hepatitis and cirrhosis? What, for example, would the preferred treatment be in the absence of biopsy data if the probability of a patient's having cirrhosis were 95 per cent?

Figure 3–13 *The preferred treatment if no biopsy were available. (The probability of cirrhosis is 0.8 and of hepatitis is 0.2.)*

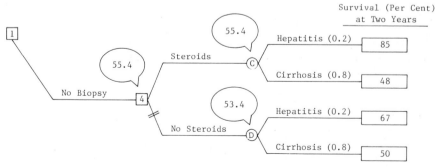

Table 3–2 shows the expected survival and preferred treatment for patients with liver disease over a range of probabilities of the two diagnoses. This table was generated by substituting the various proportions of patients with cirrhosis and with hepatitis into the decision tree of Figure 3–13 and then computing the averaged-out survival rate with and without steroids.

TABLE 3–2   PROBABILITIES OF TWO-YEAR SURVIVAL AND PREFERRED
TREATMENT FOR PATIENTS WITH CHRONIC PROGRESSIVE
LIVER FAILURE (NO BIOPSY)

PROPORTION WITH CIRRHOSIS*	SURVIVAL RATE WITH STEROIDS	SURVIVAL RATE WITHOUT STEROIDS	PREFERRED TREATMENT
0.00	0.8500	0.6700	Steroids
.01	.8463	.6683	Steroids
.05	.8315	.6615	Steroids
.10	.8130	.6530	Steroids
.20	.7760	.6360	Steroids
.50	.6650	.5850	Steroids
.80	.5540	.5340	Steroids
.89	.5207	.5187	Steroids
.90	.5170	.5170	Either
.91	.5133	.5153	No Steroids
.95	.4985	.5085	No Steroids
.99	.4837	.5017	No Steroids
1.00	.4800	.5000	No Steroids

*The remainder have hepatitis.

Note that when the rate of cirrhosis is 90 per cent (and no biopsy has been done), we would end up with the same expected survival rate regardless of the treatment chosen, and we would be indifferent as to whether we prescribed steroids. This is an example of a threshold analysis. (As an optional exercise at the end of the chapter, we ask you to prove algebraically that the two treatments have the same survival rates when the probability of cirrhosis equals 90 per cent.)

Analysis of the Optimal Strategy

Now let us return to the question of whether to perform a biopsy at General Hospital, where the proportion of such patients with cirrhosis is 80 per cent. Here we want to focus first on the biopsy branch of our decision tree in Figure 3–12. The decisions at choice nodes $\boxed{2}$ and $\boxed{3}$ are simple to make. If the biopsy specimen shows hepatitis, we will treat the condition with steroids, and if it shows cirrhosis, we will not prescribe steroids. The two-year survival rate at chance node $\circledR{B}$ becomes

$$(0.2)(0.85) + (0.8)(0.50) = 0.57.$$

Hence, if we average out further, the survival rate at node Ⓐ is

$$(0.999)(0.57) + (0.001)(0) = 0.5694,$$

or 56.94 per cent. Without the biopsy information we saw that the survival rate was 55.4 per cent (Figure 3–13). Therefore, the probability of survival on the "biopsy" branch exceeds the probability of survival on the "no biopsy" branch by

$$56.94\% - 55.4\% = 1.54\%.$$

Our conclusion from the analysis is that if 10,000 patients with chronic progressive liver failure had a liver biopsy performed prior to treatment, we would expect 154 more of them to be alive at the end of two years than if no biopsies had been performed and all patients had been given steroids.

Net Expected Value of Clinical Information

The difference between the two-year survival rates with and without a biopsy is a measure of the **net expected value of clinical information** obtained from the biopsy. Notice that the *net* expected value of test information as used here takes into consideration the mortality that is intrinsic to the use of the test. In our present example the mortality that is attributable to the liver biopsy is given as 1/1,000, and the net expected value of clinical information from the biopsy is 1.54 per cent.

Definition. The **net expected value of clinical information** obtained from a test is the difference between the averaged-out outcome value with the test and the averaged-out outcome value without the test when the risks of the test itself are taken into consideration.

Now think about the appendicitis example again. What is the net expected value of the clinical information obtained by waiting six hours? This value of observational information is completely analogous to the value of information that may be obtained from diagnostic tests. The net value of the information is the difference between the death rate following the decision to obtain the information and the death rate following the decision not to obtain the information. In this case (Figure 3–9) the net expected value of clinical information that will be gained by waiting six hours is 1.53 minus 1.40, or 0.13 *fewer* deaths per 1,000 patients. In that case, however, the information is not *perfect*, because the observation of symptoms does not reveal with certainty the true state of the patient.

THE EXPECTED VALUE OF PERFECT CLINICAL INFORMATION

The liver biopsy in this example gives *perfect* information; the biopsy tells us with *certainty* which disease the patient has. The value of this information lies in its ability to correct what would have been a suboptimal decision. We measure this value in terms of the reduction in mortality that results from the information, and we can compute it using the decision tree in Figure 3–14.

We found that the expected survival at node Ⓑ is 57.0 per cent and that the

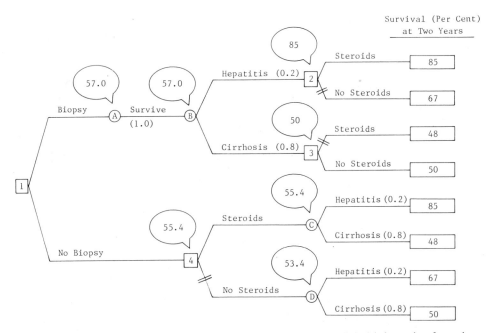

Figure 3–14 Calculation of the expected value of perfect clinical information for patients with chronic progressive liver failure.

expected survival at node 4 is 55.4 per cent. If the biopsy had no mortality associated with it, the value at node Ⓐ would equal the value at node Ⓑ, that is, 57.0 per cent. The difference between 57.0 per cent with the biopsy and 55.4 per cent without the biopsy, or 1.6 per cent survival, is the **expected value of perfect clinical information**. It is the value of the information without correcting for the risk of the diagnostic procedure. The *net* expected value of perfect clinical information in this example is 1.54 per cent, as calculated previously. The difference between 1.60 per cent and 1.54 per cent, or 0.06 deaths per 1000 patients, is a measure of the risk associated with the biopsy. But this risk is much less than the benefit (1.60 lives per 100 patients) to be gained by performing the biopsy, so the net value is positive, and the biopsy is indicated.

Definition. The **expected value of perfect clinical information** is the difference between the averaged-out outcome value with a test and the averaged-out outcome value without a test when the test reveals the true disease state with certainty and is assumed to have no risk.

Another way to get the same result in this example is to observe that the biopsy has value only if it indicates cirrhosis, because only then does it affect a decision. Steroids are the treatment of choice without a biopsy (Figure 3–13), and they are also the treatment of choice with known hepatitis. The biopsy is the cause of death in one patient in 1,000, but if the biopsy specimen shows cirrhosis in the survivors (with a probability of 0.8), then no steroids will be used, and two lives per 100 patients (50 – 48) will be saved. Thus, the expected value of the biopsy (the gross value, not the value net of its risk) is

$$(0.8) (2) = 1.6$$

lives per 100 patients, which is the same answer we derived with the aid of the decision tree.

THE DEPENDENCE OF THE EXPECTED VALUE OF PERFECT CLINICAL INFORMATION UPON UNDERLYING PROBABILITIES

We saw in Table 3–2 how the optimal survival rate and the preferred treatment change as the proportion of patients with cirrhosis varies from 0.00 to 1.00. Table 3–3 shows how the expected value of biopsy information changes as the proportion of patients with cirrhosis varies. This table is based on results from the decision tree of Figure 3–14. The expected value of biopsy information is greatest at just that probability of disease (0.9 in this case) at which the two possible treatments result in the same survival rate. (Recall that we derived this fact from our threshold analysis in the section dealing with that subject [p. 65].)

Table 3–3 also shows that the net expected value of biopsy information in our hepatitis-cirrhosis example remains positive until the very extremes of disease probabilities, at which values we would already be nearly certain prior to the biopsy results which disease was present. If we were not certain of the exact probabilities of cirrhosis or hepatitis but were quite confident of the other parameters in the problem, Table 3–3 should make us comfortable with the decision to take a biopsy specimen from all patients. We might not be able to say *exactly* how much benefit to expect, but we could be reasonably confident that the best decision strategy would be to perform a biopsy. This is another example of a **sensitivity analysis**: The validity of our conclusion is tested against a range of possible values for an uncertain probability.

TABLE 3–3 NET EXPECTED VALUE OF BIOPSY INFORMATION
(IN TERMS OF ADDED PROBABILITY OF TWO-YEAR SURVIVAL)
FOR PATIENTS WITH CHRONIC PROGRESSIVE LIVER FAILURE

PROPORTION WITH CIRRHOSIS*	SURVIVAL RATE WITH BIOPSY	SURVIVAL RATE WITHOUT BIOPSY	NET EXPECTED VALUE OF BIOPSY DATA
0.00	0.8492	0.8500	−0.0008
.01	.8457	.8463	−0.0006
.05	.8317	.8315	0.0002
.10	.8142	.8130	.0012
.20	.7792	.7760	.0032
.50	.6743	.6650	.0093
.80	.5694	.5540	.0154
.89	.5380	.5207	.0173
.90	.5345	.5170	.0175
.91	.5310	.5153	.0157
.95	.5170	.5085	.0085
.99	.5030	.5017	.0013
1.00	.4995	.5000	−0.0005

*The remainder have hepatitis.

Figure 3–15 shows a graphic analysis of the expected value and the net expected value for a hypothetical diagnostic test that carries a 5 per cent risk of mortality and that distinguishes perfectly between two possible diseases.

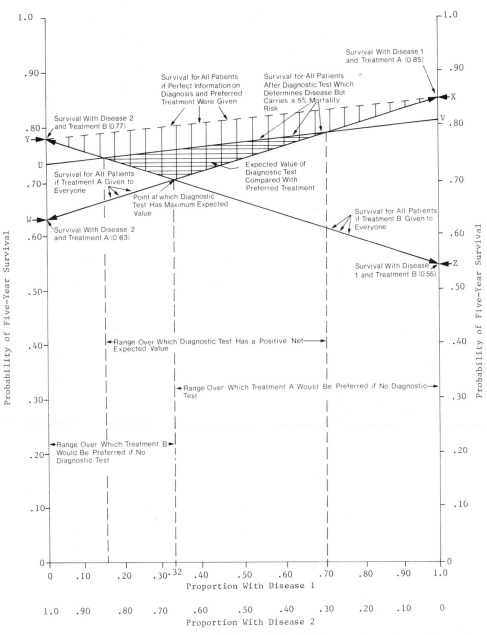

Figure 3–15 The five-year survival rate, with and without a diagnostic test that carries a five per cent risk of mortality and which distinguishes between two hypothetical diseases with differing preferred treatments. (These are shown as a function of varying proportions of

the two diseases in a population. The height of the vertically shaded area 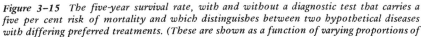 *represents*

the expected value of perfect clinical information. The height of the crosshatched area represents the net expected value of perfect clinical information.)

We assume that all patients in the population have either disease 1 or disease 2 and that the outcome of interest is five-year survival. Figure 3–15 illustrates the following principles: (1) The value, net or gross, of a diagnostic test depends on the probabilities of the diseases or conditions it distinguishes, and (2) the value, net or gross, of a diagnostic test is greatest when the probabilities of the diseases are such that one would be indifferent between the two available treatments for a randomly selected patient.

In this example, treatment A is preferred for patients with disease 1 (an 85 per cent survival rate at point X versus a 55 per cent survival rate at point Z), and treatment B is preferred for patients with disease 2 (a 77 per cent survival rate at point Y versus a 63 per cent survival rate at point W). If all patients were given treatment A, the survival rate would depend on the proportion of patients with each disease and would follow the line that ascends most steeply to the right (WX). Similarly, if all patients were given treatment B, the survival rate would correspond to the line ascending most steeply to the left (ZY). The point at which these lines cross, which is marked by the middle vertical dashed line, corresponds to the probability of disease at which the two available treatments would be equally desirable in the absence of diagnostic test information. At this point, the survival rate with either treatment is 70 per cent.

The uppermost broken line (YX) in the figure represents survival if a test could determine the correct diagnosis for all patients without subjecting the patients to risk and if the preferred treatment were given. The hypothetical diagnostic test produces perfect information but carries a 5 per cent risk of mortality. Therefore, the line indicating survival if the diagnostic test were administered to all patients is the solid line (UV), which is 95 per cent of the distance between the horizontal axis and the uppermost broken line.

The width (from top to bottom) of the vertically shaded area directly above any particular proportion of the population with the disease gives the expected value of perfect clinical information from the diagnostic test in that population. The horizontally crosshatched region spans that range in the proportion of the population with the disease over which the diagnostic test (with a 5 per cent risk) has a positive net expected value.

Notice that the gross or net expected value of the diagnostic test is greatest at that proportion of the population with the disease at which one would be indifferent between treatments in the absence of the test. This occurs in the diagram when the probability of disease 1 is approximately 0.32. At this point the survival rate with either treatment is 70 per cent if no test is done. Also at this point the survival rate if a riskless test were performed would be about 80 per cent. This difference, 10 per cent, is the maximum possible expected value of perfect information; any risk associated with the test or any shift in the proportion of patients with each disease would lower the expected value.

THE EXPECTED VALUE OF IMPERFECT CLINICAL INFORMATION: A PREVIEW

Very few tests in clinical medicine are perfect. If the liver biopsy indicated the correct diagnosis only 90 per cent of the time, it might misdiagnose 10 per cent of cirrhosis cases as hepatitis and 10 per cent of hepatitis cases as cirrhosis. In that case, the information is less valuable, but it still could have a positive value. In fact, we can calculate its expected value by methods very similar to those we have used to evaluate a "perfect" test. However, we will need to develop additional techniques before we can estimate the value of this kind of "imperfect" situation. We shall return to the problem of estimating the **expected value of clinical information** in Chapter Five.

3.7 SUMMARY OF CHAPTER THREE

The mathematical language of **probability** provides a precise way to communicate information about uncertainties in clinical decision making. The probability of an event may be viewed as the frequency with which the event occurs in a population, or the proportion in a population experiencing that event. Later we shall think of probabilities as measures of one's strength of belief that an event will occur. Probabilities for individual patients may be derived from observed proportions in the population from which the individuals are selected.

Probabilities range from 0.0 to 1.0. To this point we have used the terms **proportion, rate,** and **frequency** as synonyms for probability. Probabilities and proportions are sometimes expressed as **percentages** ranging from 0 per cent to 100 per cent. The probability of an event, E, is written as $P[E]$.

Probabilities obey the **summation principle,** which states that the sum of the probabilities of all possible occurrences of a chance event must equal 1.0, or 100 per cent. In a decision tree the summation principle implies that the probabilities of all possible states of the patient or of other relevant probabilistic events represented at a chance node must sum to 1.0.

The **joint probability** of two or more events is the probability that they will all occur. The joint probability of two events, E and F, is written as $P[E$ and $F]$ or as $P[E, F]$. Joint probabilities obey a summation principle that requires that if either event F_1 or F_2 must occur (i.e., $P[F_1] + P[F_2] = 1$), then

$$P[E, F_1] + P[E, F_2] = P[E].$$

The **conditional probability** of one event, E, given another event, F, is the probability that E will occur once it is known that F occurs. It is written as $P[E|F]$ and is read "the probability of E given F." The conditional and joint probabilities of two events are related by the formula

$$P[E, F] = P[E|F] \circ P[F].$$

Two or more events are said to be **independent** if the conditional probability of one event, given the others, does not depend on the other events. Symbolically, events E and F are independent if and only if

$$P[E|F] = P[E].$$

When events are independent, their joint probabilities obey the **product rule.**

$$P[E, F] = P[E] \cdot P[F].$$

The product rule does not hold for events that are not independent.

Averaging out is the process of calculating the probability of an event from several conditional probabilities. Specifically, if we know $P[F_1]$, $P[F_2]$, and $P[F_3]$ as well as the conditional probabilities $P[E|F_1]$, $P[E|F_2]$, and $P[E|F_3]$, then we can apply the summation principle and the definitions of joint and conditional probability to derive the probability of event E as the following weighted average:

$$P[E] = P[F_1] \cdot P[E|F_1] + P[F_2] \cdot P[E|F_2] + P[F_3] \cdot P[E|F_3].$$

To evaluate a decision tree, start at the far right, where the possible final outcomes are arrayed. **Average out** the value of all possible branches at each chance node by multiplying the probability of each branch by the value attached to it and summing the values of all branches at the node. Then **fold back** along the *one* branch from each choice node that offers the most favorable value (e.g., the highest value if it is a survival rate or the lowest value if it is a death rate). It is convenient to mark a double slash across any choice branch that has been eliminated. By this sequential process of averaging out and folding back along the branches of the decision tree, one can derive the preferred **strategy** for the clinical decision problem.

In this chapter we have restricted ourselves to a single outcome measure for any given decision problem, such as the probability of death or survival. Using techniques described in Chapter Seven, more realistic and complicated outcome measures may be employed.

Sensitivity analysis is the process of examining the validity of a particular conclusion over a range of possible estimates for a given parameter, such as a probability. **Threshold analysis** determines the value of a parameter at which the previously optimal strategy becomes no better than its nearest competitor.

The **expected value of clinical information** is the difference between the averaged-out outcome value following the strategy in which information is obtained and the averaged-out outcome value following the strategy in which information is not obtained. In this chapter we analyzed two examples, one in which the additional information was obtained from observing patients over time and the second in which the information was derived from a diagnostic biopsy. In order for a test to be of net positive value, it must satisfy a necessary and sufficient condition. The necessary condition is that at least one decision following the test must depend upon the results of the test; in other words, at least one possible test result must lead to the selection of a subsequent branch that is different from the branch that would have been selected in the absence of the test. The sufficient condition is that the average benefit from this change in decision must outweigh any risk involved in using the test.

The use of probability, especially of specific probabilities for an individual patient, is central to systematic clinical decision making. In the next three chapters, we turn to the origin and use of probabilistic information.

═══════════════════════════════

EXERCISES FOR CHAPTER THREE

EXERCISES FOR SECTION 3.2

1. *Diagnostic Tests for Renovascular Disease*

Two tests for renovascular disease in patients with hypertension are the intravenous pyelogram (IVP) and the renogram (RG). The IVP is an x-ray procedure that detects obstructions of the renal arteries; the RG is a procedure that uses radioactive isotopes to identify renovascular disease.

When an IVP is taken of hypertensive patients with known renovascular disease, the findings are abnormal (positive test results) in 78 per cent, whereas the results are positive for 85 per cent of the patients when the RG is administered. However, the results of both the IVP and the RG are positive for only 69 per cent of these patients.

a. What is the joint probability of the results of the IVP *and* the RG being positive for a hypertensive patient with renovascular disease?
b. In hypertensive patients with renovascular disease, what is the conditional probability of the result of an IVP's being positive, given a positive finding on an RG?
c. In patients with hypertension and renovascular disease, what is the conditional probability of the result of an RG's being positive, given a positive finding on an IVP?

2. *Abnormal Results in a Battery of Tests*
A battery of six laboratory tests is designed so that, in patients who have no disease, the probability of having an abnormal result on any single test is 5 per cent. The tests are independent in these patients.

a. What is the probability that in a well patient the results of all six tests will be abnormal?
b. What is the probability that in a well patient at least one of the six test results will be abnormal?

EXERCISES FOR SECTION 3.3

3. *Intravenous Pyelogram (IVP)*
Among hypertensive patients admitted to the hospital *with* renovascular disease, 78 per cent have a positive result on an IVP. Among hypertensive patients admitted *without* renovascular disease, 11 per cent have a positive result on an IVP. In a given hospital, 10 per cent of hypertensive patients admitted to the hospital have renovascular disease. What proportion of hypertensive patients admitted to the hospital would have a positive finding on an IVP?

EXERCISES FOR SECTION 3.4

4. *Disease Q*
There are two alternative treatments for disease Q: surgery and radiotherapy. You must decide whether to prescribe radiotherapy or to perform an exploratory procedure to determine whether the patient might be a candidate for surgery. The drawback of the exploratory procedure is that it compromises the effectiveness of radiotherapy.
If you choose to prescribe radiotherapy without performing an exploratory procedure, the patient has a 0.8 chance of survival.
If you choose to do the exploratory procedure, there is a 50 per cent chance that the patient's condition will be operable. In that case you still have a choice between surgery and radiotherapy. Radiotherapy following the exploratory procedure gives the patient a 60 per cent chance of survival. Surgery has a complication rate of 20 per cent; if there are complications, the chance that the patient will die is 30 per cent, but if there are no complications, the chance that the patient will die is only 5 per cent.
You want to give the patient the highest possible probability of survival. What would your best strategy be?

5. *Acute Tarkism**
Acute tarkism is a hypothetical, rapidly progressing disease with a 20 per cent chance of mortality if it is left untreated. Early and extensive surgery, which has a mortality of 0.1 for all patients, always cures acute tarkism. No other treatment is available. Assume that the only outcome about which you care is a reduction in the death rate.

---

*This problem was suggested by Donald M. Berwick, M.D.

The AT test, which identifies people with acute tarkism at a stage when surgery might help, is available. The problem with the AT test is that it sometimes indicates that a person has acute tarkism when the person is in reality perfectly well.

a. Suppose that only 40 per cent of the cases in which the test result is positive actually have the disease. Would you recommend an operation for a person whose AT test result was positive?

b. What proportion of patients with a positive AT test would have to have acute tarkism in order for you to recommend surgery for a person with a positive AT test result? (This is an example of a threshold analysis.)

EXERCISES FOR SECTION 3.6

5. *Open-Lung Biopsy for Pneumocystis*

Pneumocystis is a protozoan microorganism that is an extremely rare pathogen in humans. It is a significant threat, however, to immunosuppressed patients, including those who are treated with chemotherapy and radiation for leukemia or neoplasms. In susceptible patients, *Pneumocystis* can produce severe pneumonia with fever, diffuse pulmonary infiltrates, and hypoxemia. Unfortunately, this syndrome can have many causes in these already ill patients, and at Referral Cancer Hospital, *Pneumocystis* probably accounts for only one fifth of such cases.

Assume that an open-lung biopsy is the only good way to diagnose the presence of *Pneumocystis* and that it yields perfect information. The biopsy itself carries a significant risk of mortality; assume that it is responsible for a 4 per cent mortality in this severely ill patient population.

Assume that if this condition were left untreated it would be fatal in 90 per cent of the cases. Even in these severely ill patients whose condition is not due to *Pneumocystis*, their six-month survival rate is only 65 per cent. Although a reasonably safe drug has recently been used to treat this syndrome, at one time the preferred treatment, and the only one to be considered here, was the drug pentamidine. If it is administered to patients with *Pneumocystis*, pentamidine improves survival such that half the patients will still be alive after six months. Pentamidine is itself a very toxic drug, and if it is administered to patients without *Pneumocystis*, it reduces their six-month survival rate from 65 per cent to 63 per cent.

Draw a decision tree for patients in whom *Pneumocystis* is suspected to be the cause of their illness. Use the six-month survival rate as the outcome of concern, and answer the following questions:

a. In the absence of a biopsy, would it be better to treat the condition with pentamidine or to withhold this drug?

b. Should an open-lung biopsy be performed on patients, or should they simply be given the preferred treatment without the biopsy? What is the expected value of the perfect information obtained from the biopsy, and what is the net expected value?

c. What would the mortality from the lung biopsy itself have to be in order to make you indifferent between performing an open-lung biopsy and treating the condition without performing a biopsy?

d. If you choose the no biopsy-pentamidine strategy, you might be able to reconsider the decision to do a biopsy if the patient responds poorly to the drug. How would you restructure your decision tree to take this possibility into account?

7. *Maximum Expected Value of Clinical Information*

In the liver biopsy example (p. 63) it was asserted that the biopsy has maximum value when the probability of cirrhosis is at the level at which the two treatment alternatives (steroids and no steroids) are equally desirable. Show that the two treatment alternatives are equally desirable when the probability of cirrhosis is 90 per cent.

Chapter Four

The Use of Diagnostic Information to Revise Probabilities

4.1 CLINICAL INFORMATION AND PROBABILITY REVISION

Physicians have at their disposal an enormous variety of clinical information to serve as a guide in decision making. Some pieces of clinical information derive from diagnostic tests, which in some cases may be expensive or, as in the case of the liver biopsy example of Chapter Three, may be risky. Other valuable information can be secured simply by observing the patient or following his or her response to treatment. The purpose of clinical information, however it is obtained, is to aid the physician in making a proper diagnosis and thereby in choosing the best treatment.

The preceding chapter introduced the notion of probability and illustrated how probabilities may be used in the averaging-out-and-folding-back process to arrive at an optimal strategy of management. In this chapter we will consider how the information obtained from a diagnostic test or clinical observation relates to the probabilities in a clinical decision problem.

Consider again the liver biopsy example of Chapter Three (Figure 3–12). Now, instead of assuming that the biopsy yields perfect information as to whether the patient has hepatitis or cirrhosis, suppose more realistically that the biopsy gives valuable but not perfect diagnostic information. That is, suppose that the biopsy sometimes indicates hepatitis when, in fact, the patient has cirrhosis and that it sometimes fails to identify hepatitis when it is present.

A modified decision tree for this decision problem is shown in Figure 4–1. This decision tree incorporates the two most common kinds of clinical decisions: whether to test (node $\boxed{1}$) and whether to treat (nodes $\boxed{2}$, $\boxed{3}$, and $\boxed{4}$).

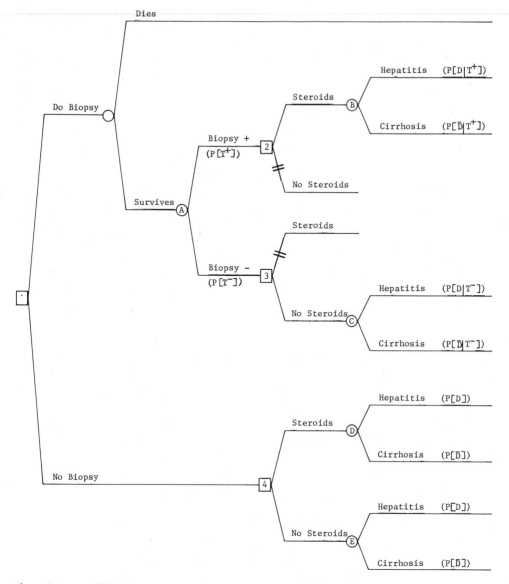

Figure 4–1 A modified decision tree for the liver biopsy problem.

The probabilities associated with the chance nodes, as indicated on the decision tree, are illustrative of three generic types. The first type of probability, the probability of a positive test result ($P[T^+]$) or a negative test result ($P[T^-]$), is found at node (A). In this context "positive" means "positive for hepatitis," which indicates the desirability of intervention with steroids. The second type of probability, the probability that the patient has the disease ($P[D]$) or does not have the disease ($P[\bar{D}]$) for which treatment might be prescribed, is represented at nodes (D) and (E). The third type of probability represented in Figure 4–1 relates to the value of the clinical information provided by the biopsy: It is the *conditional* probability that the patient either has or does not have the disease *given* the content of the clinical information. At chance node (B) the probabilities ($P[D \mid T^+]$ and $P[\bar{D} \mid T^+]$) are conditional upon a positive test result for hepatitis; at node Ⓒ the probabilities ($P[D \mid T^-]$ and $P[\bar{D} \mid T^-]$) are conditional upon a negative test result for hepatitis. We shall see in this chapter that these three types of probability are related in a very special way.

Several points are illustrated by the decision tree in Figure 4–1. The decision problem is typical in many respects of a variety of clinical decision problems. First, observe that the decision tree identifies the number and precisely defines the character of the probabilities needed to resolve the clinical issue. This focus powerfully inhibits any tendency to do too many tests or to overlook the acquisition of a crucial piece of information.

Second, note the relations that the probabilities at chance nodes Ⓑ, Ⓒ, Ⓓ, and Ⓔ bear to the clinical information obtained. At nodes Ⓓ and Ⓔ the probabilities of disease are assessed without the benefit of additional test information. They reflect the probabilities assigned to the two disease possibilities— hepatitis and cirrhosis—*before* the biopsy has been done. These probabilities, which we shall call **prior probabilities** of disease, may reflect the proportions of the population that have the two diseases. In the analysis of this example in Chapter Three, the prior probability of hepatitis was taken to be 0.2, and the prior probability of cirrhosis was 0.8. The probabilities at node Ⓑ, on the other hand, are conditional upon the result that the biopsy specimen is positive for hepatitis. At that point the probability of hepatitis is no longer 0.2; it is presumably greater than the prior probability of 0.2 because we now have the information that the biopsy specimen showed hepatitis. We will call this conditional probability of disease, given a piece of clinical information, a **posterior probability** of disease, because it is assessed *after* the result of the clinical test or observation is known. In the case analyzed in Chapter Three in which the liver biopsy was assumed to yield perfect information, the posterior probability of hepatitis, given a biopsy specimen that was positive for hepatitis, was 1.0. In actuality, this probability would be less than 1.0, although it would surely be greater than the prior probability of 0.2.

This chapter will be concerned with the process of using clinical information, such as the result of a diagnostic test, to reassess the probability that a patient has one of several possible diseases. In our conditional probability notation, we may write this probability as $P[D \mid T^+]$, which we read "the probability of disease given a positive test result." Ordinarily, estimates of such probabilities are not readily available. Instead, one is more likely to have an assessment of the probability of a positive test result among patients with the disease, or $P[T^+ \mid D]$, and some prior probability of the disease, or $P[D]$. The process of taking the test result into account by converting the prior probability, $P[D]$, to a posterior probability of disease, $P[D \mid T^+]$ or $P[D \mid T^-]$, is called **probability revision**. The major part of this chapter is devoted to techniques for using test information to revise probabilities in a consistent way.

This chapter, together with Chapters Five and Six, relates generally to the sources of information upon which clinical probabilities are based. Chapter Five expands upon the material in this chapter to permit the decision maker to assess more generally the value of clinical test information, including instances in which several tests may be used simultaneously or in which clinical tests may be repeated. The medical literature, clinical experience, and subjective judgment as sources of information upon which to base a probability assessment are all discussed in Chapter Six.

4.2 PROBABILISTICALLY DISTRIBUTED QUANTITIES*

The result of a diagnostic test, such as the measurement of diastolic blood pressure, is obviously unknown before the test is conducted. The diastolic blood pressure might be 80 mm Hg, 92 mm Hg, or any number within the possible range. To each possible test result there corresponds a probability. For example, the probability that a 50-year-old woman will have a diastolic blood pressure between 90 mm Hg and 95 mm Hg might be about 10 per cent. We shall refer to a quantity such as the level of diastolic blood pressure as a **probabilistically distributed quantity (PDQ)** and to the schedule of probabilities associated with each possible value of the PDQ as its **probability distribution.** Often we graph a probability distribution as shown in Figure 4–2.

Sometimes, as in the case of blood pressure, a PDQ takes its possible values from a continuous scale. One way to represent the probability distribution of such a quantity is by a discrete approximation, as Figure 4–2 illustrates. That is, we divide the blood pressure scale into discrete intervals (e.g., of 5 mm Hg wide) and represent the probability that the quantity will fall into each interval by the heights of the bars. Often we estimate a probability distribution from an empirical **frequency distribution,** that is, from the observed proportions of measurements of a PDQ that fall into each interval.

Another way to represent the probability distribution of a continuous PDQ is by a **probability density function,** as shown in Figure 4–3. The area under the curve, which represents a probability density function, is always defined as 1.0, indicating a probability of 1.0 that the PDQ will be somewhere along the scale (e.g., that the diastolic blood pressure will be a positive number). The probability that the PDQ will fall within any specified interval (e.g., between 90 and 95 mm Hg) is indicated by the area under the curve within the specified range. For example, in Figure 4–3 the shaded area represents the probability that the diastolic blood pressure is between 90 and 95 mm Hg; its area is approximately 10 per cent of the total area under the curve, thus denoting a probability of 0.1 for that interval.

In our discussion of test results as probabilistically distributed quantities, we shall usually characterize them by discrete probability distributions with

---

*This section provides background material on probability distributions and may be skipped or skimmed by those who are familiar with these concepts.

Figure 4–2 The probability distribution of diastolic blood pressure in 50-year-old women. (Adapted from National Center for Health Statistics, Vital and Health Statistics, Series 11, No. 5, Washington, D.C., 1964.)

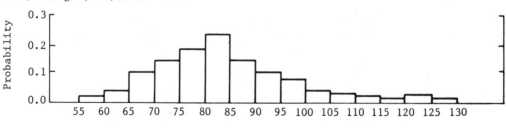

Diastolic Blood Pressure (mm Hg)

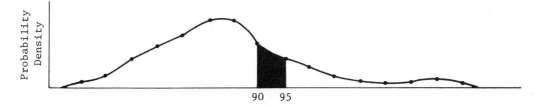

Figure 4–3 *The probability density function for diastolic blood pressure in 50-year-old women.*

appropriately defined intervals. For artistic reasons, however, we shall occasionally represent them by their continuous probability density functions. The two representations are, as Figures 4–2 and 4–3 illustrate, very similar when the range of the interval is small.

4.3 TESTS AS SEPARATORS

TESTS AND OTHER CLINICAL INFORMATION

To begin our discussion of the use of clinical information, we describe the essential properties of a test. We shall use the word *test* to refer to any means of seeking information about a patient: historical, physical, chemical, radiographic, or other. Tests provide information that can separate patients into groups with differing probabilities of disease; if the test accomplishes this separation, we can then use the test result to modify our prior expectations that a given patient has a particular disease.

Remember that a probability is really a perception of the decision maker. An individual patient either has the disease or does not. Information obtained from a test does not, of course, alter the state of the patient, but it may alter the physician's perception of how probable it is that the patient has one disease or another.

Some people distinguish between diagnostic tests and screening tests. A *diagnostic test* is performed to determine the nature of a specific complaint, symptom, or syndrome, whereas a *screening test* is performed to help identify patients at high risk for a disease. While the reasons for using these tests may differ, their essential properties for purposes of clinical decision analysis are the same. Both diagnostic and screening tests are employed to raise or lower the assessed probability that a patient has a disease, that is, to help the physician become more certain of the patient's condition.

SEPARATORS AND THE POSITIVITY CRITERION

Tests typically have two features: (1) a **separator** variable, which is a measurable property that relates to a particular disease, and (2) a **positivity criterion**, which is a particular value of the separator variable that distinguishes patients who are considered "normal" for purposes of subsequent decision making from those who are considered "diseased." If we are interested in hypertension, for example, one possible separator variable would be the average diastolic blood pressure at three successive readings, and we might choose as our positivity criterion a diastolic blood pressure of 90 mm Hg. In the diagnosis of tuberculosis, the separator variable might be the size of the indurated papule induced by injection of a small quantity of antigen into the skin, and the positivity criterion might be 10 mm. We shall demonstrate in this section how a separator variable, or a test result, may be represented as a probabilistically distributed quantity, where the probability distribution depends on the true disease state of the patient.

SGOT and Myocardial Infarction

Let us now apply the concepts of a separator variable and positivity criterion to an important contemporary clinical problem: the identification of patients who have acute myocardial infarction (MI) among all those who are seen in the emergency ward with chest pain. One separator variable for myocardial infarction is the serum level of glutamic oxaloacetic transaminase (SGOT), an enzyme that may be elevated in the presence of cardiac damage. Figure 4–4 displays the results of a study in which SGOT levels were measured in 94 patients with chest pain.* Of the 94 patients, 48 had myocardial infarction and 46 did not. The data are presented in a form that presumes that we have ascertained independently of the SGOT level whether each patient had myocardial infarction.

The horizontal axis represents the separator variable (the SGOT level), with this value increasing to the right. The separator variable is divided into intervals of 50 units/liter wide, except for the highest interval, which covers the range from 250 to 600 units/liter.

Above this axis we plot the frequency distribution of SGOT levels in patients who were subsequently proven to have acute MI. Shown on the figure are the proportions of patients whose SGOT levels fall within each interval. For example, 11 of the 48 patients with MI, or approximately 23 per cent, had SGOT levels between 50 units/liter and 100 units/liter. Below the horizontal axis, we construct an analogous frequency distribution based on the number of patients who did *not* have myocardial infarction.

Biologic variables often show a substantial spread in values for both diseased and nondiseased populations; furthermore, the values in the two groups usually overlap. This overlap makes it impossible to define a positivity criterion that distinguishes perfectly all those with a disease from all those without it. Most clinical tests share this imperfection, but it does not render them useless. Our task is to discover the positivity criterion that makes the best possible separation of those in the population who have the disease from those who do not have it. As we shall see later in this chapter (Section 4.11), the choice of an optimal positivity criterion depends on the context in which the test is to be used to reach a clinical decision.

The Implications of Choosing a Positivity Criterion

Let us arbitrarily set the positivity criterion, or **cutoff point**, for the SGOT level at 100 units/liter. Using this cutoff point, the proportion of patients with MI whose test results are positive (i.e., SGOT $\geqslant$ 100 units) is 52 per cent. This is represented in Figure 4–4 by the shaded portion of the area *above* the horizontal axis. Using the same cutoff point, the fraction of patients without MI whose test

---

*These data are adapted from Galen and Gambino,[82] although a few of the data points have been altered for pedagogic reasons.

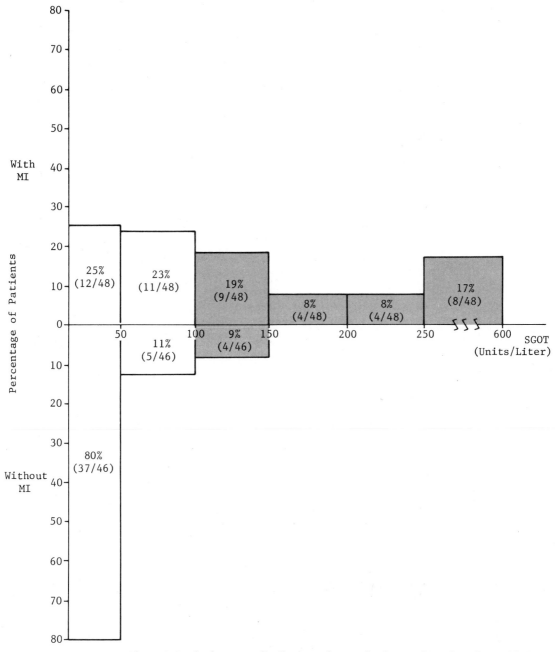

Figure 4–4 *The frequency distributions of SGOT levels at 24 hours in patients with chest pain with (above the axis) and without (below the axis) myocardial infarction (MI). (The shaded area above the horizontal axis denotes the rate of positive test results among patients with MI, assuming a positivity criterion of 100 units/liter. The shaded area below the horizontal axis denotes the rate of positive test results among patients without MI, assuming the same positivity criterion.) (Adapted in part from data of Galen and Gambino.[80])*

results are positive is 9 per cent. This is represented by the shaded portion of the area *below* the horizontal axis.

Note that if we move the cutoff point to the right, the proportion of patients without MI whose test results are positive will decrease, but so will the proportion of patients with MI whose positive test results correctly identify the condition. If we move the positivity criterion to the left, we will increase the fraction of patients whose test results are identified as positive for MI both among those with MI and among those without MI. Moving the positivity criterion always entails these trade-offs, provided that the distributions of the numbers of diseased and nondiseased individuals along the separator variable overlap.

With our positivity criterion at 100 units/liter, we have divided our study population of 94 patients into four groups: 25 whose test results are positive and who have the disease, or **true positives (TP)**; 4 whose test results are positive but who do not have the disease, or **false positives (FP)**; 23 patients who have the disease whose test results are negative, or **false negatives (FN)**; and 42 whose test results are negative and who do not have the disease, or **true negatives (TN)**. These data are expressed in tabular form using 2 X 2 tables in Table 4–1. The definitions of these four terms, which we shall use throughout the book, are as follows:

TABLE 4–1   TEST RESULTS IN A STUDY POPULATION*

	GENERAL CASE			SGOT LEVEL IN PATIENTS WITH CHEST PAIN			
Test Result	D	$\overline{D}$	Totals by Row	Test Result	MI	No MI	Totals by Row
T^+	TP	FP	TP + FP (total test positives)	SGOT $\geqslant$ 100 units/liter	25	4	29 (test positives)
T^-	FN	TN	FN + TN (total test negatives)	SGOT < 100 units/liter	23	42	65 (test negatives)
Totals by column	TP + FN (total diseased patients)	FP + TN (total nondiseased patients)		Totals by column	48 (with MI)	46 (without MI)	94 (total in study population)

*T^+ indicates the test result is positive; T^-, the test result is negative; D, the disease is present; $\overline{D}$, the disease is absent; TP, true positives; TN, true negatives; FP, false positives; FN, false negatives; and MI, myocardial infarction.

Definition. Consider a test defined by a separator variable for which a positivity criterion has been chosen and which is intended to distinguish between two disease states, D (disease present) and $\overline{D}$ (disease absent).

True positives (TP) are patients in whom the disease is present and the test result is positive.

True negatives (TN) are patients in whom the disease is absent and the test result is negative.

False positives (FP) are patients in whom the disease is absent but the test result is positive.

False negatives (FN) are patients in whom the disease is present but the test result is negative.

In Section 4.4 we use these concepts to develop an approach to probability revision.

Measurement Error

Besides the relation of biologic variables to the presence or absence of disease, test measurements themselves have two important characteristics. First, the method of measurement may introduce a systematic error, or **bias**, into the results. The analytic method in a particular laboratory for determining the SGOT level, for example, may result in adding a number to its true numerical value. We will refer to a test's freedom from bias as its **accuracy**. Even if a test is free from bias, however, random errors may be introduced each time the test is run. The freedom from random errors in the measurement may be called the **precision**, or **reliability**, of the test. Accuracy and precision will be discussed in Chapter Five. For the remainder of this chapter we shall make the simplifying assumptions that all of our tests are perfectly accurate and precise and that the variation we observe among the members of a population reflects the true state of the patients.

WHY DICHOTOMIZE THE RESULTS OF A TEST?

By selecting a positivity criterion, we simplify the remaining analysis of the decision problem by reducing the number of possible test results to two: positive and negative. The set of probabilities required for the full analysis of the decision tree is then reduced to those mentioned in Section 4.1: the probability of disease, $P[D]$; the conditional probability of disease given a positive test result, $P[D | T^+]$; the conditional probability of disease given a negative test result, $P[D | T^-]$; and the probability of a positive test result, $P[T^+]$. The probabilities of the complementary events to each of these (e.g., the probability of *no* disease, $P[\bar{D}]$) are obtained simply by subtracting each from 1.0.

Although the techniques developed in the sections that follow can be generalized to many possible test results, we introduce the methods of probability revision in the context of a test whose results have been dichotomized according to a single positivity criterion. It is common to dichotomize a continuous separator variable into "positive" and "negative" regions. This is because most medical action is dichotomous: We decide to operate or not to operate, to initiate treatment or not to initiate it. The dichotomies in our examples are therefore motivated by realism as well as by pedagogic simplicity.

The generalization of these techniques to many possible test results along a separator variable will be made in Section 4.7. In the SGOT example, instead of using a positivity criterion such as 100 units/liter to reduce the possible test results to T^+ and T^-, we might have preserved the full range of the separator variable. Then, using the discrete intervals indicated in Figure 4–4, we would want to assess the following probabilities: $P[0–49 \text{ Units}]$, $P[50–99 \text{ Units}]$, $P[100–149 \text{ Units}]$, and so on; $P[MI | 0–49 \text{ Units}]$, $P[MI | 50–99 \text{ Units}]$, $P[MI | 100–149 \text{ Units}]$, and so on; as well as $P[MI]$. In Section 4.11 we will return to the problem of choosing an "optimal" positivity criterion based on an analysis in which the full range of test results is considered.

4.4 PROBABILITY REVISION USING CONTINGENCY TABLES

THE 2 × 2 TABLE FOR SGOT AND MI

We shall use the 2 × 2 contingency tables in Table 4–1 to define some important probabilities. Using these probabilities we will introduce the concept of probability revision. Specifically, we will calculate the probability that a patient has myocardial infarction given a positive SGOT test result, or $P[D \mid T^+]$. Study Table 4–1 carefully to be sure you understand it before going on to the next section.

SOME IMPORTANT CONDITIONAL PROBABILITIES: SENSITIVITY AND SPECIFICITY

Consider the proportion of patients with MI who have a positive SGOT test result. This proportion is 25/48, or about 52 per cent. Alternatively, we could have obtained this result by adding the fractions in the shaded portion of the area above the axis in Figure 4–4. This is the probability of a positive test result given that the disease is present; it may be expressed symbolically as $P[T^+ \mid D]$. We call this probability the **true-positive rate** (*TPR*) of the test. Similarly, the proportion of patients without the disease who have a negative test result is 91 per cent, or 42/46. This probability of a negative test result given that the disease is absent is denoted by $P[T^- \mid \bar{D}]$ and is called the **true-negative rate** (*TNR*) of the test. The complement of the true-positive rate is the proportion of patients with disease who have a negative test result, or $P[T^- \mid D]$; this is called the **false-negative rate** (*FNR*) of the test. In the example the false-negative rate is 100 per cent minus 52 per cent, or 48 per cent. Finally, the complement of the true-negative rate is the proportion of patients without the disease who have a positive test result, or $P[T^+ \mid \bar{D}]$; this is called the **false-positive rate** (*FPR*) of the test and is equal to 9 per cent in our example.

Symbolically, we can define these rates as follows:

$$TPR = TP/(TP + FN); \quad FNR = FN/(TP + FN);$$
$$TNR = TN/(TN + FP); \quad FPR = FP/(TN + FP).$$

Thus, in our example the false-positive rate is $FP/(TN + FP)$, or $4/(42 + 4)$, which equals approximately 0.09.

Technically, the proportions we observe from the empirical study sample are not the actual probabilities but only estimates of the underlying probabilities. In Chapter Six we will become more careful about the distinction between observed rates and underlying probabilities.

The formal definitions of these terms are as follows:

Definition. Consider a test defined by a separator variable for which a positivity criterion has been chosen and which is intended to distinguish between two disease states, D (disease present) and $\bar{D}$ (disease absent).
The **true-positive rate** (*TPR*) is the proportion of patients with the disease who have a positive test result. It is equal to $P[T^+ \mid D]$.
The **true-negative rate** (*TNR*) is the proportion of patients without the disease who have a negative test result. It is equal to $P[T^- \mid \bar{D}]$.
The **false-positive rate** (*FPR*) is the proportion of patients without the disease who have a positive test result. It is equal to $P[T^+ \mid \bar{D}]$.
The **false-negative rate** (*FNR*) is the proportion of patients with the disease who have a negative test result. It is equal to $P[T^- \mid D]$.

Observe that the true-positive rate and the false-negative rate sum to 1.0, or 100 per cent, and that the true-negative rate and false-positive rate also sum to

1.0, or 100 per cent. An ideal test has a true-positive rate of 1.0 (and therefore a false-negative rate of 0.0) and a false-positive rate of 0.0 (and therefore a true-negative rate of 1.0).

Synonyms for the true-positive rate and the true-negative rate in common usage are, respectively, test **sensitivity** and test **specificity**. A test with a high true-positive (and low false-negative) rate is said to be a **sensitive** test; a test with a low false-positive (and high true-negative) rate is said to be a **specific** test.

Definition. The following terms are synonymous with the true-positive rate and true-negative rate, respectively:
The **sensitivity** of a test is equal to its true-positive rate, or $P[T^+ | D]$.
The **specificity** of a test is equal to its true-negative rate, or $P[T^- | \bar{D}]$.

A sensitive test is very good at detecting patients with the disease; a specific test is very good at screening out patients who do not have the disease. Remember that test sensitivity applies to patients with the disease; test specificity applies to patients without the disease. Thus, sensitivity and specificity are two separate measures: A test may have a high sensitivity and a low specificity, a low sensitivity and a high specificity, both a high sensitivity and a high specificity, or both a low sensitivity and a low specificity. The definitions of these probabilities and others to be introduced in this chapter are summarized in Table 4–2.

TABLE 4–2 PROBABILITIES ASSOCIATED WITH TESTS

COMMON NAME	MEANING	PROBABILITY NOTATION	EQUIVALENT PROBABILITIES	ESTIMATE OF PROBABILITIES FROM 2 × 2 TABLE DERIVED FROM STUDY SAMPLE
Sensitivity of test; true-positive rate (TPR)	Frequency of positive test results in those with disease	$P[T^+ | D]$	$1 - P[T^- | D]$	$TP/(TP + FN)$
False-negative rate (FNR)	Frequency of negative test results in those with disease	$P[T^- | D]$	$1 - P[T^+ | D]$	$FN/(TP + FN)$
Specificity of test; true-negative rate (TNR)	Frequency of negative test results in those without disease	$P[T^- | \bar{D}]$	$1 - P[T^+ | \bar{D}]$	$TN/(TN + FP)$
False-positive rate (FPR)	Frequency of positive test results in those without disease	$P[T^+ | \bar{D}]$	$1 - P[T^- | \bar{D}]$	$FP/(TN + FP)$
Prevalence of disease; prior probability of disease	Frequency of disease in the population	$P[D]$	$1 - P[\bar{D}]$	Requires independent estimate
Prior probability of nondisease	Frequency of nondisease in the population	$P[\bar{D}]$	$1 - P[D]$	Requires independent estimate
Predictive value positive	Frequency of disease in those with positive test results	$P[D | T^+]$	$1 - P[\bar{D} | T^+]$	Not available; requires knowledge of prevalence
Predictive value negative	Frequency of nondisease in those with negative test results	$P[\bar{D} | T^-]$	$1 - P[D | T^-]$	Not available; requires knowledge of prevalence
Test level; rate of test positives	Frequency of positive test results in the population	$P[T^+]$	$1 - P[T^-]$	Not available; requires knowledge of prevalence

POSTERIOR PROBABILITIES: THE PREDICTIVE VALUE POSITIVE AND THE PREDICTIVE VALUE NEGATIVE

Sensitivity and specificity are important characteristics of a test, but they are not the probabilities we usually need in order to decide how to treat a patient whose condition is suggestive of disease. Sensitivity, specificity, and their complements are the probabilities of test results *given* the presence or absence of disease; we usually need to know the probabilities of disease *given* positive or negative test results. In evaluating an individual patient, we can learn whether a test result is positive or negative, and from this information we can infer the probability of disease.

For a patient selected randomly from the study population upon which the estimates of sensitivity and specificity were based (Table 4–1), the probability of disease given a positive test result, $P[D \mid T^+]$, may be obtained from the 2 $\times$ 2 contingency table. This probability is calculated as $TP/(TP + FP)$, which is the proportion of those with positive test results ($TP + FP$) who also have the disease (TP). We call this the **predictive value positive** of the test.* In our study population the predictive value positive would be 25/29, or approximately 0.86. The **predictive value negative** of the test is the conditional probability of *not* having the disease given a negative test result, or $P[\overline{D} \mid T^-]$. It may be calculated as $TN/(TN + FN)$ from Table 4–1; in the example the predictive value negative in the study population is 42/65, or approximately 0.65.

Definition. Consider a test defined by a separator variable for which a positivity criterion has been chosen and which is intended to distinguish between two disease states, D (disease present) and $\overline{D}$ (disease absent).

The **predictive value positive** of the test is the probability that a patient with a positive test result actually has the disease. It is equal to $P[D \mid T^+]$.

The **predictive value negative** of the test is the probability that a patient with a negative test result actually does not have the disease. It is equal to $P[\overline{D} \mid T^-]$.

In terms of the discussion in Section 4.1, the predictive value positive and the predictive value negative are both examples of **posterior probabilities.**

We were careful to point out that the estimates of the predictive value positive and the predictive value negative obtained directly from Table 4–1 apply to the study population of 48 patients with MI and 46 patients without MI. An important practical question is whether one can use data from evaluations of a diagnostic test to estimate the predictive values of a test when it is applied to a new group of patients. Unfortunately, such a direct estimate would be misleading, unless the proportion of patients with the disease in the study population equals the proportion of patients with the disease in the population in which the test will be applied. Most diseases are relatively uncommon in the population at large; therefore, when a test is being evaluated, it is often performed on a subset of the population in which the disease is common enough to make convenient the inclusion of adequate numbers of cases. The report of such a study will give us a true picture of the fraction of patients with the disease whose test results are positive (a measure of the test's sensitivity) and the fraction of those without the disease whose test results are negative (a measure of

---

*Our terminology here follows Vecchio.[262] Some authors use other terms for this proportion, and the same is true for many other concepts defined in this book. Since there are no universally recognized conventions, we have tried to adopt the most widely used nomenclature.

the test's specificity). But it does not permit us to calculate the probability that an individual in a different population has the disease given a positive test result.

To estimate the predictive value positive and predictive value negative for our patients, we need an independent estimate of the probability of the disease in the population from which our patient is selected, an estimate of the **prior probability** of disease.

The usual relationship between a study population and the more general patient population is illustrated in Figure 4–5. We are interested in determining whether a new test, T, will be useful in the diagnosis of a disease, D, which we are able to identify by other means. We search through the total population, which is represented by the large rectangle at the left, until we find an adequate number of individuals with the disease (D). Then, as is customary in such studies, we select an approximately equal number of individuals without the disease ($\overline{D}$). This constitutes our study population (shown in the rectangle to the right), about half of whom have the disease (shaded area) and half of whom do not.

We now determine which members of our study population have positive test results (T^+) and which have negative test results (T^-); these numbers are represented by the areas of the four sectors in the rectangle at the right. We are often safe in assuming that the sensitivity and specificity (i.e., the true-positive and true-negative rates) are the same in the study population as they are in the total population. In other words, the proportion of positive results among persons with the disease, $TP/(TP + FN)$, is the same in the shaded areas of both

Figure 4–5   The relation between the distributions of test results in the total population and in the study population. (Shaded areas represent patients with the disease; + denotes that the test result is positive, and − denotes that the test result is negative.)

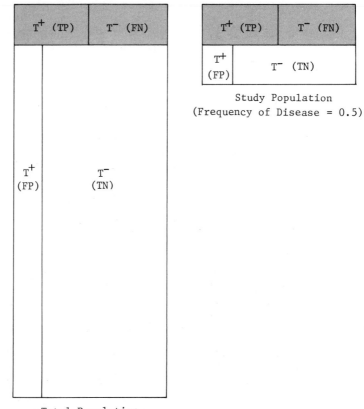

Study Population
(Frequency of Disease = 0.5)

· Total Population
(Frequency of Disease « 0.5)

rectangles of Figure 4–5. Because we selected our study population so that equal numbers of D and $\overline{D}$ individuals would be included and because the frequency of the disease is much smaller in the total population, it is apparent from the diagram that the ratio of true positives (*TP*) to all positives (*TP* + *FP*) is much smaller in the total population than in the study population.

In general, therefore, it would be wrong to infer that the probability of disease given a positive test result for an individual in the total population, $P[\text{D} \mid \text{T}^+]$, is the same as the ratio *TP/(TP* + *FP)*, which is derived from the study population. We require a procedure that will permit us to carry over our information from the study population to the total population. Such a procedure would provide us with valid estimates of two quantities: the probability that a patient with a positive test result actually has the disease (the predictive value positive) and the probability that a patient with a negative test result does not have the disease (the predictive value negative). As we shall see in the section on probability revision (p. 89), a 2 X 2 contingency table can be manipulated to revise our estimates of the probability of disease based on test results and the prior probability of disease.

PREVALENCE AND PRIOR PROBABILITY

If a patient were chosen at random from a given population, the prior probability of disease for the patient would be the disease prevalence in that population.

Definition. Disease **prevalence** is the frequency of disease in the population of interest at a given point in time.

However, patients are not selected at random. Each patient has specific characteristics, including history, physical findings, and previous test results. These characteristics along with the disease prevalence may determine the probability of disease at any point in time. This probability is conditional upon already available information and may be taken as the **prior probability** with respect to a subsequent test. For example, the prior probability that a patient has MI before the SGOT level has been determined may be based on age, blood pressure, body temperature, respiratory function, and the degree and nature of pain. In that sense, the *prior* probability is actually a *posterior* probability that is conditional upon all of these factors ($P[\text{MI} \mid$ Temperature = 99° F; BP = 160/90 mm Hg; Breathing Very Labored; Severe Continuous Chest Pain; 45-Year-Old Male]), while it is still a *prior* probability with respect to the SGOT test. The prior probability here reflects the proportion of patients with similar characteristics in whom MI would be expected.

THE RATE OF TEST POSITIVES

The graphic display of Figure 4–5 illustrates that the predictive value positive (i.e., the probability that a patient has the disease given a positive test result) depends on the disease prevalence. The same figure shows that the proportion of individuals who have positive test results also depends on the prevalence of the disease in the population. In the study population, in which the prevalence of disease is greater than it is in the total population, a greater proportion of patients will have positive test results. We will demonstrate this fact in the next section.

Definition. The **rate of test positives,** also called the **test level,** is the proportion of patients tested who have positive test results.

Before reading on, you may wish to review Table 4–2 to be sure that you know the definitions of the key probabilities associated with a test.

PROBABILITY REVISION USING THE 2 × 2 TABLE

Let us continue with the example of SGOT and myocardial infarction (Figure 4–4 and Table 4–1). Suppose that a patient in a particular hospital has a particular set of signs and symptoms and has a positive SGOT test result (using the cutoff level of 100 units/liter). The sensitivity of this test, or its true-positive rate, is 52 per cent. The specificity of this test, or its true-negative rate, is 91 per cent. What is the probability that this patient with a positive SGOT test result has MI? In other words, what is $P[D \mid T^+]$?

One way to answer this question is as follows. Using the data on the study population as displayed in Table 4–1, convert the number of patients in each cell of the 2 × 2 table to a proportion of the overall study population. Thus, for example, the 25 true positives constitute 25/94, or 26.6 per cent of the study population. These data are shown in Table 4–3.

TABLE 4–3   DISTRIBUTION OF THE STUDY POPULATION BY SGOT
TEST RESULT AND DISEASE STATUS*

| | DISEASE STATUS | | |
TEST RESULT	MI	No MI	TOTALS BY ROW
SGOT ≥ 100 units/liter	0.266	0.043	0.309
SGOT < 100 units/liter	0.244	0.447	0.691
Totals by column	0.510	0.490	1.00

*TPR = sensitivity = 0.266/0.510 = 0.52; TNR = specificity = 0.447/0.49 = 0.91.

Now we can compute the test sensitivity, or true-positive rate, from Table 4–3 just as we computed it from Table 4–1. The true-positive rate is equal to the proportion of patients with MI who have positive test results, which is 0.266/0.51, or 0.52. This is, of course, the same result we derived from the raw data in Table 4–1, because

$$\frac{0.266}{0.51} = \frac{25/94}{48/94} = \frac{25}{48}$$

$$= 0.52.$$

Similarly, the true-negative rate, or specificity, is 0.447/0.49, or 0.91, as before.

Suppose that we try to use Table 4–3 to compute the predictive value positive, or the probability of disease given a positive test result. From the top row of Table 4–3, we see that 30.9 per cent of the study population have positive test results. Of these, 26.6 per cent have MI. Therefore, we might estimate the probability of disease, given a positive test result, as 26.6 per cent/30.9 per cent, or 86 per cent.

This estimate, however, would be incorrect, because it assumes that the prevalence of the disease in the population from which this patient was selected is the same as the prevalence in the study population. The prevalence of MI in the study population is 48/94, or 51 per cent (the total of the "MI" column in Table 4–3). Suppose that this particular patient has a history, symptoms, and signs such that only 20 per cent of patients with similar findings have myocardial infarction. How does this observation modify the analysis?

The first step is to modify the column totals of Table 4–3 so that they reflect the prevalence in the population of concern. This is shown in step 1 of Figure 4–6, where the probability of MI is fixed at 20 per cent.

The second step is to use the known true-positive rate, or test sensitivity, to fill in the first column of the table (i.e., the *joint* probabilities of MI and each

Figure 4–6 The steps in probability revision for the SGOT and MI example.

Step 1: Use Prevalence to Fix Column Totals

Test Result	MI	No MI	Totals by Row
SGOT ≥ 100			
SGOT < 100			
Totals by Column	0.20	0.80	1.00

Step 2: Use Sensitivity to Fill in Disease Column

Test Result	MI	No MI	Totals by Row
SGOT ≥ 100	0.104		
SGOT < 100	0.096		
Totals by Column	0.20	0.80	1.00

Step 3: Use Specificity to Fill in Nondisease Column

Test Result	MI	No MI	Totals by Row
SGOT ≥ 100	0.104	0.072	
SGOT < 100	0.096	0.728	
Totals by Column	0.20	0.80	1.00

Step 4: Compute Row Totals

Test Result	MI	No MI	Totals by Row
SGOT ≥ 100	0.104	0.072	0.176
SGOT < 100	0.096	0.728	0.824
Totals by Column	0.20	0.80	1.00

Predictive Value Positive = 0.104/0.176 = 0.591
Predictive Value Negative = 0.728/0.824 = 0.883

possible test result). Since the true-positive rate is 52 per cent, this means that 52 per cent of 20 per cent, or 10.4 per cent, of the population have the disease *and* a positive test result. The calculation is

$$(0.52)(0.20) = 0.104.$$

Similarly, 48 per cent of those with MI have a negative test result; hence, 48 per cent of 20 per cent, or 9.6 per cent of the population, have the disease *and* a negative test result. These probabilities are indicated in step 2 of Figure 4–6.

The third step is to use the known true-negative rate, or test specificity, to fill in the second column of the table (i.e., the joint probabilities of no MI and each possible test result). Since the true-negative rate is 91 per cent, this means that

$$(0.91)(0.8) = 0.728,$$

or 72.8 per cent, of the population have no MI and a negative test result and that

$$(0.09)(0.8) = 0.072,$$

or 7.2 per cent, of the population have no MI and a positive test result. These probabilities are indicated in step 3 of Figure 4–6.

Finally, we complete the 2 × 2 table by filling in the rate of test positives and the rate of test negatives. These are simply the totals across the rows.

With the 2 × 2 table completed, we can compute the probability of MI given a positive SGOT test result in this population. Of the 17.6 per cent with positive test results, 10.4 per cent have MI and the remaining 7.2 per cent do not. Therefore, 0.104/0.176, or approximately 59.1 per cent, of patients with positive SGOT test results in our population actually have myocardial infarction. This is the correct estimate of the predictive value positive. Contrast this result with the 86 per cent that was obtained by implicitly assuming a disease prevalence of 51 per cent (Table 4–3) rather than a prevalence of 20 per cent (Figure 4–6). Clearly, the prevalence makes a difference!

The process we have just worked through is called **probability revision**. We start with a **prior probability** of MI, which in this case is 0.20. We observe a test result, which in this example is a positive SGOT test result. We revise the probability to obtain a **posterior probability** of MI given the positive test result. In this example the posterior probability is 59.1 per cent. This is the predictive value positive of this test in this particular population.

The method illustrated in Figure 4–6 can also be used to compute the predictive value negative, or the probability that a patient with a negative test result does not have MI. In Figure 4–6, step 4, the probability of a negative test result is 82.4 per cent. Included among these patients with a negative test result are 72.8 per cent who do not have MI. Therefore, the predictive value negative of the test in this population is 0.728/0.824, or approximately 0.883. This leaves a probability of MI, given a negative test result, of 1.000 minus 0.883, or 0.117.

To summarize the results for this example, we have revised our prior probability of MI as follows:

1. Without an SGOT test, we would assess $P[MI] = 0.20$.
2. If the SGOT test result is positive, we derive $P[MI \mid SGOT^+] = 0.591$.
3. If the SGOT test result is negative, we derive $P[MI \mid SGOT^-] = 0.117$.

In the next section we offer an alternative approach to probability revision, using the mathematics of probability as developed in Section 3.2. We shall demonstrate that this device, known as **Bayes' formula,** is numerically equivalent to the method that uses contingency tables, although it may be easier to use in some circumstances.

4.5 BAYES' FORMULA

A REVIEW OF PROBABILITY NOTATION

The manipulation of a contingency table and probability notation can be combined to yield an important generalization for the revision of prior probabilities. Let us review the notation introduced in Chapter Three.

Recall that the expression $P[A]$ indicates the probability of event or condition A; $P[A|B]$ denotes the probability of A contingent upon the presence of B; and $P[A, B]$ stands for the probability of the joint occurrence of both A and B. The term $P[D]$, therefore, simply means the probability of disease, or the prevalence; $P[T^+|D]$ denotes the probability that an individual has a positive test result given the presence of disease, which is a relation we expressed earlier in this chapter as the test sensitivity; and $P[T^+, D]$ means the probability of both a positive test result and the presence of disease.

With this notation in mind, let us return to the example of SGOT and myocardial infarction.

BAYES' FORMULA AND THE SGOT EXAMPLE

Our plan is to work through the steps of Figure 4–6, in which we calculated the revised probability of myocardial infarction given a positive SGOT test result (i.e., ≥ 100 units/liter). We shall derive Bayes' formula by expressing each step in probability notation.

Recall that we start with a patient for whom the prior probability of MI is assessed to be 20 per cent. We observe a positive SGOT test result as defined in Figure 4–4. What is the revised probability of MI given the positive SGOT test result?

Refer to Figure 4–6 as we carry out the steps of the probability-revision process.

Step 1. We specified the prior probability of disease, $P[D]$. In this example, $P[D]$ equals 0.2.

Step 2. We calculated the joint probability of disease and a positive test result, $P[T^+, D]$. We did this by multiplying the prior probability of disease, $P[D]$, by the true-positive rate, $P[T^+|D]$. That is,

$$P[T^+, D] = P[T^+|D] \cdot P[D]. \qquad (4–1)$$

This is the same formula we used to relate joint probabilities and conditional probabilities in Chapter Three, Equation 3–1 of Section 3.2.

In this example, $P[T^+|D]$ equals 0.52. Therefore, we found that

$$P[T^+, D] = (0.52)(0.2) = 0.104$$

as indicated in step 2 of Figure 4–6.

Step 3. We repeated the process of step 2 for the nondiseased patients. We calculated the joint probability of no disease and a positive test result, $P[T^+, \overline{D}]$, by multiplying the probability of no disease, $P[\overline{D}]$, by the false-positive rate, $P[T^+ | \overline{D}]$. That is,

$$P[T^+, \overline{D}] = P[T^+ | \overline{D}] \cdot P[\overline{D}]. \tag{4–2}$$

In the example, $P[T^+ | \overline{D}]$ equals 0.09, and $P[\overline{D}]$ equals 0.8. Therefore, we found that

$$P[T^+, \overline{D}] = (0.09)(0.8) = 0.072$$

as indicated in step 3 of Figure 4–6.

Step 4. We calculated the probability of a positive test result, $P[T^+]$, by summing across the rows of the table. Using our notation, the calculation was

$$P[T^+] = P[T^+, D] + P[T^+, \overline{D}]. \tag{4–3}$$

Equation 4–3 is an application of the summation principle for joint probabilities, which we saw in Chapter Three.

In the example,

$$P[T^+] = 0.104 + 0.072 = 0.176.$$

Thus, 17.6 per cent of test results would be positive.

Let us now express Equation 4–3 in terms of the probabilities with which we started, namely, the prevalence, the true-positive rate, and the false-positive rate. We do this by substituting the formulas for $P[T^+, D]$ and $P[T^+, \overline{D}]$ from Equations 4–1 and 4–2 into Equation 4–3. This gives us

$$P[T^+] = P[T^+ | D] \cdot P[D] + P[T^+ | \overline{D}] \cdot P[\overline{D}]. \tag{4–4}$$

Equation 4–4 is an application of averaging out, as developed in Chapter Three. In other words, the rate of test positives, or the overall fraction with positive test results, is a weighted average of the fraction of patients with disease whose test results are positive and the fraction of patients without disease whose test results are positive. The rarer the disease, the less weight the formula gives to those with disease and positive test results.

Final Step. Last, we calculated the probability of disease given a positive test result by dividing the probability of a positive test result *and* disease, 0.104, by the probability of a positive test result, 0.176, to derive the predictive value positive:

$$P[D | T^+] = 0.104/0.176 = 0.591.$$

Using probability notation, we employed the relation

$$P[D | T^+] = \frac{P[T^+, D]}{P[T^+]}. \tag{4–5}$$

Now, substituting Equation 4–4 for $P[T^+]$ and substituting Equation 4–1 for $P[T^+, D]$, we finally arrive at an important expression,

Bayes' formula (positive test result)

$$P[D \mid T^+] = \frac{P[T^+ \mid D] \cdot P[D]}{P[T^+ \mid D] \cdot P[D] + P[T^+ \mid \overline{D}] \cdot P[\overline{D}]} \qquad (4\text{--}6)$$

Bayes' formula also applies to the calculation of the probability of disease given a negative test result:

Bayes' formula (negative test result)

$$P[D \mid T^-] = \frac{P[T^- \mid D] \cdot P[D]}{P[T^- \mid D] \cdot P[D] + P[T^- \mid \overline{D}] \cdot P[\overline{D}]} \qquad (4\text{--}7)$$

To verify that Bayes' formula works in our example, let us calculate $P[D \mid T^+]$ and $P[D \mid T^-]$ using the formula directly. We find that

$$P[D \mid T^+] = \frac{(0.52)(0.2)}{(0.52)(0.2) + (0.09)(0.8)} = 0.591,$$

and that

$$P[D \mid T^-] = \frac{(0.48)(0.2)}{(0.48)(0.2) + (0.91)(0.8)} = 0.117.$$

Both of these agree with the results we obtained in the analysis using 2 × 2 tables.

Equations 4–6 and 4–7 are both forms of **Bayes' formula** (also called **Bayes' theorem**).* They consist of two kinds of terms: prior probabilities of disease or nondisease and information about the characteristics of a given test in individuals with and without disease, or a test's true-positive and false-positive rates. This information is combined to yield a new probability of the presence of disease in the patient who is the subject of the test. It is in this sense that we refer to test results as revising or modifying our prior probabilities of disease.

We began this analysis in response to the question, What is the probability of disease in an individual with a positive test result? The result is given in Bayes' formula by the ratio of the number of individuals who have the disease and whose test results are positive to the number of all those individuals whose test results are positive.

---

*Bayes' theorem was developed by the eighteenth-century mathematician Reverend Thomas Bayes.[11]

4.6 PROBABILITY REVISION BY INVERTING PROBABILITY TREES

In this section we offer an alternative approach to probability revision using probability trees. The method is equivalent to that which uses contingency tables and to Bayes' formula. You might wonder why we introduce yet another equivalent device for revising probabilities. The answer is that, although in most problems the contingency table method or Bayes' formula will be easy to apply, there will be more complicated problems in which they may be cumbersome and confusing. This method of "tree inversion" is, we think, virtually fail-safe. Later on we give an example for which Bayes' formula, unless expertly applied, can lead one astray, but for which the tree-inversion method is straightforward. We begin, however, with an easy example.

BATTERED AND ABUSED CHILDREN

We have seen that we cannot, in general, estimate correctly for the total population either the disease rate among individuals whose test results are positive, $P[D|T^+]$, or the disease rate among those whose test results are negative, $P[D|T^-]$, solely on the basis of information derived from a study population. Moreover, we cannot estimate, in general, the test-positive fraction in the population, $P[T^+]$, again because the prevalence of individuals with the disease is usually different in the study and the total population. Furthermore, study results showing a test to have a fairly high true-positive rate and a fairly low false-positive rate may lead us to a mistakenly high expectation of disease among persons in the general population whose test results are positive. The following example illustrates these points and introduces the technique of tree inversion.

Physical abuse of children by their parents is a serious public health problem. The potential damage caused by allowing a case of child abuse to go undetected is great, but the costs of falsely accusing a parent are also high. As the pediatrician responsible for a school health program, should you institute a screening program of physical examinations to detect abused children? Clearly, your response will depend to a large extent on the fraction of children with positive test results who are actually being abused.

The experience of school officials indicates that a careful physical examination will detect 95 per cent of battered children (i.e., a false-negative rate of 5 per cent), with a false-positive rate of only 10 per cent. The best information suggests that 3 per cent of school children in an average American city are being abused by their parents.

Before continuing, we suggest that you reread the preceding paragraph and, *without* using pencil and paper, make a mental estimate of the probability that a child with a positive test result is, in fact, battered. Do not try to use Bayes' formula, and make your guess before proceeding to the next paragraph.

Most people who are unfamiliar with the material in this chapter tend to guess that the probability is between 50 per cent and 90 per cent. We will now check this prediction against that derived from a more rigorous approach to the revision of prior probabilities.

One way to look at the problem is to use a 2 × 2 table, as shown in Table 4–4. Imagine that we have an unselected group of 10,000 schoolchildren. Our prior

TABLE 4–4 2 × 2 CONTINGENCY TABLE ANALYSIS FOR THE
CHILD ABUSE EXAMPLE

| | DISEASE STATUS | | |
TEST RESULT	Abused	Not Abused	TOTALS BY ROW
Positive	285 (2.85%)	970 (9.7%)	1,255 (12.55%)
Negative	15 (0.15%)	8,730 (87.3%)	8,745 (87.45%)
Totals by column	300 (3%)	9,700 (97%)	10,000 (100%)

information that 3 per cent are being abused tells us that 300 children in the group are battered. Of these 300, we will be able to detect by our physical examination some 95 per cent, or 285 children. The remaining 9,700 children, who will be similarly examined, are subject to a false-positive rate of detection of 10 per cent, so we will identify another 970 children who appear to us to be battered on the basis of our test, which in this case is the physical examination. We wish to know the probability that a child whose test result is positive is being abused, which is given by 285/(285 + 970), or 23 per cent; this figure is very different from the usual intuitive estimate.

A second way to approach the problem is to use Bayes' formula. Letting D denote the "disease" (child abuse) and T^+ and T^- denote positive and negative test results, we apply Bayes' formula (Equation 4–6):

$$P[D|T^+] = \frac{P[T^+|D] \cdot P[D]}{P[T^+|D] \cdot P[D] + P[T^+|\overline{D}] \cdot P[\overline{D}]}$$

$$= \frac{(0.95)(0.03)}{(0.95)(0.03) + (0.10)(0.97)}$$

$$= \frac{0.0285}{0.0285 + 0.097}$$

$$= 0.23,$$

which agrees with our estimate from the 2 × 2 table.

By utilizing the familiar decision tree in a new way, we can put the same problem in an alternative form. In Figure 4–7 the probability tree starts with the chance node describing the possible states of the children, D and $\overline{D}$, and then, contingent upon each, a chance node describing the test possibilities, T^+ and T^-. Bearing in mind that the sum of probabilities of all of the alternatives at a chance node must equal 1.0, we can use the information given in the statement of the problem to fill in the values as shown in Figure 4–7. Then we can calculate the probability of each joint outcome as its path probability, i.e., the product of the probabilities along the path leading to each outcome. For example, the probability of *both* D and T^+ (an abused child *and* a positive test result) is given by (0.03)(0.95), or 0.0285, as shown in the uppermost branch in the figure.

We know that the overall probability of a sequence of chance events is

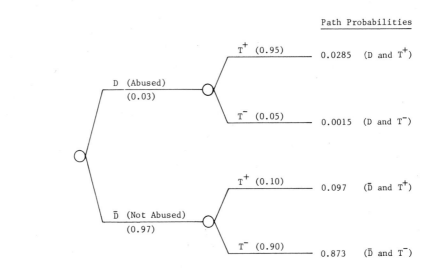

Path Probabilities

Figure 4-7 *A probability tree and the calculation of path probabilities for the child abuse example.*

independent of the order in which the events occur (Chapter Three, Section 3.2). This means that we can "invert" the order of the chance nodes and preserve the path probabilities that we calculated in the previous step. This maneuver is illustrated in Figure 4-8.

We are now in a position to estimate the probability that a child whose test result is positive is actually abused. This conditional probability is denoted by x in the lower half of Figure 4-8. We recognize it as the *predictive value positive* of the test. Similarly, we may want to know the probability that a child whose test result is negative is abused (denoted by y in the figure). Once we know the path probabilities, we have all the information we need in order to compute these conditional probabilities.

The calculation is shown in Figure 4-9. First, we can easily fill in the probabilities at node Ⓐ. They must equal the sums of the path probabilities emanating from the respective branches. Thus, the probability of a positive test result is calculated as

$$P[T^+] = 0.0285 + 0.097 = 0.1255.$$

The next step is to fill in the missing unknowns, x and y. Since the product of the probabilities along a path must equal the path probability,

$$(0.1255)\,(x) = 0.0285$$

and

$$(0.8745)\,(y) = 0.0015.$$

It follows that

$$x = 0.0285/0.1255 = 0.23,$$

so that $P[\text{Abused} \mid \text{Test Positive}]$ equals 0.23. This is the 23 per cent we calculated from the 2 × 2 table (Table 4-4) and from Bayes' formula: If a child's test

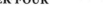

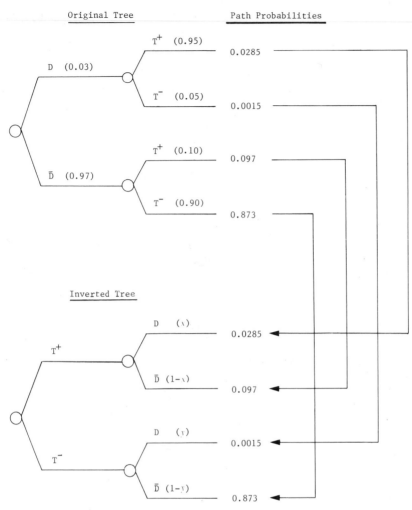

Figure 4–8 *Inverting the probability tree.*

result is positive, there is a 23 per cent chance that it is the result of physical abuse. A positive test result permits us to revise our probability estimate from a *prior probability* of 3 per cent to a *posterior probability* of 23 per cent.

Calculating the other probabilities in the same way yields the complete inverted probability tree at the bottom of Figure 4–9. Thus, the predictive value positive is 0.23, but the predictive value negative is 0.998. With a negative test result, we revise our probability that a child is abused from a *prior probability* of 3 per cent to a *posterior probability* of 0.2 per cent.

We can now return to the original problem of whether to recommend the institution of a screening program of physical examinations to detect abused children in the schools. The relevant decision tree is shown in Figure 4–10. The ultimate decision maker is the school board, and they call upon you as the pediatrician responsible for the school health program for advice. The outcomes that are likely to have the greatest impact are the relative numbers of justifiably and unjustifiably angry parents and the relative numbers of cases of abuse that are detected and undetected. Note that if you decide to screen, you will want to know the fraction of children with positive test results and the fraction with negative test results, as required at the first chance node on

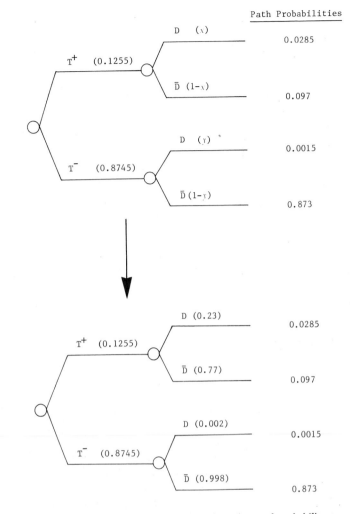

Figure 4–9   Filling in the probabilities in an inverted probability tree.

the upper branch of Figure 4–10. If a child's test result is positive, then an interview with the parents will follow. You will want to know the respective rates of abuse and nonabuse among the test-positive and test-negative children, which are to be inserted after the second chance node in the upper branch.

The procedures of probability revision lead to the probabilities shown in Figure 4–10. These estimates indicate that slightly more than three sets of parents will be made justifiably angry by an incorrect diagnosis of child battering for each set of abusive parents interviewed. This would be the adverse consequence of a program that would detect 95 per cent of abused children (the sensitivity of the test). The school board might well consider this program unfair to too many parents to justify its adoption.

USING A TREATMENT OF LIMITED EFFICACY TO DIAGNOSE A DISEASE

We now offer an example in which Bayes' formula may lead to confusion, but in which tree inversion is straightforward. Consider a patient who may or

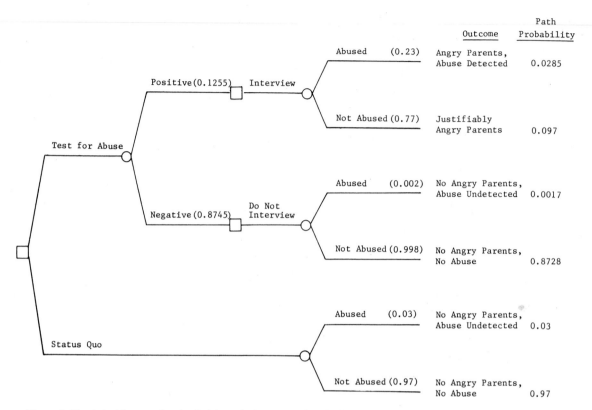

Figure 4–10 *A decision tree for the decision whether to test for child abuse.*

may not have a disease. If the patient does not have the disease, the symptoms will disappear spontaneously within three days. If the patient has the disease, the symptoms will disappear within three days only if effective treatment is administered. There is only one available treatment, and it is known that this treatment is 100 per cent effective in patients who do not have a genetic trait called factor X. The treatment is totally ineffective in persons who have factor X. Studies have shown that 50 per cent of the population has factor X; if a patient has factor X and the disease, the symptoms will always persist beyond three days. The prevalence of the disease is 20 per cent, irrespective of whether factor X is present.

The problem is as follows: You administer the treatment, and the patient's symptoms disappear within three days. What is your revised probability that the patient had the disease?

We suggest that you try to solve this problem using Bayes' formula. After a few minutes, continue reading on.

The tree inversion process for this example is shown in Figure 4–11. At the top of the figure the probability tree displays the information given. The path probabilities are calculated in the usual way as the products of the probabilities along each path.

Note that this tree has three levels of branching instead of the two levels we have seen in the past. This is part of the reason why Bayes' formula is tricky to use in this problem.

Next, we invert the tree as shown at the bottom of Figure 4–11. The order of branching selected in the inverted tree is determined by the answer we seek: the probability of disease conditional upon the disappearance of symptoms. We observe the "test result" first — in this case, whether the symptoms persist.

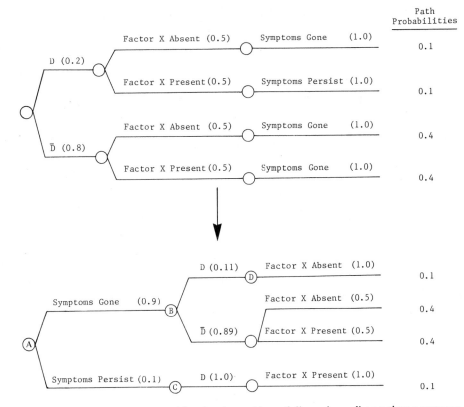

Figure 4–11 Probability revision for the problem of diagnosing a disease given a response to a treatment of limited efficacy.

We are interested in knowing the probability of disease given this result. Finally, to complete the tree, we indicate whether the patient has factor X.

The path probabilities from the top of the tree are then transferred to the corresponding paths at the bottom, as shown. We can then fill in the branch probabilities from left to right.

The probability of "symptoms gone" (at Ⓐ) is the sum of the path probabilities emanating from that branch, or

$$0.1 + 0.4 + 0.4 = 0.9.$$

The probability that the symptoms persist is therefore 0.1.

Then we move on to the next branching points (at Ⓑ and Ⓒ). At Ⓒ the only possibility is disease, so the probability of this branch is 1.0. At Ⓑ there are two possibilities. The probability of disease at this point can be obtained easily by looking ahead to Ⓓ, where the probability of the single branch, "factor X absent," must be 1.0. The product of the probabilities along the upper path, "symptoms gone," disease present ("D"), and "factor X absent," must equal the path probability of 0.1. Denote the unknown $P[D|\text{Symptoms Gone}]$ at Ⓑ by the symbol x. Then,

$$(0.9)\,(x)\,(1.0) = 0.1,$$

or, solving for x,

$$x = 0.1/0.9 = 0.11.$$

Hence, the revised probability of disease given that the symptoms have disappeared is 11 per cent, compared with a prior probability of 20 per cent.

The rest of the probabilities in the inverted tree are shown in Figure 4–11.

Thus, we have solved our original problem using the method of tree inversion. How would Bayes' formula work in this case? The problem is difficult, because it requires the introduction of the concept of a conditional probability of disease given a *joint* event, for example,

$$P[\text{Symptoms Gone} | \text{Disease Present, Factor X Absent}].$$

Bayes' formula is constructed as follows:

$$P[D | \text{Symptoms Gone}] = \frac{P[\text{Symptoms Gone} | D] \cdot P[D]}{P[\text{Symptoms Gone} | D] \cdot P[D] + P[\text{Symptoms Gone} | \overline{D}] \cdot P[\overline{D}]} . \quad (4-8)$$

By an adaptation of the summation principle for joint probabilities, it can be shown that

$$P[\text{Symptoms Gone} | D] = P[\text{Symptoms Gone} | D, \text{X Absent}] \cdot P[\text{X Absent}]$$
$$+ P[\text{Symptoms Gone} | D, \text{X Present}] \cdot P[\text{X Present}].$$

Hence,

$$P[\text{Symptoms Gone} | D] = (1.0)(0.5) + (0.0)(0.5)$$
$$= 0.5.$$

Also, we know that if the disease is absent, the symptoms will disappear:

$$P[\text{Symptoms Gone} | \overline{D}] = 1.0.$$

If we substitute the terms into Equation 4–8, we derive the result:

$$P[D | \text{Symptoms Gone}] = \frac{(0.5)(0.2)}{(0.5)(0.2) + (1.0)(0.8)}$$
$$= \frac{0.1}{0.1 + 0.8}$$
$$= 0.11.$$

If you thought this was a tricky application of Bayes' formula, you are right. The method of tree inversion, however, eliminates much of the opportunity for error. In most examples, Bayes' formula or contingency tables will work smoothly. If ever the answer eludes you, however, tree inversion is virtually guaranteed to deliver a solution.

4.7 BAYES' FORMULA WITH MANY POSSIBLE TEST RESULTS

In demonstrating probability revision, and Bayes' formula in particular, we have thus far assumed a dichotomous test result. That is, we have assumed that a positivity criterion has been applied and that there are two possible test results: positive (T^+) and negative (T^-). Bayes' formula also applies in the more general situation in which a range of test results along a continuum is possible. In this section we develop that generalization, using the example of SGOT and myocardial infarction.

Consider Figure 4–4, which shows the probability distribution of test results for patients with and without MI. We shall use the notation $P[100{-}149|D]$ to denote the probability of an SGOT level of between 100 and 149 units/liter, given that the patient has the disease (MI).

Instead of describing the test by its sensitivity and specificity, which would require us to impose a positivity criterion, we describe the complete probability distribution of test results, as shown in Table 4–5. Thus, the probability of an SGOT level between 100 and 149 units/liter in patients with MI, $P[100{-}149|D]$, is 19 per cent, and the probability of the same level in patients without MI, $P[100{-}149|\overline{D}]$, is 9 per cent.

TABLE 4–5 PROBABILITIES ASSOCIATED WITH SGOT LEVELS IN THE DIAGNOSIS OF MI IN PATIENTS WITH CHEST PAIN*

PROBABILITIES FOR PATIENTS WITH DISEASE		PROBABILITIES FOR PATIENTS WITHOUT DISEASE	
$P[0{-}49 \mid D]$	= 0.19	$P[0{-}49 \mid \overline{D}]$	= 0.80
$P[50{-}99 \mid D]$	= 0.29	$P[50{-}99 \mid \overline{D}]$	= 0.11
$P[100{-}149 \mid D]$	= 0.19	$P[100{-}149 \mid \overline{D}]$	= 0.09
$P[150{-}199 \mid D]$	= 0.08	$P[150{-}199 \mid \overline{D}]$	= 0.00
$P[200{-}249 \mid D]$	= 0.08	$P[200{-}249 \mid \overline{D}]$	= 0.00
$P[\geqslant 250 \mid D]$	= 0.17	$P[\geqslant 250 \mid \overline{D}]$	= 0.00
Totals	1.00		1.00

*Modified from data of Galen and Gambino.[82]

Suppose we have a patient with an SGOT level of 125 units/liter. We assign a prior probability of MI of 20 per cent. What is the revised probability given the SGOT level?

The answer follows from Bayes' formula. We know that the probability of this test result, given MI, is

$$P[100{-}149|D] = 0.19.$$

The probability of both this result *and* MI is

$$P[100{-}149|D] \cdot P[D] = (0.19)(0.2)$$

$$= 0.038.$$

The probability of both this result *and* no MI is

$$P[100\text{–}149|\overline{D}] \cdot P[\overline{D}] = (0.09)\,(0.8)$$

$$= 0.072.$$

Therefore, the overall probability of this SGOT result is

$$P[100\text{–}149] = P[100\text{–}149|D] \cdot P[D] + P[100\text{–}149|\overline{D}] \cdot P[\overline{D}]$$

$$= 0.038 + 0.072$$

$$= 0.11.$$

The conditional probability of MI given an SGOT level between 100 and 149 units/liter is, therefore,

$$P[D|100\text{–}149] = \frac{P[100\text{–}149,\, D]}{P[100\text{–}149]}$$

$$= \frac{P[100\text{–}149|D] \cdot P[D]}{P[100\text{–}149]}$$

$$= \frac{0.038}{0.11}$$

$$= 0.345,$$

or 34.5 per cent. This is the revised probability of disease given this particular test result.

In general, if R is any test result (in the example above, R was an SGOT level of between 100 and 149 units/liter), then Bayes' formula applies, as in Equations 4–6 and 4–7, but with the result R in place of T^+ or T^-. The expression is

---

Bayes' formula (general test result)

$$P[D|R] = \frac{P[R|D] \cdot P[D]}{P[R|D] \cdot P[D] + P[R|\overline{D}] \cdot P[\overline{D}]} \qquad (4\text{–}9)$$

If the test result is dichotomized according to a positivity criterion, then there are only two possibilities for R: T^+ or T^-. In that case, Equation 4–9 is the same as Equation 4–6 or 4–7.

Note also that since the denominator of the formula in Equation 4–9 is simply the probability of test result R, we may write

$$P[D|R] = \frac{P[R|D] \cdot P[D]}{P[R]}. \qquad (4\text{–}10)$$

4.8 THE ODDS–LIKELIHOOD RATIO FORM
OF BAYES' FORMULA

Bayes' formula, even in the dichotomous (disease versus nondisease) situation, is too involved to work in your head. And tree inversion requires a piece of paper. Sometimes you will want to get a quick estimate of revised probabilities in a few seconds. You can do this with another version of Bayes' formula that some people find easier to use mentally.

This version of Bayes' formula is also instructive in that it highlights the relations between the prior and posterior probabilities in a revealing way. It makes use of the concepts of **odds** and **likelihood ratio**, which we define at this point.

ODDS

If the probability that an event will occur is p, then the probability that it will not occur is $1 - p$. An event that has a 42 per cent chance of occurring has a corresponding 58 per cent chance of not occurring. The ratio of p to $1 - p$, or $p/(1 - p)$, is called the **odds favoring** the occurrence of an event and is another way of quantifying the likelihood of an event. The **odds against** the occurrence of an event can be expressed as $(1 - p)/p$.

Definition. Suppose that the probability of an event is p. Then we define the following:
Odds favoring the event: $p/(1 - p)$.
Odds against the event: $(1 - p)/p$.

If an event has a 0.20 probability of occurrence, the odds favoring are 0.2/0.8, or 1/4, and the odds against are 0.8/0.2, or 4 (sometimes written 4:1 and read "four to one"). If an event has a 50 per cent chance of occurrence, then odds favoring and odds against are both 0.5/0.5, or 1:1, which are called even odds. As probability varies from 0.0 to 1.0, the corresponding odds favoring range from 0 to infinity, and the odds against range from infinity to 0. The relationship of odds and probability may be shown graphically as in Figure 4–12, where each unit on the vertical axis increases by a multiple of 10.

The relation between odds against (O_A) and probability is expressed by

$$O_A = \frac{1 - p}{p}.$$

We can also reverse the calculation if we know the odds and want to determine the probability by using the relation

$$p = \frac{1}{1 + O_A}.$$

In a horse race, the odds given each horse are odds against that horse winning. Thus, if a horse is given odds of 4:1, its probability of winning is 20 per cent, because $0.2 = 1/(1 + 4)$.

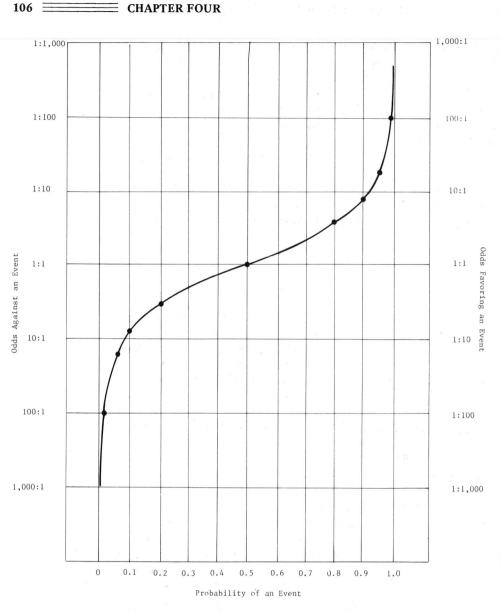

Figure 4–12 *The relation between odds and probability.*

PROBABILITY REVISION USING ODDS

Look back at Equation 4–10. Now consider the analogue of this equation for the nondiseased state:

$$P[\overline{D}|R] = \frac{P[R|\overline{D}] \cdot P[\overline{D}]}{P[R]} .$$

(4–11)

If we divide Equation 4–10 by Equation 4–11, we get the simple formula

Bayes' formula (odds-likelihood ratio form)	$\dfrac{P[D \mid R]}{P[\bar{D} \mid R]}$	$= \dfrac{P[D]}{P[\bar{D}]}$	$\cdot \dfrac{P[R \mid D]}{P[R \mid \bar{D}]}.$	(4–12)
	(posterior odds)	**(prior odds)**	**(likelihood ratio)**	

This version of Bayes' formula is expressed in terms of *odds* rather than *probabilities*. Remember that the odds favoring an event with a probability of p equals $p/(1 - p)$. The first ratio on the right-hand side of the equation, $P[D]/P[\bar{D}]$, is therefore the **prior odds** favoring disease. For example, if we started with a prior probability $P[D]$ equal to 0.1, the prior odds would be 0.1/0.9, or 1/9. The ratio on the far left, $P[D \mid R]/P[\bar{D} \mid R]$, is the **posterior odds** given the test result; it is the odds corresponding to the posterior probability $P[D \mid R]$.

To obtain the posterior odds according to Equation 4–12, we multiply the prior odds by a ratio called the **likelihood ratio**. This ratio is the relative likelihood of the occurrence of the observed test result among diseased and non-diseased patients.

Definition. The **likelihood ratio** associated with a test result is the ratio of its probability of occurrence if the disease is present to its probability of occurrence if the disease is absent:

$$\text{Likelihood ratio} = \frac{P[R \mid D]}{P[R \mid \bar{D}]}.$$

Table 4-6 summarizes the elements of the odds–likelihood ratio formulation of Bayes' theorem.

TABLE 4–6 PROBABILITY RATIOS ASSOCIATED WITH TESTS

COMMON NAME	MEANING	RATIO
Prior odds favoring disease	Ratio of disease frequency to non-disease frequency in population	$\dfrac{P[D]}{P[\bar{D}]}$
Posterior odds favoring disease (in patients with a particular test result)	Ratio of disease frequency to non-disease frequency in those with a particular test result	$\dfrac{P[D \mid R]}{P[\bar{D} \mid R]}$
Test-likelihood ratio (among patients with a particular test result)	Ratio of the frequency of a particular test result in those with disease to its frequency in those without disease	$\dfrac{P[R \mid D]}{P[R \mid \bar{D}]}$

The likelihood ratio for a positive test result (T^+) in a dichotomous test is the true-positive rate, $P[T^+ \mid D]$, divided by the false-positive rate, $P[T^+ \mid \bar{D}]$.

Yet another version of Bayes' formula may be obtained by converting Equation 4–12 from an expression of posterior *odds* to an expression of posterior *probability*. It can be shown by simple algebra and by using the relation between odds and probability that

$$P[D \mid R] = \frac{1}{1 + \dfrac{P[\bar{D}]}{P[D]} \cdot \dfrac{P[R \mid \bar{D}]}{P[R \mid D]}}.$$

The two ratios in the denominator are the prior odds *against* disease ($P[\overline{D}]/P[D]$) and the reciprocal of the likelihood ratio ($P[R|\overline{D}]/P[R|D]$).

THE LIKELIHOOD RATIO AS A MEASURE OF THE DIAGNOSTIC INFORMATION OF A TEST

Equation 4–12 shows that a test result modifies the probability of disease only if the likelihood ratio is different from 1.0. If the likelihood ratio is equal to 1.0, then the posterior odds equal the prior odds, and therefore the posterior probability equals the prior probability of disease. If all possible results of a test have likelihood ratios equal to 1.0 (i.e., each test result is as likely to occur in the presence or absence of disease), then it follows that the test conveys no diagnostic information.

USING THE ODDS-LIKELIHOOD FORM TO MENTALLY REVISE PROBABILITIES

To show how easy it is to use the odds-likelihood form of Bayes' formula, one of the authors of this book recalls the following episode:

"When my wife thought she had become pregnant for the first time, about three years ago, she went to her gynecologist to have a pregnancy test. Although she felt as she thought she *would* feel if she were to become pregnant, the test was negative. She was naturally disappointed and asked her doctor whether the test could be wrong. He told her that about 10 per cent of pregnant women have a negative result on the first pregnancy test. I met her at the doctor's office and found her disheartened by the doctor's report.

"I asked her how likely she had thought it that she was pregnant before the test, and she said, 'I was very sure.' I said, 'You mean maybe 95 per cent?', and she said, 'Yes, about 95 per cent.' I assumed that the false-positive rate was virtually nil, and calculated in my head the posterior probability using the odds-likelihood formulation. Since the prior odds favoring were about 20:1 and the likelihood ratio for a negative result about 1:10, I immediately calculated the posterior odds favoring pregnancy as (20)(1/10), or 2. This was easy for me to convert in my head to a posterior probability of about 2/3. With this conclusion, reached in a matter of seconds, I was able to reassure myself as well as my wife. Our first child is now just over two years old."

Even though the prior odds used in this illustration were rounded off (from 19:1 to 20:1), this author got a serviceable approximation in a matter of seconds. In a patient-care setting, a pocket calculator can provide a more exact and secure estimate in as little time.

USING THE ODDS-LIKELIHOOD FORM TO CHOOSE A POSITIVITY CRITERION

Later in this chapter we will return to the odds-likelihood version of Bayes' formula when we discuss the choice of a positivity criterion for a test. Up to this point we have assumed the positivity criterion to be given. In general, we shall see that choosing a positivity criterion is tantamount to choosing a value of the likelihood ratio for the cutoff point on the separator scale. With that preview, we leave this subject until Section 4.11 and turn to the use of Bayes' formula in differential diagnosis.

4.9 A GENERALIZATION OF BAYES' FORMULA TO MORE THAN TWO HEALTH STATES

In the preceding sections we learned how we might use the result of a single test to revise our prior probability that a patient has or does not have a particular disease. More commonly, we are faced with the task of revising our probabilities with respect to several alternative diagnoses for an individual patient using the results of several tests. How can we apply our methodology to this more complicated situation? In this section we generalize Bayes' formula to accommodate several possible diagnoses. In Chapter Five (Section 5.3) we will address probability revision when the results of several tests are available.

REBOUND TENDERNESS AND ABDOMINAL PAIN

A common example, which we have presented earlier, is the differential diagnosis of acute abdominal pain. Let us assume that in the population of patients seen in our emergency ward, the overwhelming majority of individuals with this complaint are suffering from one of three problems: acute appendicitis (App), acute pancreatitis (Panc), or nonspecific abdominal pain (NSAP). In this simplified example, the physician caring for the patient with acute abdominal pain is confronted with the decision of whether to operate now or to perform a test in an effort to distinguish among the three diagnostic alternatives.

The physician structures the problem as shown in Figure 4–13. Note in the upper branch that although the finding of a positive or a negative test result is followed by a decision node, the test result itself is the determinant of the action to operate or not to operate. We anticipate that 30 per cent of patients with acute abdominal pain will have appendicitis, 5 per cent will have pancreatitis, and 65 per cent will have NSAP.[241]

Our clinical test will be to see if the patient demonstrates rebound tenderness. This sign is elicited by pressing down slowly on the patient's abdomen and then suddenly releasing the pressure. In the presence of peritoneal irritation, release is accompanied by a brief episode of sharp pain, which is usually localized to the site of irritation. Studies indicate that 80 per cent of patients with appendicitis, 15 per cent of patients with pancreatitis, and 20 per cent of patients with NSAP have rebound tenderness.[241]

As was true in the preceding examples of probability revision, the information we are likely to be given is not in the form needed to address the problem of clinical management. Since surgery is generally not indicated for either pancreatitis or NSAP but is indicated for appendicitis, we would like to know the probability that a patient with rebound tenderness has appendicitis as compared with the probability that the patient has one of the other two conditions.

We can conveniently structure our information about the diagnostic problem in the form of a 2 X 3 contingency table, as shown in Table 4–7. We fill in the table just as in Figure 4–6. First, we fill in the prevalences as the column totals. Next, we fill in the values for one column at a time by multiplying the probability of a disease state by the probability of each test result given that disease state. For example, the probability of appendicitis *and* a positive test result is equal to the probability of appendicitis (0.30) times the probability of a positive test result *given* appendicitis (0.80), or 0.24. Next, we fill in the overall probabilities of each possible test result as the totals for the rows. Finally, we compute

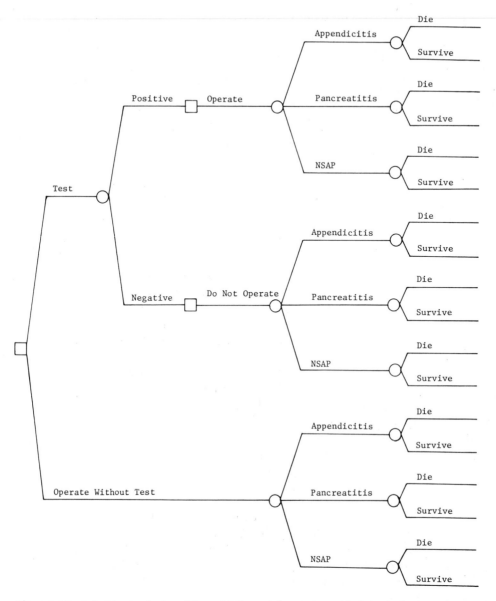

Figure 4–13 *A decision to obtain a differential diagnosis in a patient with abdominal pain.*

TABLE 4–7 PROBABILITY REVISION IN THE CASE OF THREE POSSIBLE
DISEASE STATES USING A CONTINGENCY TABLE

TEST RESULT	DISEASE STATUS			TOTALS BY ROW
	Appendicitis	Pancreatitis	NSAP*	
Positive	0.24	0.0075	0.13	0.3775
Negative	0.06	0.0425	0.52	0.6225
Totals by column	0.30	0.05	0.65	1.00

*NSAP indicates nonspecific abdominal pain.

the probability of appendicitis given the presence of rebound tenderness as the joint probability of appendicitis and a positive test result (0.24) divided by the overall probability of a positive test finding (0.3775). The result is 0.24/0.3775, or 0.64.

Three different diagnoses can also be accommodated easily in the format of Bayes' formula. The probability of appendicitis given rebound tenderness equals the probability of appendicitis and rebound tenderness divided by the overall probability of having rebound tenderness. Then, using the laws of probability, we have

$$P[\text{App}|\text{T}^+] = \frac{P[\text{T}^+|\text{App}] \cdot P[\text{App}]}{P[\text{T}^+|\text{App}] \cdot P[\text{App}] + P[\text{T}^+|\text{Panc}] \cdot P[\text{Panc}] + P[\text{T}^+|\text{NSAP}] \cdot P[\text{NSAP}]} \qquad (4-13)$$

In the example,

$$P[\text{App}|\text{T}^+] = \frac{(0.8)(0.3)}{(0.8)(0.3) + (0.15)(0.05) + (0.20)(0.65)} = 0.64.$$

A GENERALIZATION OF BAYES' FORMULA TO SEVERAL DISEASE STATES*

In general, suppose we wish to assign probabilities to each of three disease states: D_1, D_2, and D_3. One of these states represents the "normal," or non-diseased, state, so that we may use the symbol $\overline{D}$ in place of D_3 to denote the absence of disease. Now we are given the probabilities of observing a particular test result, R, given each disease state. That is, we know $P[R|D_1]$, $P[R|D_2]$, and $P[R|\overline{D}]$. We also know the prevalences $P[D_1]$ and $P[D_2]$; therefore, $P[\overline{D}]$ can be calculated from the summation principle:

$$P[\overline{D}] = 1 - P[D_1] - P[D_2].$$

What is the revised probability of each disease, given test result R?

Bayes' formula states that

$$P[D_1|R] = \frac{P[R|D_1] \cdot P[D_1]}{P[R|D_1] \cdot P[D_1] + P[R|D_2] \cdot P[D_2] + P[R|\overline{D}] \cdot P[\overline{D}]} \qquad (4-14)$$

where R represents the presence of rebound tenderness (T^+), and D_1, D_2, and $\overline{D}$ represent appendicitis, pancreatitis, and NSAP, respectively. This equation is the same as Equation 4–13. Similarly,

$$P[D_2|R] = \frac{P[R|D_2] \cdot P[D_2]}{P[R|D_1] \cdot P[D_1] + P[R|D_2] \cdot P[D_2] + P[R|\overline{D}] \cdot P[\overline{D}]} \qquad (4-15)$$

and

---

*This section is not essential to what follows and may be skipped without loss of continuity.

$$P[\overline{D}|R] = \frac{P[R|\overline{D}] \cdot P[\overline{D}]}{P[R|D_1] \cdot P[D_1] + P[R|D_2] \cdot P[D_2] + P[R|\overline{D}] \cdot P[\overline{D}]} \cdot \qquad (4\text{-}16)$$

Equations 4–14 through 4–16 thus generalize Bayes' formula to three disease states.

More generally, in the case of n possible diseases (D_1, D_2, ..., D_n), the posterior probability of any one disease (D_i) given a test result (R) would be:

$$P[D_i|R] = \frac{P[R|D_i] \cdot P[D_i]}{P[R|D_1] \cdot P[D_1] + \ldots + P[R|D_i] \cdot P[D_i] + \ldots + P[R|D_n] \cdot P[D_n]} \cdot$$

4.10 ERRORS IN PROBABILISTIC CLINICAL REASONING

The justification for using Bayes' formula instead of, or as a supplement to, unaided clinical reasoning is that it can improve one's ability to make clinical inferences. Psychologists have found that most people, including physicians, are poor intuitive statisticians.[61, 237, 260] In particular, they have found that, unaided by Bayes' formula, people make several common errors in revising probabilities. All physicians, whether they know Bayes' formula or not, should be aware of these pitfalls. In discussing them, we shall occasionally refer to the clinical episode that was presented in Chapter Two, Section 2.3.

OVEREMPHASIZING POSITIVE OR EQUIVOCAL FINDINGS

Clinical findings usually bear probabilistic relations to disease. Only rarely is a sign or a symptom pathognomonic of disease; that is, rarely will a test satisfy the condition $P[D|T^+] = 1.0$. More commonly, signs and symptoms are associated with several diseases, and diagnostic judgments are reached by weighing and combining evidence.

One pitfall in clinical reasoning is the discounting of evidence that fails to confirm one's favored diagnostic hypothesis on the grounds that there is only a probabilistic relation between evidence and hypotheses and that a perfect match is not to be expected. This error is equivalent to overemphasizing data that affirm a hypothesis and slighting data that tend to disconfirm it.

In the clinical vignette presented in Chapter Two, the intern's conviction that the correct diagnosis is amebic dysentery leads him to emphasize the history of a recent trip to Jamaica and the presence of amebae in the stool culture and to slight the evidence that disproves his hypothesis, such as the presence of pain in the right lower quadrant of the abdomen and the possibility that "anyone who has spent time in Jamaica would show amebae in the stool."

Another illustration of this pitfall is found in a classic study of clinical inference.[238] A group of nurses were presented with a series of cases in which the presence or absence of a particular symptom was associated equally often with the presence or absence of a particular diagnosis. Each of the four possible combinations occurred 25 per cent of the time in a series of brief case descriptions, so that the true-positive and false-positive rates of this symptom in relation to the disease were both 0.5. These nurses nonetheless concluded that the symptom was diagnostically helpful; that is, that its true-positive rate and true-negative rate both exceeded 50 per cent. They could, of course, point to many instances in the series to support this erroneous conclusion. Equally numerous instances of a lack of association between the symptom and the disease were forgotten or neglected.

The error made here was to focus excessively on the relatively high frequency of the symptom among the diseased, $P[T^+|D]$, when attention should have properly been directed to that frequency in relation to the probability of observing that finding in nondiseased persons, $P[T^+|\overline{D}]$. The diagnostic information from a test depends on the likelihood ratio, $P[T^+|D]/P[T^+|\overline{D}]$, not simply on its probability given a particular condition. Indeed, the most frequently observed error in the interpretation of clinical data is to overestimate the likelihood ratio and treat a finding that is really noncontributory as if it had relevance for a particular diagnosis.[61] This is a difficult point to remember in informal clinical information processing, and Bayes' formula makes it explicit.

MISINTERPRETING NEGATIVE FINDINGS

One mistake in interpreting the absence of a positive test result is illustrated in the brief discussion of Rovsing's sign in the clinical episode. The intern rules out appendicitis because the sign is absent; his reasoning hinges on equating $P[D|T^+]$ with $P[\overline{D}|T^-]$. Because the presence of Rovsing's sign points unequivocally toward appendicitis, he erroneously concludes that the sign's absence rules out the disease. Another way of expressing the intern's error is that he treats a perfectly specific test as if it were perfectly sensitive. The surgeon is more logically consistent and points out that the conditional probability of Rovsing's sign is very low, given either the presence or absence of appendicitis; therefore, its absence proves nothing. Exercise 1 at the end of this chapter deals with this point.

THE LIMITATIONS OF THE PHYSICIAN AS OBSERVER

In discussing probability revision, we have presumed the accuracy of test results and other observations of patients. Physicians, as all humans, have limitations as observers. Among the factors contributing to observer error are (1) the degree of ambiguity in the presence or character of the observation; (2) the conditions under which the observation is made (e.g., jaundice is more visible in sunlight than under incandescent light); (3) the physical and emotional state of the physician observer; (4) the expectations of the physician before making the observation; and (5) the influence of peers who are making the same observation. The best strategy can work no better than the data base on which it depends. We have little to say in this book about improved means of observing patients and gathering information about them. Yet, errors in observation impede good patient care just as ineffective decision making does.

4.11 THE CHOICE OF A POSITIVITY CRITERION

Throughout the discussion of tests and their use in revising prior probabilities, we have assumed that the tests were perfectly reliable and accurate and that we knew when a test result was positive, that is, we knew where along the separator variable the positivity criterion for each test should be placed. This section examines the latter assumption. We shall look at the consequences of alternative locations of the positivity criterion, or cutoff point, along the separator variable, develop a method for comparing the performance of tests or observers, and, finally, show how the decision-analytic approach may be used to arrive at the optimal value of a positivity criterion. We begin with a clinical example.

TONOMETRY AND GLAUCOMA

Glaucoma is a condition of the eye in which vision is impaired; it is often (but not always) associated with higher than average intraocular pressure. It is thought that the high pressure gradually cuts off the blood supply to the optic nerve in some patients, which leads to blindness. In a small proportion of cases, an anatomic defect affects fluid outflow from the eye chamber, but in a majority of cases there is no obvious reason for the high pressure (chronic simple glaucoma). Regardless of the mechanism, it is a fact that persons with high intraocular pressure (IOP) have a higher prevalence of blindness and a higher risk of developing blindness in the future. Chronic simple glaucoma accounts for 12 per cent of all blindness in the United States.

Ophthalmologists believe that it is important to start treating this disease early because the prognosis for persons treated early is much better than the prognosis for those who are first treated when the blindness is already well established.

The pressure in a patient's eye can be measured by a nonspecialist quite simply with a clinical instrument called the Schiötz tonometer. Anesthetic drops are placed in the patient's eye, and the instrument is gently applied. An indicator on a dial measures the intraocular pressure according to the resistance that is met.

Suppose that IOP, as measured by Schiötz tonometry, were distributed according to the hypothetical frequency distribution shown in Figure 4–14. We use the same format that we used for the SGOT level in Figure 4–4. The distribution of IOP among patients with glaucoma is represented above the horizontal axis; the distribution of IOP among patients without glaucoma is shown below the axis. For example, the probability that a patient with glaucoma has a reading on the Schiötz tonometer between 4 and 5 is 0.181, whereas the probability that a patient without glaucoma has a reading in that range is only 0.005. (Note, as IOP *decreases,* the Schiötz score *increases.*)

The clinical problem is the establishment of a positivity criterion. What Schiötz score should be considered the boundary between "positive" and "negative"? We will return to this problem shortly in the section on choosing the best cutoff point (p. 121). First, however, we develop some additional ways to describe the properties of a clinical test, such as the test to measure the SGOT level and Schiötz tonometry.

THE RECEIVER-OPERATING CHARACTERISTIC (ROC)*

In our earlier discussion of the SGOT example, we considered the relations

---

*This section is not essential to what follows and may be skipped or skimmed without loss of continuity.

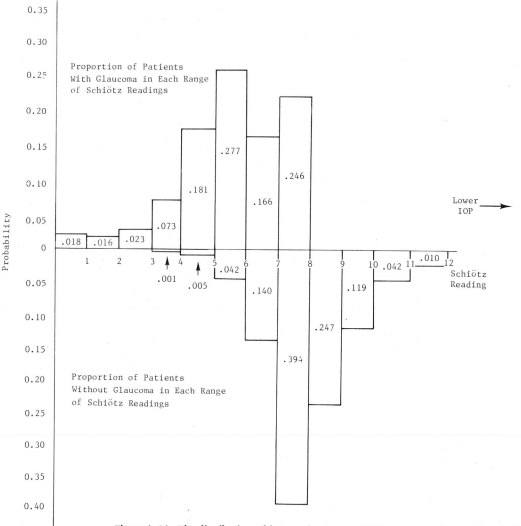

Figure 4–14 *The distribution of intraocular pressure (IOP) among patients with and without glaucoma.*

among true positives *(TP)*, false negatives *(FN)*, true negatives *(TN)*, and false positives *(FP)* at the single arbitrary level of the separator variable. Figures 4–4 and 4–14 suggest that if we were to move the positivity criterion from the left to the right along the separator variable, we could generate a series of 2 × 2 tables. One example of such a table was given in Table 4–3 for the SGOT test. In general, the true-positive rate, false-negative rate, false-positive rate, and true-negative rate would vary with the position of the cutoff point.

A 2 × 2 table expressing the results of a test as a function of the positivity criterion has some redundant elements because *TPR* plus *FNR* equals 1 and *TNR* plus *FPR* equals 1 (Table 4–2). These relationships enable us to obtain the same information about the test using only one term from each of the two equations, for example, the *TPR* and the *FPR* (or, equivalently, the *TPR* and the *TNR* — the sensitivity and specificity). Since our ultimate objective is to use the test to separate individuals who have the disease from those who do not, we could specify the change in the *TPR* and the *FPR* in relation to a series of cutoff points. It is simpler, however, and equivalent to plot the way in which the *TPR* and the *FPR* change with respect to each other as the positivity criterion is varied.

Imagine a test — the results of which are distributed for D and $\bar{D}$ individuals along the separator variable, as shown for test A in the upper left panel of Figure 4–15. For every value of the positivity criterion, equal proportions of the D and $\bar{D}$ individuals are test positive. An alternative way of expressing the performance of the test is shown in the lower left panel of the same figure, in which the *TPR* is plotted against the *FPR* for all possible values of the cutoff point for test A. We derive the lower curve for test A as follows. For each possible positivity criterion, *x*, record the *TPR* as the area to the right of the cutoff point above the axis, and record the *FPR* as the area to the right of the cutoff point below the axis. In the figure, for test A, point A corresponds to a *TPR* of 0.5 and a *FPR* of 0.5; this corresponds to point A′ in the lower left panel. Since the value of the *TPR* equals that of the *FPR* throughout the range of test A, the relation is described by the 45-degree line of identity. Earlier in this chapter we indicated that a test was an observation performed for the purpose of separating subjects into groups with differing probabilities of disease. Test A is worthless because it does not differentiate patients who have the disease from those who do not.

Now consider test B, whose performance is represented by the upper middle panel of Figure 4–15. It is evident that there exists a range of positivity criteria (point C, for example), that achieve perfect separation of D and $\bar{D}$ individuals.

Figure 4–15 *The distribution of test results and receiver-operating characteristic (ROC) curves for various tests. (The upper panels show the probability density functions for various test results for diseased and nondiseased patients. The lower panels show the corresponding ROC curves.)*

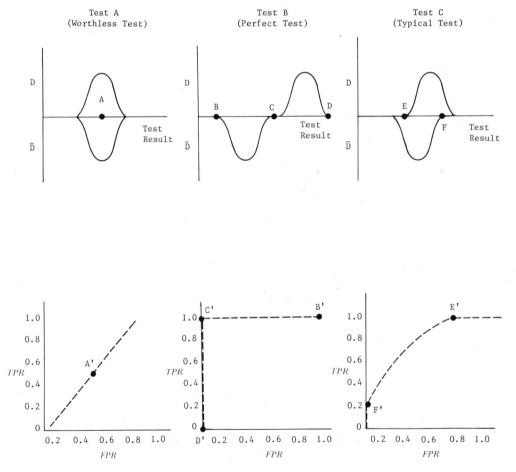

If we now imagine the cutoff point moving through all possible values of the separator variable while we observe the changes in the *FPR* and the *TPR*, we can construct the relation shown in the lower middle panel of the figure. The figure illustrates that it is possible to set the cutoff point for this particular test such that it will detect 100 per cent of D individuals without identifying as test positive any individuals who are $\overline{D}$; this is represented at point C′. This special relation between the *TPR* and the *FPR* establishes that the test is a perfect one.

A more realistic characterization of the performance of clinical tests is shown in the upper right panel of Figure 4–15. Here, although there is clearly a range of cutoff points that will separate individuals into groups with differing probabilities of disease and nondisease (between E and F), no positivity criterion will identify all D individuals as test positive without erroneously identifying some $\overline{D}$ individuals as test positive. The relation between the *TPR* and the *FPR* for test C is plotted in the lower right panel of the figure; as we might expect, the curve is intermediate between that of the worthless test shown in A and the perfect test shown in B.

To illustrate how test performance can be plotted as the relation between the true-positive rate and the false-positive rate, we have taken the hypothetical data concerning Schiötz tonometry as presented in Figure 4–14 and replotted the results as shown in Figure 4–16. For reference to Figure 4–14, we have identified each point in Figure 4–16 by the corresponding Schiötz score used as the cutoff point. For example, with a cutoff score of 6, the *TPR* is the probability to the left of 6 above the axis in Figure 4–14, and the *FPR* is the corresponding area below the axis. Hence, at the cutoff score of 6,

$$TPR = 0.018 + 0.016 + 0.023 + 0.073 + 0.181 + 0.277 = 0.588$$

Figure 4–16 Graph of the true-positive rate (TPR) versus the false-positive rate (FPR) for the Schiötz results given in Figure 4–14.

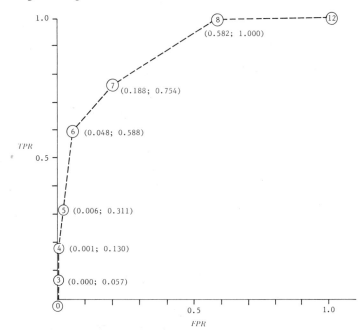

and

$$FPR = 0.001 + 0.005 + 0.042 = 0.048.$$

Because of the aggregation of the original data, we can compute only the discrete points on the curve, and these have been connected with a dashed line. As the positivity criterion for glaucoma becomes more stringent (i.e., as we require lower Schiötz scores before considering the test result positive for glaucoma), the curve sweeps from the upper right down to the lower left.

The description of test performance as the relation between the true-positive rate and the false-positive rate is called a **receiver-operating characteristic (ROC) curve**. Although these curves were originally developed for other purposes, they are useful for evaluating clinical observations and tests and for comparing clinical decision makers. ROC curves show the discriminative ability of a test (or, more precisely, of a test and its observer) by the position of the full curve in a graph plotting the relation between the *TPR* and the *FPR*. The farther upward and to the left the curve lies in the diagram, the better is the test, as is shown in Figure 4-17. The ROC graph also distinguishes that inherent discriminative ability of the test from the user's choice of a positivity criterion, which is indicated by any particular point on the curve.

Information on tests in the medical literature can often be represented on a ROC graph. Consider again the problem of acute abdominal pain in which the differential diagnosis involves appendicitis, for which early surgical intervention is indicated, and a series of alternative diagnoses (here combined into the category of nonspecific abdominal pain), for which surgical intervention is

Figure 4–17 A comparison of tests using their ROC curves.

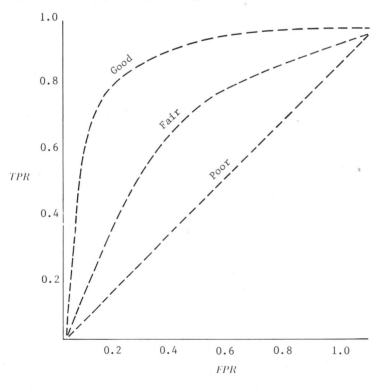

undesirable. In this example the percentage of true positives (the *TPR*) represents the proportion of patients with appendicitis who underwent a timely operation, and the percentage of false positives (the *FPR*) represents the proportion of patients who underwent an operation but who proved not to have appendicitis.

The results of studies conducted in two university hospitals are shown in Figure 4–18. In one study by White,* surgeons in the pediatric unit were operating at point W_1, which is close to the 45-degree line of nondiscrimination. White assumed that the pressure of other responsibilities interfered with appropriate decision making and adopted a special policy allowing any patient whose

---

*Cited in Neutra.[181]

Figure 4–18 *The experiences of investigators in two hospitals in diagnosing appendicitis. (Modified from Neutra.[181])*

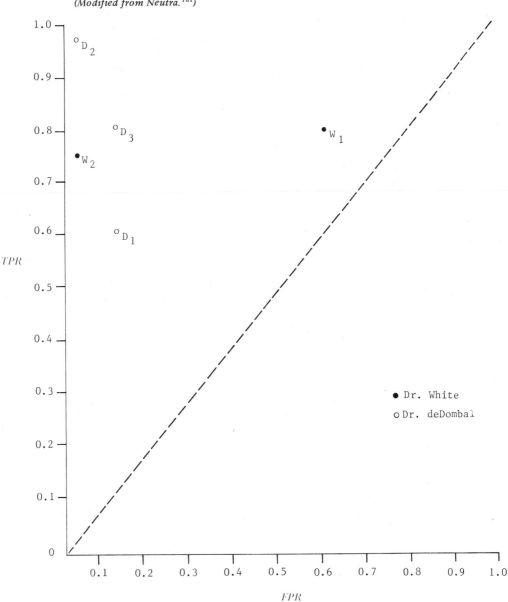

diagnosis was uncertain to be kept in the emergency unit for several hours of close observation. In effect, he substituted this new "test" for the old. Coincident with this change, there was a dramatic decrease in the FPR, with no significant change in the TPR, and performance shifted to point W_2.

Another experience has been reported by deDombal and colleagues[55] in a study that we will discuss further in Chapter Nine. These investigators initially found surgeons to be operating at point D_1 in Figure 4–18. They then initiated an experiment in which the surgeons knew that their diagnostic performance was being compared with that of a computer, although they were unaware of the diagnosis generated by the computer. During this phase of the experiment, there was a simultaneous decrease in the FPR and an increase in the TPR, which is expressed at the operating point D_2. One year after the experiment, performance had shifted back to point D_3.

RANKING TESTS *

In the preceding examples, each point represents a single positivity criterion, but we lack information regarding the entire ROC curves. Are we in a position to infer anything about the relative merits of the procedures used to arrive at the decisions represented by points D_1 and D_2? Since in any one ROC curve there is always a trade-off between the TPR and the FPR, it is clear that D_1 cannot lie on the same ROC curve as D_2. Thus, the difference in the two points is not simply due to the choice of a positivity criterion. Since D_2 lies to the left of and higher than D_1, the test procedure that resulted in the performance at D_2 was different from and *superior* to the procedure that resulted in the performance indicated by D_1.

We can now summarize the material of the previous section in a form that provides us with a method for ranking the merit of individual tests in revising a given prior probability. Imagine that we have collected from the literature reports of four different diagnostic tests — B, C, D, and E — for the same condition and that we propose to compare them with the present standard test, A. The reports include information from which we can calculate the true-positive and false-positive rates at a specified cutoff point, but, as is almost always the case, they do not include sufficient information to construct the full ROC curves.

We begin by constructing a coordinate system in Figure 4–19, with its origin at the pair of values for the TPR and the FPR that symbolize the performance of test A in the ROC plane. Test C falls in the right lower quadrant of this new coordinate system; from what we already know of the shape of ROC curves, the curve indicating the performance of test C will lie below and to the right of the ROC curve passing through point A. Assuming other things, such as costs and risks, to be the same in both tests, we may safely conclude, then, that test A is superior to test C. Similarly, test B, which is indicated by the ROC curve that passes through point B, must be better than test A, which is represented by the ROC curve that passes through point A.

The relative merits of tests D and E are less clear. Given what we already know of the general shape of ROC curves and our limited information about

---

*This section is not essential to what follows and may be skipped or skimmed without loss of continuity.

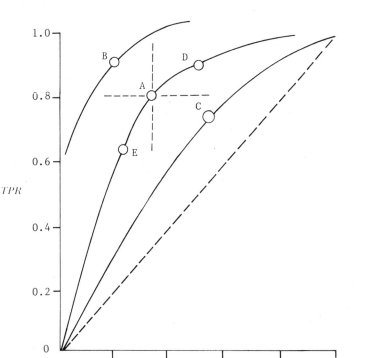

Figure 4–19 A format for ranking tests.

tests D and E, it is possible that points E, A, and D lie on the same ROC curve and that the differences in the values of the *TPR* and the *FPR* result only from the particular choices of the cutoff points used in the three reports. From the standpoint of an analysis based on the ROC curve, points E, A, and D could belong to the same test, with each point representing a different trade-off between test sensitivity and specificity. In contrast to points B and C, which the ROC analysis unambiguously demonstrates to be superior and inferior, respectively, to A, the approach by itself does not permit conclusions as to the relative merits of operating at point E, A, or D.

In order to determine an optimal positivity criterion, we need to consider the outcomes associated with the use of a test. A method for incorporating this information into the choice is developed in the next section, in which glaucoma is used as the example.

CHOOSING THE BEST CUTOFF POINT

It would seem desirable to let a variety of properly weighted factors determine the positivity criterion for a given test, such as Schiötz tonometry. Imagine for a moment that glaucoma were rare, that is, that it had a low prior probability, and that the treatments required were both expensive and hazardous. These circumstances would make it more desirable to set a relatively stringent cutoff point, which is farther to the left in Figure 4–14, in an effort to minimize the number of false positives. Alternatively, if glaucoma were relatively common, as it is in elderly persons with impaired visual acuity, as well as serious if left untreated, we would prefer to shift our operating position more to the right in order to increase test sensitivity and reduce the number of false negatives. (Remember that the lower the Schiötz score, that is, the farther it is to the left, the stronger is the evidence for glaucoma.)

We can identify a number of variables to consider in our choice of a cutoff point: the prior probability of disease, the distributions of test results of patients with and without disease along the separator variable, and the outcomes associated with each of the states identified by the test, that is, *FP, TP, FN,* and *TN.* Intuitively, at least, we should seek a cutoff point that balances the risk of false negatives and false positives.

Analysis of the Cutoff Problem

The structure of the problem is shown in the form of the familiar separator variable diagram and a decision tree in Figure 4–20. The decision is whether to designate a particular test score, X, as either positive (T^+) or negative (T^-). As usual, D and $\bar{\text{D}}$ stand for individuals with and without the disease. Test outcomes are denoted by *TP, FP, FN,* and *TN,* with the prefix *C* indicating

Figure 4–20 *Decision analysis for the choice of a test's positivity criterion. (CTP indicates consequences of a true positive; CFP, consequences of a false positive; CFN, consequences of a false negative; and CTN, consequences of a true negative.)*

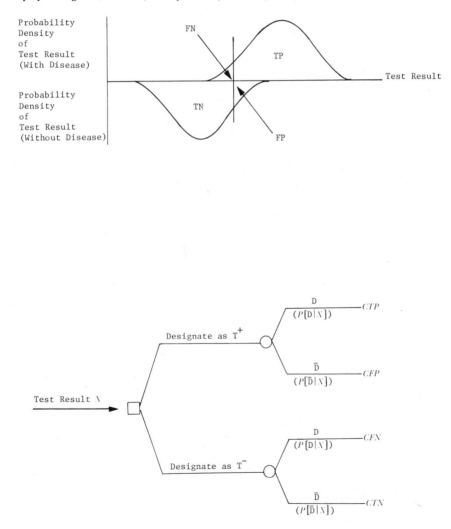

the consequences of that test result. These consequences may be measured in terms of mortality or whatever outcome measure is being averaged out. For example, if the disease is appendicitis and the "test" is the set of criteria upon which the decision to operate is based, then these consequences could correspond to the death rates under the various possible combinations of disease state and decisions concerning whether to operate.

For most distributions of test results for diseased and nondiseased individuals along the separator variable, for example, for those shown in the upper panel of Figure 4–20, the value of X that causes us to be indifferent between the two branches of the decision tree (i.e., between calling the results of the test positive or negative) will be the optimal cutoff point. Notice that any potential cutoff point can be defined in terms of the test result likelihood ratio at that point $(P[X|D]/P[X|\overline{D}])$. Our objective, then, is to find that test result X (or, equivalently, that likelihood ratio, $P[X|D]/P[X|\overline{D}]$) for which the decision to call the test result positive yields precisely the same averaged-out value as the decision to call the test result negative.

The averaged-out value for the test-positive branch, T^+, is the sum of the products of probabilities and outcome values of each branch beyond the chance node, or

$$CTP \cdot P[D|X] + CFP \cdot P[\overline{D}|X]. \qquad (4\text{–}17)$$

Similarly, for the test-negative branch, T^-, the averaged-out value is

$$CFN \cdot P[D|X] + CTN \cdot P[\overline{D}|X]. \qquad (4\text{–}18)$$

If we set Equation 4–17 equal to Equation 4–18, we obtain the following relationship

$$\frac{P[D|X]}{P[\overline{D}|X]} = \frac{CTN - CFP}{CTP - CFN}. \qquad (4\text{–}19)$$

Because the left-hand side of Equation 4–19 indicates the posterior odds, we can use the odds-likelihood form of Bayes' formula that we derived earlier:

$$\frac{P[D|X]}{P[\overline{D}|X]} = \frac{P[D]}{P[\overline{D}]} \cdot \frac{P[X|D]}{P[X|\overline{D}]}. \qquad (4\text{–}20)$$

When we substitute the terms of Equation 4–20 into Equation 4–19 and change their order, we obtain the final results:

$$\frac{P[X|D]}{P[X|\overline{D}]} = \frac{P[\overline{D}]}{P[D]} \cdot \frac{CTN - CFP}{CTP - CFN}. \qquad (4\text{–}21)$$

The equation tells us that the positivity criterion, expressed as the likelihood ratio, is the product of the ratio of the prior probabilities of nondisease and disease and the ratio of the net consequences of nondisease and disease.* This result fulfills our intuitive expectations that the positivity criterion should be

---

*It can be shown mathematically that the slope of the ROC curve at any given point is equal to the likelihood ratio at that point. See McNeil et al.[165]

influenced by the prior odds of disease, the outcomes associated with alternative test results in diseased and nondiseased individuals, and the shape of the distributions of the probabilities of both types of individuals along the separator variable.

Application to Schiötz Tonometry and Glaucoma

Let us apply this method to the choice of a positivity criterion for Schiötz tonometry.

First, using Figure 4–14, consider the implications of a positivity criterion of 4.5; that is, suppose we consider all scores above 4.5 (i.e., lower IOP) to be *negative* and all scores below 4.5 (i.e., higher IOP) to be *positive.* The likelihood ratio corresponding to this test result is equal to

$$\frac{P[4.0 - 4.9 \,|\, \text{Glaucoma}]}{P[4.0 - 4.9 \,|\, \text{No Glaucoma}]} = \frac{0.181}{0.005}$$

$$= 36.2.$$

This becomes the left-hand side of Equation 4–21, the criterion for an optimal cutoff point.

Next, suppose that we are using Schiötz tonometry in a population in which the prevalence of glaucoma is 4 per cent; hence, the prior odds against glaucoma are

$$\frac{P[\text{No Glaucoma}]}{P[\text{Glaucoma}]} = \frac{0.96}{0.04}$$

$$= 24.$$

This enters the right-hand side of Equation 4–21 as the prior odds ratio, $P[\overline{D}]/P[D]$.

Given the prior odds and the likelihood ratio at the chosen cutoff level of 4.5, what would have to be true of the ratio of net consequences,

$$\frac{CTN - CFP}{CTP - CFN},$$

in order that this cutoff level be optimal? If we denote this ratio by r and use Equation 4–21 and the quantities calculated previously, we obtain

$$36.2 = 24 \cdot r$$

or

$$r \cong 1.5.$$

The cutoff level of 4.5 on the Schiötz scale, therefore, is optimal if the difference in benefit between a true negative and a false positive is 1.5 times as great as the difference in benefit between a true positive and a false negative. This would mean that the value of avoiding a false positive is 1.5 times the value of avoiding a false negative.

This, however, does not seem correct in the case of glaucoma. The risk associated with an undetected case is very great. Moreover, treatment is not that invasive. If anything, we would expect the ratio of net consequences to be *less* than 1.0; that is, it is worse to fail to detect a case of glaucoma than to incorrectly identify a nondiseased person as having glaucoma. Therefore, we want to detect relatively more patients with the disease. To do this, we should shift the positivity criterion in the direction of increasing the true-positive rate, or to the right.

Guided by these considerations, suppose we try a cutoff value of 6.5 on the Schiötz scale. Then the likelihood ratio is

$$\frac{P[6.0-6.9 \mid \text{Glaucoma}]}{P[6.0-6.9 \mid \text{No Glaucoma}]} = \frac{0.166}{0.140}$$

$$= 1.19.$$

The prior odds against glaucoma remain 24, so according to Equation 4–21 we have

$$1.19 = 24 \cdot \frac{CTN - CFP}{CTP - CFN},$$

or

$$\frac{CTN - CFP}{CTP - CFN} = 0.05.$$

Thus, the cutoff of 6.5 on the Schiötz scale is optimal if it is 20 times worse in terms of net risk to fail to identify a case of glaucoma than to administer treatment to a patient who does not actually have glaucoma. This is a matter of value judgment, but this result seems plausible. Thus, we might reasonably choose 6.5 as the positivity criterion.

Suppose that we are screening for glaucoma in a population in which the prevalence of the disease is only 0.4 per cent, or one tenth of the prevalence in the original population. For example, we might be screening a younger population in which the disease is less common. In this case the prior odds against the disease have increased, thus increasing the value of the right-hand side of Equation 4–21. If we assume the same ratio of net consequences, the only way to restore the equality in the formula is to increase the value of the left-hand side of the equation—the likelihood ratio. If we increase the likelihood ratio in Figure 4–14, we must move the cutoff value to the left, to a *more* stringent criterion.

Rules of Thumb in Choosing a Positivity Criterion

A variety of methods to determine positivity criteria for clinical tests are currently in use, but these are deficient in several respects. In one approach, patients without a particular disease are tested, and the results are distributed along the separator variable. The mean and standard deviation are then calculated. Finally, a zone that is two standard deviations above and below the mean is considered to define the "normal" range. This approach fails to consider the rarity or frequency of the disease and the distribution of test results of patients who have the disease and ignores the impact of false-positive or false-negative errors.

Another common approach is to choose a point on the separator variable that will identify 95 per cent of individuals with the disease as test positive. This was the origin of the traditional criterion that an induration of 10 mm or more defines a positive tuberculin test. This method of selection, however, ignores the distribution of test results in those without the disease, the prevalence of the disease, and all consequences but those that are due to false-negative error.

The expression that defines an optimal positivity criterion (Equation 4–21) leads to several rules of thumb for the adjustment of the cutoff point in response to changes in the consequences of a test result and in the prevalence of disease:

1. Cutoff points should be responsive to changes in the consequences of different test results (i.e., *TP, FP, TN, FN*). If the adverse consequences of false negatives *increase* relative to the adverse consequences of false positives, the cutoff point should be shifted in the direction of *lesser* stringency. If the adverse consequences of false negatives *decrease* relative to the adverse consequences of false positives, the cutoff point should be shifted in the direction of *greater* stringency. Both shifts serve to reduce the probability of the worse error.

2. As the prevalence of a disease *decreases*, the cutoff point should shift in the direction of *greater* stringency, thus reducing the number of false *positives*. Conversely, as the prevalence *increases*, the cutoff point should shift in the direction of *lesser* stringency, thus reducing the number of false *negatives*.

4.12 SUMMARY OF CHAPTER FOUR

This chapter has described the use of clinical information to revise probabilities of disease as needed in the solution of clinical problems.

A **test** result may be described in terms of where it falls along a **separator variable**. The **positivity criterion** for the separator variable divides the test population into *TP, FP, TN,* and *FN* categories. The test **sensitivity**, or **true-positive rate**, is the probability that a patient with a disease will have a positive test result; the test **specificity**, or **true-negative rate**, is the probability that a patient without a disease will have a negative test result. Although test sensitivity and specificity convey important information about a test, they alone are not sufficient to determine the probability of disease in tested patients. That probability depends as well on the **prevalence** or **prior probability of disease** in a population, $P[D]$. We call the probability of disease given a positive test result the **predictive value positive** of the test. The probability of not having the disease given a negative result is called the **predictive value negative** of the test.

The process by which test results are used to modify prior probabilities is called **probability revision**. This can be accomplished by manipulating contingency tables or by using **Bayes' formula**. Bayes' formula can be used to revise prior probabilities when several diagnoses are considered and several tests are included.

A derivative formulation of Bayes' theorem states that the **posterior odds** equal the **prior odds** times the test **likelihood ratio**. Probabilities can also be revised by "inverting" the appropriate decision tree.

The **receiver-operating characteristic (ROC)*** curve is a useful way of describ-

---

*The contents of this paragraph were covered in an optional section.

ing test or observer performance. ROC diagrams may be used to rank the merits of alternative tests or the skills of different observers.

A decision-analytic approach can be used to derive an optimal positivity criterion for a test. The cutoff point, which is defined in terms of the test likelihood ratio, depends upon the ratio of prior probabilities of nondisease and disease in the population and the ratio of consequences of false-positive ($CTN - CFP$) and false-negative ($CTP - CFN$) test results.

New terms that were introduced in this chapter are summarized in Tables 4–2 and 4–6.

EXERCISES FOR CHAPTER FOUR

EXERCISES FOR SECTION 4.4

1. *Rovsing's Sign*
Assume that Rovsing's sign is a perfectly specific test for appendicitis; its presence confirms appendicitis beyond doubt. It is, however, rarely present.

For this problem, assume that the probability of appendicitis is 0.16 for the patient under consideration. Also assume that the probability of Rovsing's sign in appendicitis is 0.0001 but that it never occurs unless appendicitis is present.

Use 2 X 2 contingency tables as needed to answer the following questions:

a. Given that a patient has appendicitis, what is the probability that the patient exhibits Rovsing's sign?
b. Given that a patient does *not* have appendicitis, what is the probability that the patient exhibits Rovsing's sign?
c. Given that a patient exhibits Rovsing's sign, what is the probability that the patient has appendicitis?
d. Given that a patient does *not* exhibit Rovsing's sign, what is the probability that the patient has appendicitis?

2. *Screening for Breast Cancer*
A breast cancer screening program using mammography would detect 67 per cent of women with undiagnosed cancer of the breast and would falsely detect as positive only 1 per cent of those without cancer. It is estimated that 0.3 per cent of women who are screened have undetected cancer.

a. Estimate in your head the probability that a woman with a positive test result (an abnormal mammogram) actually has breast cancer. (No computations; use your intuition!)
b. Now calculate (i) the probability that a woman does not have cancer if the test result is negative and (ii) the probability that a woman has cancer if the test result is positive.

EXERCISES FOR SECTION 4.5

3. *Rovsing's Sign*
Answer the questions in Exercise 1 for Section 4.4 using Bayes' formula.

4. *Screening for Breast Cancer*
Answer the questions in Exercise 2 for Section 4.4 using Bayes' formula.

5. *Appendicitis Among Aborigines*
Appendicitis is very unusual among a group of aborigines; it occurs once in every million cases of acute abdominal pain. An aborigine is seen by you with

pain in the right lower portion of the abdomen, rigid muscles of the right lower quadrant of the abdomen, and a high white blood cell count. An epidemiologist has given you the following table:

	Appendicitis	Other Abdominal Pain
Percentage with these symptoms	80%	1%
Percentage with other symptoms	20%	99%

What cause of his pain is more likely—appendicitis or "other abdominal pain"? Use Bayes' formula to compute your revised probability that this patient has appendicitis.

6. *Intravenous Pyelogram*
The prevalence of renovascular disease (RVD) among hypertensive patients in your clinic is 10 per cent. The intravenous pyelogram (IVP) has a true-positive rate of 78 per cent and a false-positive rate of 11 per cent in detecting RVD among those with hypertension.

a. Use Bayes' formula to calculate the probability that a patient with a positive test result (an abnormal IVP) has RVD.
b. Use Bayes' formula to calculate the probability that a patient with a negative test result (a normal IVP) has RVD.

EXERCISES FOR SECTION 4.6

7. *Child Abuse*
A screen for child abuse has a true-positive rate of 95 per cent and a false-positive rate of 10 per cent. What is the probability that a child with a positive test result is abused if

a. the prevalence of abuse is 3 per cent?
b. the prevalence of abuse is 0.3 per cent?
c. the prevalence of abuse is 0.03 per cent?

8. *A Treatment of Limited Efficacy*
Recall the problem of diagnosing a disease by observing the patient's response to a treatment of limited efficacy (p. 99). The physician assesses that there is a 50 per cent chance that the patient is missing factor X, in which case the treatment relieves the symptoms, and a 20 per cent chance that the patient has the disease. The treatment is administered and the symptoms disappear.
The analysis in the text showed that the revised probability that the patient has the disease is 11 per cent. What is the revised probability that the patient has factor X?

EXERCISE FOR SECTION 4.9

9. *The Observation of Patients With Abdominal Pain*
In this problem you are asked to derive some of the conditional probabilities that we used in the analysis of whether to wait six hours before deciding whether to operate on patients with equivocal signs and symptoms of appendicitis.
The probability that the patient has appendicitis is 0.16. If the patient does have appendicitis, there is a 0.1875 chance that the appendix has already perforated; if you wait six hours, this probability increases to 0.24.
If the appendix has perforated by the end of six hours, there is a 0.84 chance that the symptoms will have gotten worse and a 0.16 chance that they will have stayed the same. If the appendix is inflamed but has not perforated by the end of six hours, there is a 0.8 chance that the symptoms will have gotten worse and a 0.2 chance that they will have stayed the same. If the appendix is

not diseased, there is a 0.39 chance that the symptoms will remain the same for six hours and a 0.61 chance that they will improve.

a. Calculate the probability that the patient has a perforated appendix at the beginning of the six hours.
b. Calculate the probability that the patient will have a perforated appendix if you wait six hours.
c. Calculate the probability that the patient's symptoms will
   i.   get worse,
   ii.   stay the same,
   iii.   get better.
d. Calculate the conditional probability that the patient has a perforated appendix if the symptoms
   i.   get worse,
   ii.   stay the same,
   iii.   get better.
e. Calculate the conditional probability that the patient has an inflamed appendix after six hours if the symptoms
   i.   get worse,
   ii.   stay the same,
   iii.   get better.

When you have finished, compare your answers to the probabilities on the decision tree in Chapter Three, Figure 3–5.

EXERCISES FOR SECTION 4.11

10. *Appendectomy in the Old and the Young*
    Surgeons are concerned with the proper indication for appendectomy in elderly patients, because their conditions differ from those of younger patients with abdominal pain in a number of important ways. First, older persons with appendicitis are said to display milder symptoms than younger patients, and their condition is therefore more easily confused with nonspecific abdominal pain than is the case for younger patients. Second, appendicitis is far less common in older people. Finally, the mortality in cases in which the appendix perforates compared with that in cases in which a nondiseased appendix is removed differs in older people from that in younger people. Consider the following figures for younger and older patients:[115]

Mortality	Ages 30–49	Over Age 49
In patients in whom a perforated appendix is removed	13.8/1,000	67.3/1,000
In patients in whom an inflamed appendix is removed	0.9/1,000	5.7/1,000
In patients in whom a nondiseased appendix is removed	0.7/1,000	4.0/1,000

Assume that the death rates in this table accurately reflect the consequences of false-negative, true-positive, and false-positive classifications of patients. This provides the information you would need in order to move the cutoff point for interpreting signs and symptoms in younger patients to a more appropriate one for older patients. We are dealing with the cutoff point on a hypothetical separator variable based on signs, symptoms, and laboratory tests. Your objective is to minimize the death rate.

a. Describe in terms of the concepts developed in this chapter the specific factors that might make the cutoff point different for older people than for younger people. How does the value of each factor differ for older as compared with younger people?
b. How does the value of each factor (taken singly and holding others constant)

affect the optimal cutoff point for older as compared with younger people?

c. The preceding description contains both quantitative and qualitative information. Itemize the additional quantitative information that you would need in order to choose the optimal cutoff point to minimize the death rate.

11. *ROC Curves**

The ROC curve plots the true-positive rate versus the false-positive rate, and, as explained in Section 4.11, it describes the full performance of a test because of the following relations: *TPR* plus *FNR* equals 1, and *TNR* plus *FPR* equals 1. One might with equal validity describe the performance of a test as the *TPR* plotted against the *TNR*, the *FNR* against the *TNR*, or even the *FNR* against the *FPR*.

Consider the general shape of the ROC curve, which sweeps up from the lower left to the upper right. What would the general shape be if the *TPR* were plotted against the *TNR*?

---

*This problem relates to the optional section on the receiver-operating characteristic (p. 114).

Chapter Five

The Value of
Clinical Information

5.1 AN ANALYSIS OF THE DECISION TO TEST

One of the most frequent decisions a physician makes is whether to order a test. What should a physician think about when contemplating the use of a diagnostic test? In this chapter we will extend our analysis of the value and the choice of diagnostic tests.

Two concepts developed thus far are especially pertinent in considering diagnostic tests. One is **probability revision,** which was presented in Chapter Four. A diagnostic test is used by the clinician to gain greater certainty as to the patient's condition. In the terms we presented in Chapter Four, a test provides information that can be used to reassess the probabilities assigned to possible disease states. Before the test is ordered, the physician implicitly or explicitly associates a set of prior probabilities with the possible disease states; each possible test result, then, leads to a revision of those probabilities. The value of a diagnostic test depends, in large part, on its ability to achieve separation among the diagnostic alternatives, that is, on the extent to which different test results lead to different sets of posterior probabilities for the possible disease states. The ultimate value of a diagnostic test depends, however, on its potential for changing a subsequent therapeutic decision concerning the patient.

The second concept introduced thus far that is relevant to making decisions about tests is the **expected value of clinical information.** In Chapter Three we defined a special case of this concept in which we considered a test that provided perfect discrimination among disease states. Using the example of the liver biopsy for hepatitis and cirrhosis, we defined the **expected value of perfect clinical information** as the difference between the outcome rate (e.g., the death rate) when the treatment decision must be made without the information and the outcome rate when the treatment decision can be made contingent upon the test result. Recall also that when some risk is inherent in a test procedure, that risk must be taken into account in calculating the *net* expected value of clinical information.

Our objective in this chapter is to expand upon the concepts of probability revision and the expected value of clinical information so that they apply more generally to clinical situations in which diagnostic testing decisions are made. Most diagnostic tests do not provide perfect information, as we assumed in our analysis of the liver biopsy example in Chapter Three, nor are they free of measurement error, as we have assumed thus far. Moreover, physicians rarely order a single test; findings from panels of multiple tests and repetitions of the same test often constitute the information base upon which a physician tries to reach a diagnosis, or, in the language of clinical decision analysis, revises the probabilities of disease. In this chapter, therefore, we consider the following topics:

Tests That Provide Imperfect Information.   Tests that are not perfect and that are subject to measurement error are not as valuable as perfect tests, but they may still be of value. In Section 5–2 we describe the sources of error in a test and then generalize the concept of the expected value of clinical information to apply to imperfect tests. The objective is to provide the clinician with a basis for discriminating between tests that are valuable despite their errors and tests whose errors render them useless in a given clinical context.

Multiple Tests.   The differential diagnosis of disease is seldom carried out by the use of a single test. The concept of a diagnostic work-up involving many tests is commonplace in medicine. In Chapter Four we generalized the method of probability revision to the case in which a single test was used to discriminate among several possible diseases. Here we generalize to situations in which several test results must be combined. For example, in the diagnosis of myocardial infarction, a physician might order a test not only to measure the level of SGOT but also to measure the level of lactic dehydrogenase (LDH) and creatine phosphokinase (CPK), all three of which are enzymes whose increased level in the blood suggests tissue damage. In the diagnosis of kidney disease, a physician might order tests to measure both serum creatinine and blood urea nitrogen (BUN) levels. In the diagnosis of appendicitis, the physician observes many symptoms and signs. An objective of Section 5–3, in which the methods of probability revision are extended to the case of multiple tests, is to give the clinician insights into the circumstances under which a second or third test can be of either substantial incremental value or little, if any, incremental value.

Repeated Tests.   Just as many tests may be ordered in batteries, individual tests may be repeated in order to expand the information base for decision making. Sometimes such repetition has value; other times it does not. In Section 5–4 we apply the concepts that were developed earlier in the chapter to analyze the clinical decision to repeat a test.

5.2 TESTS THAT DO NOT GIVE PERFECT INFORMATION

Almost no diagnostic test yields perfect information; that is, only rarely does a test result identify with certainty which disease the patient has. Part of the imperfect nature of a test lies in its inability to discriminate absolutely among disease states, as we have seen in our examples of SGOT and myocardial infarction and Schiötz tonometry and glaucoma. Adding to the imperfection of a test is the fact that the underlying physical parameter (e.g., the SGOT concentration or the intraocular pressure) may not be measured perfectly by the instruments available. In this section we define some terminology that will enable us to discuss these different kinds of test errors and then consider them in the evaluation of testing decisions. Next, we generalize the methods of probability revision to tests that are subject to measurement error. Then, we present a generalized concept of the **expected value of clinical information,** with which we develop further insights into the conditions under which a clinician can expect a test to be of value in caring for a patient.

DISCRIMINATION, PRECISION, AND ACCURACY

Discrimination

When we introduced the notion of a **separator variable** in Chapter Four, we showed how results from a test can be represented as a probability distribution under each possible disease state. Figure 4–4 is such a representation of the level of SGOT in relation to the presence or absence of myocardial infarction; Figure 4–14 provided a comparable representation of intraocular pressure in relation to glaucoma.

Let us suppose for a moment that both of the tests described in those figures were free of measurement error, that is, that the tests measure, respectively, the *true* level of SGOT in the blood and the *true* intraocular pressure. In that case the extent to which the probability distribution above the axis and the probability distribution below the axis fail to overlap reflects the ability of the test to discriminate between the disease states.

A "perfect" test is one for which the conditional probability distributions of the separator variable (that is, conditional upon the disease states) do not overlap at all. Test B of Figure 4–15 is such a test; any result to the right of point C indicates with certainty the absence of disease. A dichotomous (one scored positive or negative) perfect test has a sensitivity of 1.0 and a specificity of 1.0.

In general, we may refer to the ability of a separator variable, exclusive of errors in measurement, to separate disease states as its **discrimination.** The errors introduced by measurement are described next.

Precision

An observed test result may differ from the underlying true value because of either of two kinds of measurement error, which we shall call **imprecision** and **inaccuracy.**

Precision, or test-retest **reliability,** refers to the tendency of repeated measurements on the same sample to yield the same result. For example, suppose a serum sample contains a glucose concentration of 100 mg/100 ml. If an analyzer runs six determinations on the sample and the results are 99, 102, 100, 100, 101, and 98, the test is more precise than if the results are 112, 88, 125, 105, 75, and 95.

Let us now explore the effects of imprecision on the shape of the distribution of test results. Assume that we have a group of patients for whom the true value of a test on a particular separator variable is known to be 100. (Assume that we have independently verified this value.) We now use an imprecise test instrument to reevaluate this group of patients. The distribution of the measured variable might be as shown in the lower panel of Figure 5–1. The degree of "spread," or random error, around the true value of 100 is a measure of the imprecision of the test.*

More generally, assume that we have a population of patients the true test values for which are known to be distributed along a particular separator variable, as shown in the upper panel of Figure 5–2. We now test individuals at random and in large numbers from that population, using the imprecise test characterized in Figure 5–1. For each value in the upper panel, the test yields a distribution spread around that value, as is shown in Figure 5–1. The aggregate effect on the distribution of the measured test results is shown in the lower panel of Figure 5–2. A comparison of the two distribution curves in Figure 5–2 indicates that the spread of results on our retest of the sample population is substantially broader than is the test variable in the population from which we

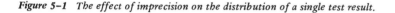

*Statisticians sometimes use the variance or standard deviation of a test as a measure of its imprecision.

Figure 5–1   The effect of imprecision on the distribution of a single test result.

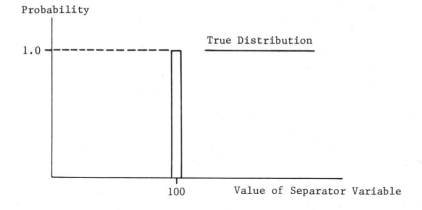

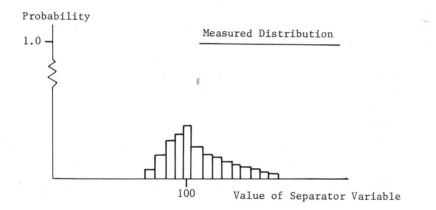

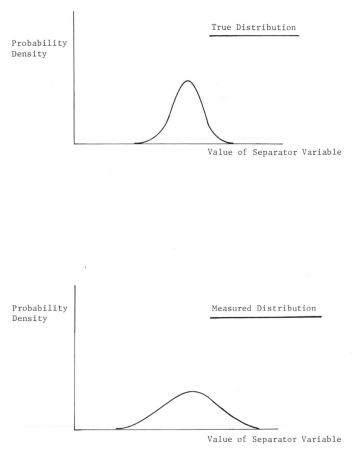

Figure 5–2 *The effect of imprecision on the distribution of test values.*

selected our large sample. The absence of spread or random error in the test results is the measure of their precision or reliability.

In practice, when one observes a particular distribution of results along a separator variable, it is not possible to discern the effect of imprecision on the true distribution. The effect of imprecision can be revealed only by comparing the distribution with that obtained by using a more precise measure.

The consequences of imprecision in a test used as a separator are illustrated in Figure 5–3. The upper panel shows the distribution of test values for individuals with (D) and without ($\overline{D}$) the disease along the separator variable for a completely precise test. It is apparent that the test results achieve relatively good separation of the D and $\overline{D}$ populations; it has good discrimination. The consequence of performing this test in a manner that decreases its precision is shown in the lower panel. The spread of results for both the D and $\overline{D}$ groups along the separator variable is increased, and there is now a zone of overlap that includes more individuals from each group. Clearly, the separating capability of the test is decreased. As precision decreases, the distributions of test results for D and $\overline{D}$ individuals tend to become indistinguishable, and the test has diminishing value in revising prior probabilities.

For real tests the observed distributions of values for D and $\overline{D}$ individuals along the separator variable depend both upon the true distribution of values in the population and on the precision of the test itself. Increasing imprecision would make the observed distributions resemble more closely those in the lower

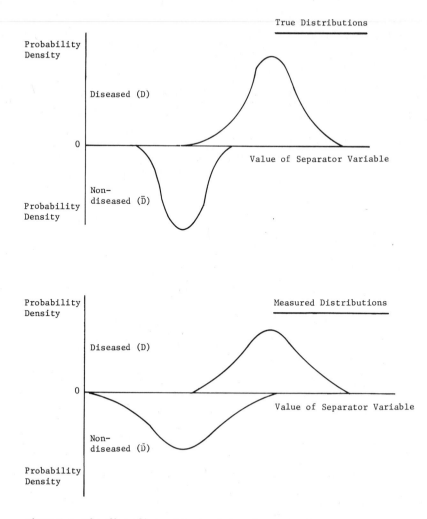

Figure 5–3 *The effect of imprecision in a test used as a separator.*

panel of Figure 5–3. Even for a test that is relatively imprecise, however, if a suitable cutoff point divides the population into groups with differing probabilities of disease, the test may retain value in revising prior probabilities of disease. We shall see an example of this in the section on probability revision for tests with measurement error (p. 139).

Most physicians are aware that findings from the medical history, the physical examination, and laboratory tests show variation when repeated by the same or different observers or laboratories. A recent review documents the degree of variation for some widely used observations, emphasizes the lack of information about variations in many other important clinical observations, and concludes that there is "little room for complacency" regarding the "reliability of clinical data, methods and judgments."[137]

The precision, or reliability, of some tests may be improved by rigorous standardization. When all practicable steps have been taken to improve the reliability of a test, the effects of residual imprecision can often be mitigated by repetition of the test. We will return to the issue of assessing the value of repeating a diagnostic test in Section 5.4.

Accuracy

The **accuracy** of a test refers to the tendency of test measurements to center around the true value of the separator variable. Consider the example of the analyzer that is being used to measure the true serum glucose level of 100 mg/100 ml. The analyzer that yielded the six measurements of 99, 102, 100, 100, 101, and 98 is fairly accurate because the results center around the true value of 100.* By contrast, if a second analyzer is miscalibrated so that it produces six readings of 105 mg/100 ml on the same sample, this test is not very accurate.

A test may be accurate but imprecise, or it may be very precise yet inaccurate. For example, the miscalibrated analyzer that always reads 5 mg/100 ml higher than the true value is inaccurate but very precise.

The meaning of test accuracy is illustrated in Figure 5–4. The distribution of true values of the separator variable for our population is shown in the upper panel, while the distribution of the results of an inaccurate test applied to a large number of individuals is shown in the lower panel. Two features of the distribution of the test results are noteworthy. First, the spread of values in the

---

*In statistical terms, a test's accuracy is measured by the proximity of its mean value to the true value. In the example given, the sample mean is (99 + 102 + 100 + 100 + 101 + 98)/6 = 100.

Figure 5–4 The effect of inaccuracy on the distribution of test values.

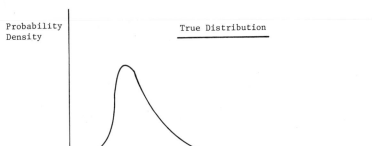

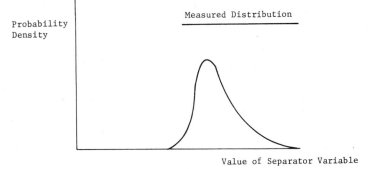

lower panel is no greater than that in the upper panel; the test procedure is perfectly precise. Second, the distribution of values in the lower panel is shifted to the right, indicating the presence of a systematic error, or inaccuracy, in the test procedure. Sometimes we refer to such a systematic error as a test's **bias**.

The upper panel of Figure 5–5 shows the distribution of unbiased (i.e., accurate) test results for D and $\overline{D}$ individuals along the separator variable, with an optimum positivity criterion chosen by the method described in Chapter Four, Section 4–11. If an inaccurate test is applied to a similar population, its results are distributed as shown in the lower panel of the figure. The use of the standard cutoff point now yields a different set of relations among the number of true-positive (*TP*), false-positive (*FP*), true-negative (*TN*), and false-negative (*FN*) individuals and, therefore, no longer achieves the best separation of individuals with and without the disease.

Figure 5–5 *The effect of inaccuracy in a test used as a separator. (TP indicates true positives; FP, false positives; TN, true negatives. and FN, false negatives.)*

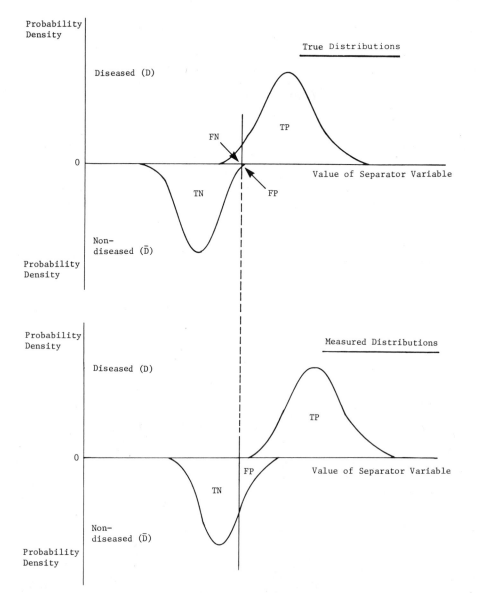

The component of error in the result of an inaccurate but precise test is not random; in fact, it is the same from one test to another. For this reason, repetition of the test produces no improvement in test performance as it does in the case of an imprecise test.

PROBABILITY REVISION FOR TESTS WITH MEASUREMENT ERROR: IMPRECISE MEASUREMENT OF THE SGOT LEVEL AND MYOCARDIAL INFARCTION

In Chapter Four, we showed how the result of a diagnostic test can be used to revise the probabilities of disease states. The examples used were tests that were assumed to be free of measurement error (i.e., perfectly precise and accurate). In this section we demonstrate that it is possible to generalize the methods of probability revision to imprecise or inaccurate tests, without requiring any new, more complex analytical machinery. The approaches using Bayes' formula and probability tree inversion apply perfectly well to tests with measurement error.

Consider once again the example of SGOT and myocardial infarction (MI) from Chapter Four. Suppose that the "true" probability distributions of SGOT values among patients with and without MI are given in Figure 4–4. These are the true values in the sense that they are measured by an ideal (perfectly precise and accurate) procedure. For example, the probability of a true SGOT level between 100 and 149 units/liter in a patient with MI is 0.19, and the probability of a true SGOT level between 100 and 149 units/liter in a patient without MI is 0.09.

Suppose that a perfectly precise test yields an SGOT level in the range of 100 to 149 units/liter. What is the revised probability that the patient has MI? Using Bayes' formula, we obtain

$$P[\text{MI}|\,100\text{–}149] = \frac{P[100\text{–}149|\text{MI}] \cdot P[\text{MI}]}{P[100\text{–}149|\text{MI}] \cdot P[\text{MI}] + P[100\text{–}149|\overline{\text{MI}}] \cdot P[\overline{\text{MI}}]}$$

$$= \frac{(0.19)\,(0.2)}{(0.19)\,(0.2) + (0.09)\,(0.8)}$$

$$= \frac{0.038}{0.038 + 0.072}$$

$$= 0.345.$$

Hence, an SGOT level in that range would lead us to revise the probability of MI from 20 per cent to 34.5 per cent.

Now, let us suppose that our SGOT measurement is imprecise, as follows: If the *true* value lies in a particular interval, there is a 0.6 probability that the *measured* value will lie in the same interval; however, there is a 0.2 probability that the measured value will be one interval lower and a 0.2 probability that the measured value will be one interval higher than the true value. (In case the true value is at either extreme, such as between 0 and 49 or 250 and 600 units/liter, assume a 0.8 probability that the measured value will be equal to the true value and a 0.2 probability that the measured value will be one interval off.) For example, suppose the true SGOT level is between 150 and 199 units/liter. Then the test result will be distributed as follows, conditional upon that true value: a probability of 0.2 between 100 and 149 units/liter; a probability of 0.6 between 150 and 199 units/liter; and a probability of 0.2 between 200 and 249 units/liter.

Given the data in Figure 4–4 and the properties of our imprecise test for the measurement of the SGOT level, we can derive the probability distributions of the measured test results. For example, what is the probability of a measured value between 100 and 149 units/liter in a patient with MI? The answer is contained in the probability tree in Figure 5–6. The probability of a measured value between 100 and 149 units/liter in a patient with MI is the sum of the path probabilities corresponding to "measured SGOT 100–149" conditional upon MI, or

$$0.046 + 0.114 + 0.016 = 0.176.$$

We can derive the probability of each *measured* SGOT value conditional upon MI or no MI using similar calculations. The results are shown in Table 5–1.

We are now in a position to calculate the revised probability of MI given a measured SGOT level in each interval. For example, in Table 5–1 we find that the probability of a measured SGOT level between 100 and 149 units/liter in patients with MI is 0.176 and the probability of a measured SGOT level between 100 and 149 units/liter in patients without MI is 0.076. Hence, the revised

Figure 5–6　*A probability tree for the imprecise SGOT test.*

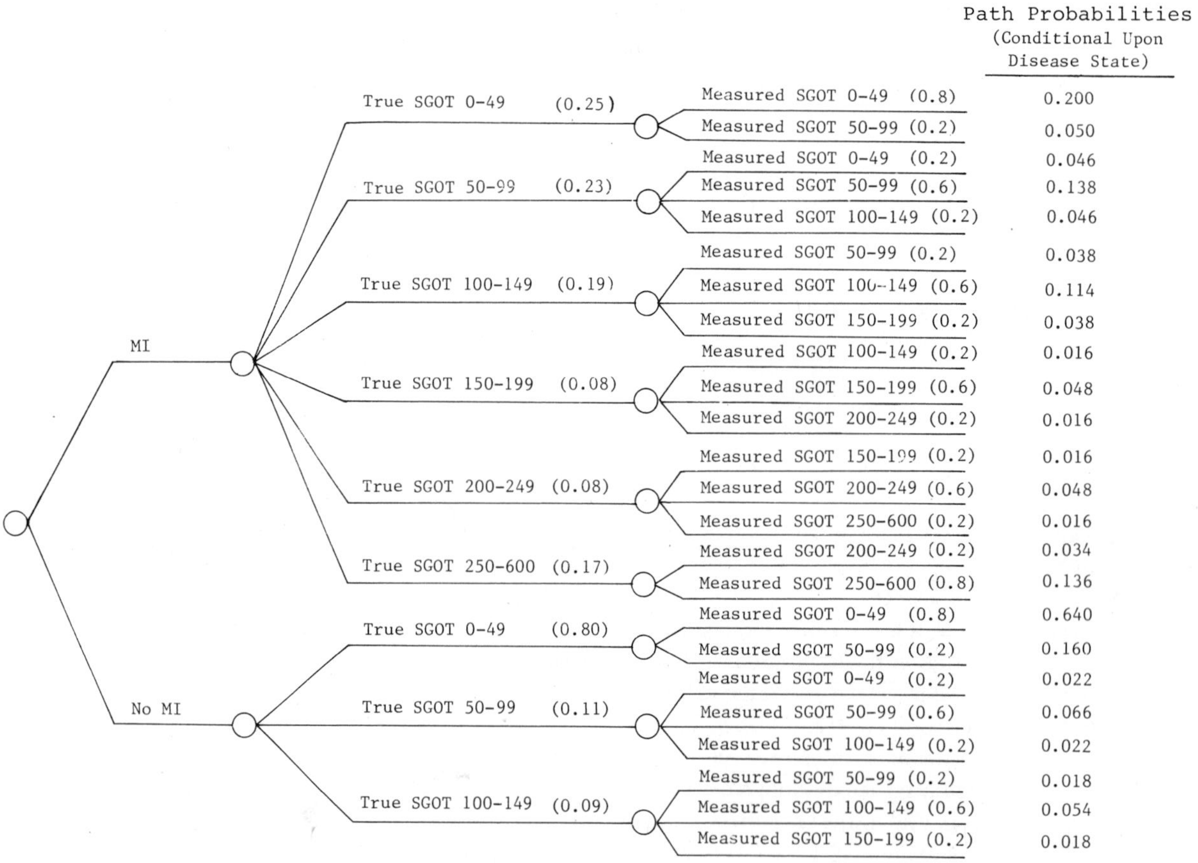

	Path Probabilities (Conditional Upon Disease State)
True SGOT 0–49 (0.25) → Measured SGOT 0–49 (0.8)	0.200
Measured SGOT 50–99 (0.2)	0.050
Measured SGOT 0–49 (0.2)	0.046
True SGOT 50–99 (0.23) → Measured SGOT 50–99 (0.6)	0.138
Measured SGOT 100–149 (0.2)	0.046
Measured SGOT 50–99 (0.2)	0.038
True SGOT 100–149 (0.19) → Measured SGOT 100–149 (0.6)	0.114
Measured SGOT 150–199 (0.2)	0.038
Measured SGOT 100–149 (0.2)	0.016
True SGOT 150–199 (0.08) → Measured SGOT 150–199 (0.6)	0.048
Measured SGOT 200–249 (0.2)	0.016
Measured SGOT 150–199 (0.2)	0.016
True SGOT 200–249 (0.08) → Measured SGOT 200–249 (0.6)	0.048
Measured SGOT 250–600 (0.2)	0.016
True SGOT 250–600 (0.17) → Measured SGOT 200–249 (0.2)	0.034
Measured SGOT 250–600 (0.8)	0.136
True SGOT 0–49 (0.80) → Measured SGOT 0–49 (0.8)	0.640
Measured SGOT 50–99 (0.2)	0.160
Measured SGOT 0–49 (0.2)	0.022
True SGOT 50–99 (0.11) → Measured SGOT 50–99 (0.6)	0.066
Measured SGOT 100–149 (0.2)	0.022
Measured SGOT 50–99 (0.2)	0.018
True SGOT 100–149 (0.09) → Measured SGOT 100–149 (0.6)	0.054
Measured SGOT 150–199 (0.2)	0.018

MI / No MI

TABLE 5–1   PROBABILITIES OF MEASURED SGOT LEVELS GIVEN THE
PRESENCE OR ABSENCE OF MI

| | DISEASE STATUS | |
MEASURED SGOT LEVEL (Units/Liter)	MI	No MI
0–49	0.246	0.662
50–99	0.226	0.244
100–149	0.176	0.076
150–199	0.102	0.018
200–249	0.098	0
250–600	0.152	0
Totals	1.000	1.000

probability of MI given a measured SGOT level between 100 and 149 units/liter
can be derived from Bayes' formula as follows:

$$P[MI|100–149] = \frac{P[100–149|MI] \cdot P[MI]}{P[100–149|MI] \cdot P[MI] + P[100–149|\overline{MI}] \cdot P[\overline{MI}]}$$

$$= \frac{(0.176)(0.2)}{(0.176)(0.2) + (0.076)(0.8)}$$

$$= 0.367.$$

Hence, if the measured SGOT level is between 100 and 149 units/liter, we revise
our probability of MI from 20 per cent to 36.7 per cent. The revised probability
for the perfectly precise SGOT test in this interval was calculated previously as
34.5 per cent.

The revised probabilities for SGOT results in each interval for both the
perfectly precise SGOT test and the imprecise SGOT test are shown in Table 5–2.
Note that with the perfectly precise SGOT test, a level of 150 units/liter or
higher leads, in our example, to a certain diagnosis of MI. With an imprecise
SGOT test, however, the probability of MI is increased to only 58.6 per cent
if the measured result is between 150 and 199 units/liter. When using a test that
is subject to imprecision, the physician should exercise more caution in reaching
a diagnosis on the basis of a single test result.

Over the full range of SGOT values, we observe in Table 5–2 that the revised
probabilities using the imprecise test have changed, but not so dramatically
that the test is rendered useless. It is important, however, for a physician to be
aware of a test's imprecision when revising probabilities of disease based on its
results.

THE EXPECTED VALUE OF IMPERFECT CLINICAL
INFORMATION

In Chapter Three we introduced the concept of the **expected value of perfect
clinical information.** This was defined as the difference between the expected

TABLE 5–2 REVISED PROBABILITIES OF MYOCARDIAL INFARCTION USING EITHER A PERFECTLY PRECISE SGOT TEST* OR AN IMPRECISE SGOT TEST†

SGOT LEVEL (Units/Liter)	P [MI	SGOT LEVEL, PRECISE TEST]	P [MI	SGOT LEVEL, IMPRECISE TEST]
0–49	0.072	0.085
50–99	0.343	0.188
100–149	0.345	0.367
150–199	1.000	0.586
200–249	1.000	1.000
250–600	1.000	1.000

*See Figure 4–4.
†See Table 5–1.

outcome for the strategy with the perfect test and the expected outcome for the strategy without the test. We showed how to calculate the expected value of perfect clinical information using the example of the liver biopsy to discriminate between hepatitis and cirrhosis.

With the background on probability revision gained from Chapter Four, we move on to the evaluation of tests that do not give perfect information because of imperfect test discrimination or because of inaccuracy or imprecision in the test measurement. Typically, a given positivity criterion will be associated with both false positives and false negatives. What is the expected value of this kind of imperfect clinical information? How can the decision maker compare the expected value with the risks (and costs) of collecting the information and thereby decide whether the test should be performed?

In this section we develop the general concept of the **expected value of clinical information (EVCI).** Then, we demonstrate how the physician can use decision analysis to help decide whether a test should be done, that is, whether the expected value of its information exceeds the risk of obtaining it.

Recall the liver biopsy decision in Chapter Three, Section 3–6. Instead of assuming that the biopsy is a perfect discriminator between hepatitis and cirrhosis, assume that there are errors. In particular, assume that in the presence of hepatitis the test will fail to identify the disease 10 per cent of the time and that in the presence of cirrhosis the test will incorrectly diagnose hepatitis five per cent of the time. The source of the error could be a combination of observation error, faulty equipment or laboratory procedures, or inherent limitations of the test in detecting disease.

The choice between this imperfect biopsy and no biopsy is displayed in the decision tree of Figure 5–7. The tree introduces an alternative, but numerically equivalent, way of representing the "survives" or "dies" chance node following the performance of a test that carries some risk of death. The risk is displayed compactly by the "toll gate" symbol along the "imperfect biopsy" branch. The toll gate (⌐) means if this branch is chosen, the survival rate must be reduced by the proportion of individuals who die from the procedure. In this case, the "toll" is one death per 1,000 patients who undergo the biopsy. This means that when you have averaged out and folded back to point Ⓐ, before folding back to the beginning of the tree, subtract 0.001 times the survival rate at point Ⓐ to give the *net* survival rate for the imperfect biopsy strategy. Thus, if the

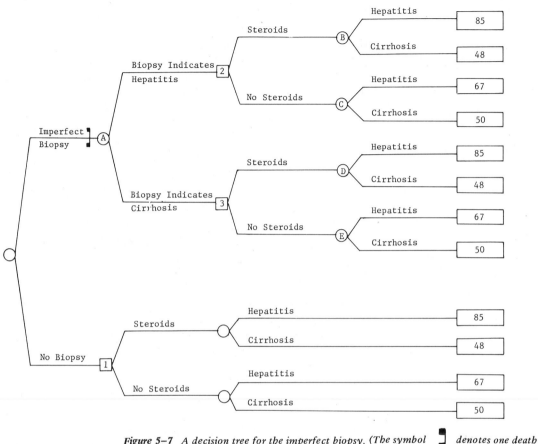

Survival (per cent)

Figure 5-7 A decision tree for the imperfect biopsy. (The symbol ▮ denotes one death per 1,000 patients who undergo the biopsy.)

survival rate at (A) were 50 per cent, we would subtract (0.001) (50), or 0.05 per cent, from 50 per cent to yield a net survival rate of 49.95 per cent. This would then be compared with the survival rate at [1] to fold back the final step and choose between performing a biopsy and not performing a biopsy. Note, however, that this toll gate notation could be applied just as easily in the case of perfect information as it is in this example of imperfect information. Note also that in actuality the toll might include an economic cost. We do not consider such costs here, but in Chapter Eight you will see how such costs might also be introduced into the analysis in deciding whether to perform the test.

The only substantive difference between Figure 5-7 and Figure 3-12 is that the test in Figure 5-7 is not perfect. The chance node at (A), which describes the possible test results, does not branch into "hepatitis" and "cirrhosis" but instead into "biopsy indicates hepatitis" and "biopsy indicates cirrhosis." The reason is that the test does not determine with certainty which disease is present. We must make the treatment decision at [2] or [3] on the basis of the test result, although we are aware that the test finding may be wrong. Following our decision, the outcome is determined by which disease is actually present.

Now let us begin to insert the probabilities in the decision tree. The probabilities at (A), for example, are

$$P[\text{Biopsy Indicates Hepatitis}]$$

and

$$P[\text{Biopsy Indicates Cirrhosis}] .$$

We recognize these as variations of the test level and its complement, or $P[T^+]$ and $P[T^-]$. The probabilities at both Ⓑ and Ⓒ are

$$P[\text{Hepatitis} | \text{Biopsy Indicates Hepatitis}]$$

and

$$P[\text{Cirrhosis} | \text{Biopsy Indicates Hepatitis}] ;$$

and the probabilities at Ⓓ and Ⓔ are conditional on "biopsy indicates cirrhosis." These are, respectively, analogous to the predictive value positive, $P[D|T^+]$, and the predictive value negative, $P[\overline{D}|T^-]$. As usual, however, we do not have the probabilities in this form. Instead, we have the prevalence,

$$P[\text{Hepatitis}] = 0.2,$$

and we have the analogues of sensitivity and specificity,

$$P[\text{Biopsy Indicates Hepatitis} | \text{Hepatitis}] = 0.9$$

and

$$P[\text{Biopsy Indicates Cirrhosis} | \text{Cirrhosis}] = 0.95.$$

As in the many examples we encountered in Chapter Four, we must use a 2 × 2 contingency table, Bayes' formula, or an inverted probability tree to obtain the probabilities we need.

In Figure 5–8 we display the probability revision by the method of tree inversion. At the top of the figure we show the probabilities in the form in which they are available. For example, the probability of hepatitis is 0.2, and if hepatitis is present, the biopsy will indicate this with a probability of 0.9. The path probability of the event that hepatitis is present *and* that the test will denote this is thus

$$(0.2) (0.9) = 0.18$$

as indicated in the figure. Before examining the bottom half of Figure 5–8, you might wish to try inverting the tree yourself, just as we did in Chapter Four. The correct probabilities are shown on the inverted tree in the lower half of Figure 5–8.

Now we can fill in all of the probabilities at the chance nodes in Figure 5–7. This leads us to Figure 5–9, which is the full decision tree for this example. For comparative purposes, the perfect biopsy from Figure 3–12 is included as an option. Make sure that you understand the sources of all the probabilities on the tree.

The results of the averaging-out-and-folding-back process are shown in Figure 5–9. The process is straightforward. For the perfect biopsy, steroids are indicated if the biopsy specimen shows hepatitis; otherwise they are not. The expected

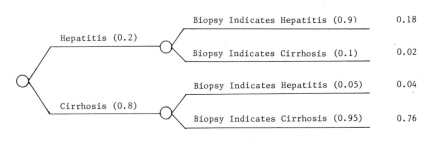

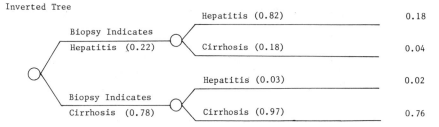

Figure 5-8 Probability revision for the imperfect biopsy. (Assumptions are as follows: P[Biopsy Indicates Hepatitis | Hepatitis] equals 0.90; p[Hepatitis] equals 0.20; P[Biopsy Indicates Cirrhosis | Cirrhosis] equals 0.95; and P[Cirrhosis] equals 0.80.)

Figure 5-9 The expected value of clinical information for the imperfect biopsy. The expected value of perfect clinical information is 57.0 per cent minus 55.4 per cent, which equals 1.6 per cent increase in the survival rate. The expected value of imperfect clinical information is 56.6 per cent minus 55.4 per cent, which equals 1.2 per cent increase in the survival rate. The expected cost of information is a decline in the survival rate of 0.057 per cent.

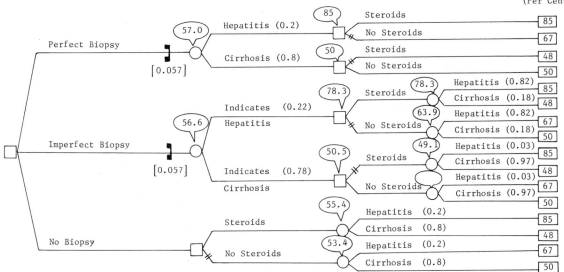

survival rate with the perfect biopsy (*before* considering mortality that is attributable to the biopsy) is 57.0 per cent. The reduction in the survival rate owing to the biopsy is

$$(0.001)(57.0) = 0.057\%$$

as indicated at the toll gate symbol.

For the imperfect biopsy, the analysis shows that steroids are indicated if the biopsy specimen shows hepatitis but not if the biopsy specimen reveals cirrhosis. The expected survival rate with the imperfect biopsy (*before* subtracting the mortality that is due to the biopsy) is 56.6 per cent, which is slightly less than that with the perfect biopsy.

When no biopsy is performed, steroids are the treatment of choice, and the expected value is a survival rate of 55.4 per cent, which is less than that associated with either a perfect or an imperfect biopsy.

Now let us calculate the **expected value of clinical information (EVCI)** for the imperfect biopsy and compare it with the EVCI for the perfect biopsy. We will begin by restating the general definition of the EVCI.

Definition. The **expected value of clinical information (EVCI)** of a test is the difference between the averaged-out outcome value when the test is performed and the averaged-out outcome value when the test is not performed.

The EVCI for the perfect biopsy, which we calculated in Chapter Three, Section 3.6, is the difference between the expected survival rate with the perfect biopsy (57.0 per cent) and the expected survival rate without a biopsy (55.4 per cent), or 1.6 per cent. To obtain the *net* expected value of the perfect biopsy, we subtract the mortality that is due to the biopsy itself, that is, 0.057 per cent, or about 0.06 per cent. The difference,

$$1.6\% - 0.06\%$$

or 1.54 per cent, is the *net* EVCI. This, of course, is the same result we arrived at in Chapter Three.

The EVCI for the imperfect biopsy is the difference between 56.6 per cent and 55.4 per cent, or 1.2 per cent. When we subtract the mortality of approximately 0.06 per cent that is due to the biopsy, we get a *net* EVCI of

$$1.2\% - 0.06\%$$

or 1.14 per cent. Since the EVCI of the imperfect biopsy is greater than the mortality from the procedure, we conclude that the imperfect biopsy is better than no biopsy at all. It is not, however, better than the perfect biopsy, which has a higher EVCI (1.6 versus 1.2 per cent) but approximately the same risk (a 0.06 per cent decrease in the survival rate).

If a higher mortality were associated with the perfect biopsy, for example, one in 100 patients instead of one in 1,000, then its toll would increase tenfold to about 0.6 per cent, and its net EVCI would be approximately

$$1.6\% - 0.6\%$$

or 1.0 per cent. This would compare unfavorably with the 1.14 per cent for the imperfect biopsy. Sometimes we would prefer a test with reduced discrimination (or precision, or accuracy) if its risks are lower than those of a more informative test.

TESTS WHOSE RESULTS HAVE NO CLINICAL VALUE

Under what conditions might a test have no value and thus be contraindicated if it entails even the slightest risk? We provided some guidance to answering this question in Chapter Three, but the conditions warranting a test bear review in light of the material introduced in Chapters Four and Five.

A *necessary* condition for a test to have positive value, or an EVCI of greater than 0, is that it contain some information. A test contains some information unless its results are *independent* of the disease in question. Suppose that $P[T^+|D]$ equals 0.2 and that $P[T^+|\overline{D}]$ equals 0.2. In this case the positive test result occurs with the same probability whether or not the disease is present. (A somewhat fanciful example would be an "eye test" to distinguish hepatitis from cirrhosis; if the patient has blue eyes, call it hepatitis; otherwise, call it cirrhosis.) In our example, suppose the pathologist reports the presence of hepatitis with a probability of x, regardless of whether hepatitis or cirrhosis is present. Since the likelihood ratio for this test result is 1.0, the posterior odds favoring hepatitis are the same as the prior odds, regardless of what the pathologist reports.

Any test whose results are independent of the disease is an obviously useless test. However, a lack of independence between the test results and the disease does not guarantee an EVCI of greater than 0. A *sufficient* condition for a test to have a positive EVCI is that the preferred decision change following some results of the test.

Consider, for example, the imperfect biopsy example in Figure 5–9. The patient in this case, however, has a much higher prior probability of hepatitis, for example, 0.6. Perhaps this patient has a history of disease that is more indicative of chronic hepatitis than would otherwise be the case.

The analysis of probabilities for this new case is left as an exercise at the end of the chapter. The result is that the higher prior probability leads to a predictive value of the "biopsy indicates hepatitis" result that is much higher than in the original case — 0.96 versus 0.82. The predictive value of the "biopsy indicates cirrhosis" result is lower — 0.86 versus 0.97.

The full analysis is shown in Figure 5–10. Notice the outcome for the "imperfect biopsy" branch. If the biopsy specimen shows hepatitis, steroids are indicated because the survival rate with steroids is 83.5 per cent as compared with 66.3 per cent without steroids. But if the biopsy specimen indicates cirrhosis, steroids are still preferred — 53.2 per cent versus 52.4 per cent. This is so because the prior probability of hepatitis was so much higher than in the previous case. Thus, steroids are preferred regardless of the biopsy results, and we expect the biopsy to have no effect on subsequent decisions. Setting aside the possible prognostic value of the test information and ignoring possible research benefits, we conclude that the biopsy has no value. In fact, this is revealed by the analysis. The expected value with the biopsy is 70.2 per cent, which is the same as the value with no biopsy. Its EVCI is therefore 0. Its *net* EVCI is actually *negative* because of the 0.07 per cent mortality that is attributable to the biopsy. Therefore, the imperfect biopsy should not be done in this case.

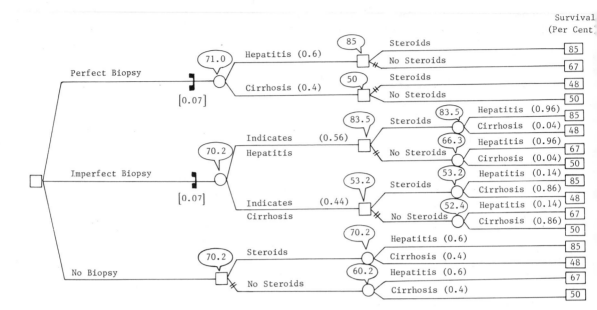

Figure 5-10 *The expected value of clinical information for the imperfect biopsy in a patient who is likely to have hepatitis (P[Hepatitis] equals 0.6). The expected value of perfect clinical information is 71.0 per cent minus 70.2 per cent, which equals a 0.8 per cent increase in the survival rate. The expected value of imperfect clinical information is zero, because the treatment decision is not affected by the information.*

This finding can be generalized as was stated in Chapter Three. If a test has no effect on any subsequent decision (and no prognostic or research benefits), then its expected value of clinical information is 0, and its net EVCI will be negative if it involves any risk at all. Note that our analysis considers only the potential benefit and risk to an individual patient; the economic costs of medical actions are discussed in Chapter Eight.

In summary, two *necessary* conditions for a test to be of value to the patient are the following:

1. It must convey information in the sense that it can change some probabilities.
2. Its result must be able to change the probabilities enough to affect a subsequent decision.

Strictly speaking, the second condition may not be necessary if prognostic information from the test is itself of sufficient value to the patient.

These necessary conditions apply to imperfect as well as perfect tests. If these conditions are not fulfilled, no test can be justified, at least in terms of outcome to the patient. Furthermore, for a test to be worthwhile, a *sufficient* condition is that its EVCI outweigh any risk from the test itself.

5.3 THE VALUE OF MULTIPLE TESTS

In clinical practice, choices among alternative diagnoses are seldom made on the basis of a single test. How great an advantage is gained by the use of a battery of tests to obtain information on the probability of a disease? How does the advantage depend upon the specific properties of the tests? These and related questions are the subject of this section.

PROBABILITY REVISION USING MORE THAN ONE TEST

To introduce the problem of probability revision using the results of several tests, we offer an example to which we shall return later in this section.

The Diagnosis of Renovascular Disease in a Hypertensive Patient

About 10 per cent of patients with high blood pressure who are seen at an urban teaching hospital clinic have renovascular disease (RVD). It is important to diagnose RVD because it can often be corrected surgically. It is also important to minimize the number of false positives, because such patients would be subjected unnecessarily to renal arteriography, an x-ray procedure that confirms the presence or absence of RVD but at some risk to the patient.

In this teaching hospital, two diagnostic tests are available to determine the presence of RVD. One is the intravenous pyelogram (IVP), another x-ray procedure. The other is the renogram (RG), a procedure involving the use of radioactive isotopes. A positivity criterion has been established for each test, and individuals from a study population have been separated by disease status into the usual 2 X 2 tables, with the probabilities for each test shown in Table 5–3. The true-positive rate for the IVP is 78 per cent and the true-positive rate for the RG is 85 per cent.

TABLE 5–3   PROBABILITIES OF TEST RESULTS FOR THE INTRAVENOUS PYELOGRAM AND RENOGRAM IN THE DIAGNOSIS OF RENOVASCULAR DISEASE*

| | DISEASE STATUS | |
TEST RESULT	RVD	$\overline{\text{RVD}}$
IVP$^+$	0.78	0.78
IVP$^-$	0.22	0.89
RG$^+$	0.85	0.10
RG$^-$	0.15	0.90

*Source: McNeil et al.[167] RVD indicates renovascular disease; IVP, intravenous pyelogram; and RG, renogram.

An IVP and an RG are obtained, and the results of both are abnormal (positive). What is the revised probability that the patient has RVD? How does this revised probability compare with what the revised probability would have been if only the IVP had been ordered? How does it compare with what the revised probability would have been if only the RG had been ordered?

The answers to these questions will tell us much about the value of multiple tests to determine the presence of a disease. If the revised probability of disease is higher when both test results are positive than it is when either test result alone is positive, then ordering both tests may have some value. If, however, the revised probability of disease is only slightly different when both test findings are positive or negative than it is when either test result alone is positive or negative, then the value of ordering both tests is more questionable.

To begin to analyze the tests, let us assume a prior probability of disease of 0.10 and use the techniques with which we are already familiar to compute

revised probabilities for each test separately. For the IVP, the revised probabilities are as follows:

$$P[RVD|IVP^+] = \frac{P[IVP^+|RVD] \cdot P[RVD]}{P[IVP^+|RVD] \cdot P[RVD] + P[IVP^+|\overline{RVD}] \cdot P[\overline{RVD}]}$$

$$= \frac{(0.78)(0.1)}{(0.78)(0.1) + (0.11)(0.9)}$$

$$= 0.441;$$

and

$$P[RVD|IVP^-] = \frac{P[IVP^-|RVD] \cdot P[RVD]}{P[IVP^-|RVD] \cdot P[RVD] + P[IVP^-|\overline{RVD}] \cdot P[\overline{RVD}]}$$

$$= \frac{(0.22)(0.1)}{(0.22)(0.1) + (0.89)(0.9)}$$

$$= 0.027.$$

For the RG we obtain

$$P[RVD|RG^+] = 0.486$$

and

$$P[RVD|RG^-] = 0.018.$$

Hence, we see that the RG has both a higher predictive value positive (48.6 per
cent versus 44.1 per cent) and a higher predictive value negative (98.2 per cent
versus 97.3 per cent) than the IVP. But what are the advantages of using *both*
tests?

Suppose that we apply Bayes' formula to revise the probability of disease
given that *both* test results are positive. We do this by treating the joint event
(RG^+, IVP^+) as if it were a single test result, as follows:

$$P[RVD|RG^+, IVP^+] =$$

$$\frac{P[RG^+, IVP^+|RVD] \cdot P[RVD]}{P[RG^+_1 IVP^+|RVD] \cdot P[RVD] + P[RG^+_1 IVP^+|\overline{RVD}] \cdot P[\overline{RVD}]} . \qquad (5-1)$$

Hence, we have simply applied Bayes' formula but substituted for the test
result the *joint* test result (RG^+, IVP^+).

How do we proceed from Equation 5–1? We know the values for $P[RVD]$
and $P[\overline{RVD}]$, which are 0.1 and 0.9, respectively. But the conditional probabilities in the formula are not immediately available to us from the data in Table
5–3. That is, we know the probability of RG^+ given the presence or absence of
disease ($P[RG^+|RVD]$ and $P[RG^+|\overline{RVD}]$), and we know the probability of
IVP^+ given the presence or absence of disease ($P[IVP^+|RVD]$ and $P[IVP^+|$
$\overline{RVD}]$). But we do not know the probability of IVP^+ *and* RG^+ given the presence of disease or the probability of IVP^+ *and* RG^+ given the absence of disease. One way to obtain those needed probabilities is to make an assumption

called **conditional independence.** We develop this assumption and its use in probability revision before returning to the problem of assessing the value of tests for renovascular disease.

Conditional Independence

Recall from Chapter Two that two events are **independent** if their joint probability equals the product of their individual probabilities:

$$P[E, F] = P[E] \cdot P[F].$$

The example of the sex of fraternal twins was given in Chapter Two; the probability of two boys is equal to

$$P[Boy, Boy] = P[Boy] \cdot P[Boy]$$
$$= (1/2)(1/2)$$
$$= 1/4.$$

It is possible to multiply the two individual probabilities to yield the joint probability because the sex of one twin is independent of the sex of the other. In other words, knowledge that the first twin is a boy does not influence the probability that the second twin is a boy.

Now we can generalize the concept of independence to situations in which all events are conditional upon some underlying event, or state, such as the presence of a disease. Suppose we have two tests, T_1 and T_2, that are applied in a subpopulation *known* to have a disease, D. Suppose further that knowing the result of T_1 *in this subpopulation* does not influence the probabilities assigned to the result of T_2 *in this subpopulation.* Then we shall say that the two tests are **conditionally independent given D.**

When two tests are conditionally independent, the **multiplication rule for joint probabilities** applies: If T_1 and T_2 are conditionally independent given disease D, then

$$P[T_1^+, T_2^+ | D] = P[T_1^+ | D] \cdot P[T_2^+ | D]. \qquad (5\text{--}2)$$

Note in Equation 5–2 that every probability in the formula is conditional upon disease D. For our purposes we will use the multiplication rule as a definition of conditional independence.

Definition. Two tests, T_1 and T_2, are said to be **conditionally independent given disease D** if the multiplication rule for joint probabilities (Equation 5–2) holds true for all possible test results, e.g., R_1 and R_2, in patients with the disease:

$$P[R_1, R_2 | D] = P[R_1 | D] \cdot P[R_2 | D]. \qquad (5\text{--}3)$$

Two observations are in order before we turn to some examples. First, if Equation 5–2 holds true for a dichotomous test, then it is possible to use the summation principle to show that

$$P[T_1^+, T_2^- | D] = P[T_1^+ | D] \cdot P[T_2^- | D],$$

$$P[T_1^-, T_2^+|D] = P[T_1^-|D] \cdot P[T_2^+|D],$$

and

$$P[T_1^-, T_2^-|D] = P[T_1^-|D] \cdot P[T_2^-|D].$$

Hence, Equation 5–2 is sufficient to establish conditional independence for tests T_1 and T_2.

The second observation is that conditional independence given the presence of disease (D) does *not* guarantee conditional independence in the absence of disease ($\overline{D}$) and vice versa. Equations 5–2 and 5–3 might apply, but their analogues with $\overline{D}$ substituted for D might not. We shall see an example of the importance of this observation later in this section.

We now give an example of conditional independence.

Example: Symptoms and Signs of Appendicitis. In the diagnosis of appendicitis, several symptoms and signs may be noted by the physician. Among these are pain in the right lower quadrant of the abdomen (RLQ), rebound tenderness (Reb), rectal tenderness (Rect), and severe pain (Sev). The conditional probabilities of each of these in patients with appendicitis (App) or nonspecific abdominal pain (NSAP) are given in Table 5–4.

TABLE 5–4 PROBABILITIES OF FOUR COMMON SYMPTOMS OR SIGNS
IN APPENDICITIS AND NONSPECIFIC ABDOMINAL PAIN*

SYMPTOM OR SIGN	PROBABILITY IN APPENDICITIS	PROBABILITY IN NSAP
Right lower quadrant pain	0.74	0.29
Rebound tenderness	0.95	0.26
Rectal tenderness	0.43	0.16
Severe pain	0.39	0.19

*Modified from Neutra.[181] The data are based on Staniland et al.[241] NSAP indicates nonspecific abdominal pain.

If we assume conditional independence, we can calculate the probability of any combination of the presence or absence of these symptoms and signs in patients with or without appendicitis. For example, suppose that we want to know the probability of RLQ$^+$, Reb$^+$, Rect$^-$, and Sev$^-$ in patients with and without appendicitis. Assuming conditional independence given appendicitis, we have

$$P[RLQ^+, Reb^+, Rect^-, Sev^-|App] = P[RLQ^+|App] \cdot P[Reb^+|App] \cdot$$
$$P[Rect^-|App] \cdot P[Sev^-|App]$$

$$= (0.74)(0.95)(0.57)(0.61)$$

$$= 0.244.$$

Assuming conditional independence given NSAP, we have

$$P[RLQ^+, Reb^+, Rect^-, Sev^-|NSAP] = P[RLQ^+|NSAP] \cdot P[Reb^+|NSAP] \cdot$$
$$P[Rect^-|NSAP] \cdot P[Sev^-|NSAP]$$

$$= (0.29)(0.26)(0.84)(0.81)$$

$$= 0.051.$$

Hence, we conclude that this combination of symptoms and signs is 24.4 per cent likely in appendicitis and only 5.1 per cent likely in NSAP.

Probability Revision When Tests Are Conditionally Independent

The assumption of conditional independence simplifies considerably the task of revising probabilities using multiple tests. In fact, by assuming conditional independence we would be able to use the individual test data in Table 5–3 to solve our problem of probability revision for the IVP and the RG. But let us first briefly reconsider the appendicitis example.

Symptoms and Signs of Appendicitis. Suppose we observe the combination of symptoms and signs described in the previous section, namely, $(RLQ^+, Reb^+, Rect^-, Sev^-)$. What is the revised probability of appendicitis given a prior probability of 16 per cent? If we are willing to assume conditional independence both given appendicitis *and* given NSAP, the calculation using Bayes' formula is straightforward:

$$P[App|RLQ^+, Reb^+, Rect^-, Sev^-] = \frac{P[RLQ^+, Reb^+, Rect^-, Sev^-|App] \cdot P[App]}{P[RLQ^+, Reb^+, Rect^-, Sev^-|App] \cdot P[App] + P[RLQ^+, Reb^+, Rect^-, Sev^-|NSAP] \cdot P[NSAP]}$$

$$= \frac{(0.244)(0.16)}{(0.244)(0.16) + (0.051)(0.84)}$$

$$= 0.477.$$

The assumptions of conditional independence permitted us to use the probability 0.244 for the combination of symptoms and signs given appendicitis and the probability 0.051 for the same combination given NSAP; both of these probabilities were calculated in the preceding section on conditional independence (p. 151).

The Diagnosis of Renovascular Disease. We return now to the problem with which we introduced the topic of probability revision using multiple tests: the diagnosis of renovascular disease using the intravenous pyelogram and the renogram. We want to revise our prior probability of 10 per cent given that both test results are positive. We wrote Bayes' formula in Equation 5–1 but were stymied because we did not have assessments of the probabilities of the joint test result (RG^+, IVP^+) among patients with or without the disease.

We might consider using the assumption of conditional independence to overcome this obstacle. In particular, let us assume that the results of the RG and the IVP are conditionally independent given the presence or absence of disease. This means, for example, that if we have a patient who is known to have RVD and we know that the result of the IVP is positive, then our assessment of the probability that the RG is also positive is unaffected; it remains at 0.85 (Table 5–3).

Having made this assumption, we proceed as follows:

$P[RVD|RG^+, IVP^+]$

$$= \frac{P[RG^+, IVP^+|RVD] \cdot P[RVD]}{P[RG^+, IVP^+|RVD] \cdot P[RVD] + P[RG^+, IVP^+|\overline{RVD}] \cdot P[\overline{RVD}]}$$

$$= \frac{P[RG^+|RVD] \cdot P[IVP^+|RVD] \cdot P[RVD]}{P[RG^+|RVD] \cdot P[IVP^+|RVD] \cdot P[RVD] + P[RG^+|\overline{RVD}] \cdot P[IVP^+|\overline{RVD}] \cdot P[\overline{RVD}]}$$

(by assuming conditional independence)

$$= \frac{(0.85)\,(0.78)\,(0.1)}{(0.85)\,(0.78)\,(0.1) + (0.10)\,(0.11)\,(0.9)}$$

$$= 0.870.$$

Hence, we would revise our probability of disease from 10 per cent all the way up to 87 per cent if both test results were positive. This compares with revised probabilities of 44.1 per cent for a positive IVP finding alone and 48.6 per cent for a positive RG finding alone. It would seem that much is to be gained by using the tests in combination.

But is it valid to assume conditional independence between the IVP and the RG? What would be the revised probabilities if conditional independence does not hold? We will deal with these questions in the next section. First, however, we generalize from what we have learned in the case of conditional independence.

General Properties of Revised Probabilities With Conditionally Independent Tests. The results in the previous examples indicate that the simultaneous use of two conditionally independent tests permits us to assign a higher probability of disease to the individual who has two positive test results than we could achieve with the use of either test alone. This outcome is a general property of using batteries of conditionally independent tests for the same disease. It can be proven that

$$P[D\,|\,T_1^{+},\,T_2^{+}] > P[D\,|\,T_1^{+}]$$

if the tests are conditionally independent.

The proof is as follows. Earlier in this section we indicated that conditional independence of test results justified the multiplication rule (Equation 5–2). If we substitute Equation 5–2 into Bayes' formula, we get

$$P[D\,|\,T_1^{+},\,T_2^{+}]$$

$$= \frac{P[T_1^{+}|D] \cdot P[T_2^{+}|D] \cdot P[D]}{P[T_1^{+}|D] \cdot P[T_2^{+}|D] \cdot P[D] + P[T_1^{+}|\overline{D}] \cdot P[T_2^{+}|\overline{D}] \cdot P[\overline{D}]}.$$

Dividing the numerator and the denominator by $P[T_2^{+}|D]$, we arrive at

$$P[D\,|\,T_1^{+},\,T_2^{+}] = \frac{P[T_1^{+}|D] \cdot P[D]}{P[T_1^{+}|D] \cdot P[D] + P[T_1^{+}|\overline{D}] \cdot \left(\dfrac{P[T_2^{+}|\overline{D}]}{P[T_2^{+}|D]}\right) \cdot P[\overline{D}]}.$$

By the definition of a positive test, the term

$$\left(\frac{P[T_2^{+}|\overline{D}]}{P[T_2^{+}|D]}\right)$$

in the denominator must be less than one. That is, the probability of a test defined as positive will always be less in the $\overline{D}$ population that it will be among D individuals. But note that the second equation differs from the usual Bayes expression for $P[D\,|\,T_1^{+}]$ only by the aforementioned term. Since the denominator of the second equation is reduced by its presence, the value of the entire right-hand side must be increased. It follows, therefore, that

$$P[D\,|\,T_1^{+},\,T_2^{+}] > P[D\,|\,T_1^{+}]$$

if the tests are conditionally independent.

On occasion the tests that are performed in the evaluation of a possible diagnosis do not have the property of conditional independence. Intuitively, one might suspect that tests that show some degree of positive correlation would have a less dramatic effect on the revised probability of disease than those that are independent. This issue is the subject of the following section.

Probability Revision When Tests Are *Not* Conditionally Independent

It is possible to avoid making unnecessary assumptions about conditional independence if one has data in the form required by Equation 5–1, namely, the conditional probabilities of the *joint* occurrence of test results given the disease state. In the case of the RG and the IVP, such data happen to be available.

The Diagnosis of Renovascular Disease. In revising the probability of renovascular disease using the IVP and the RG, we have to this point used the data in Table 5–3 and assumed conditional independence. Consider now the data in Table 5–5, which are much more comprehensive. In particular, these data provide the information we need to revise the probability of disease without making any additional assumptions. For example, the table reveals that

$$P[\text{RG}^+, \text{IVP}^+ | \text{RVD}] = 0.69$$

and

$$P[\text{RG}^+, \text{IVP}^+ | \overline{\text{RVD}}] = 0.08.$$

TABLE 5–5 PROBABILITIES OF JOINT TEST RESULTS OF THE INTRAVENOUS PYELOGRAM AND RENOGRAM IN THE DIAGNOSIS OF RENOVASCULAR DISEASE*

TEST RESULT	RVD			$\overline{\text{RVD}}$		
	IVP$^+$	IVP$^-$	Row Totals	IVP$^+$	IVP$^-$	Row Totals
RG$^+$	0.69	0.16	0.85	0.08	0.02	0.10
RG$^-$	0.09	0.06	0.15	0.03	0.87	0.90
Column totals	0.78	0.22	1.00	0.11	0.89	1.00

*Source: McNeil et al.[167] The cutoff point assumed for the renogram corresponds to the less stringent criterion analyzed in the original article. RVD indicates renovascular disease; IVP, intravenous pyelogram; and RG, renogram.

Notice also that the row totals and column totals in Table 5–5 agree with the data in Table 5–3; for example, the probability of a positive IVP finding in patients with disease is 0.78.

We are in a position to apply Equation 5–1.

$P[\text{RVD} | \text{RG}^+, \text{IVP}^+]$

$$= \frac{P[\text{RG}^+, \text{IVP}^+ | \text{RVD}] \cdot P[\text{RVD}]}{P[\text{RG}^+, \text{IVP}^+ | \text{RVD}] \cdot P[\text{RVD}] + P[\text{RG}^+, \text{IVP}^+ | \overline{\text{RVD}}] \cdot P[\overline{\text{RVD}}]}$$

$$= \frac{(0.69)(0.1)}{(0.69)(0.1) + (0.08)(0.9)}$$

$$= 0.489.$$

The revised probability of disease is only 48.9 per cent in this situation compared with 87.0 per cent when conditional independence is assumed. Even more startling, perhaps, is that the revised probability of disease with a positive IVP result *alone* was 44.1 per cent and that the revised probability of disease with a positive RG result *alone* was 48.6 per cent. This analysis surely calls into question the value of using *both* tests.

An examination of Table 5–5 reveals where the assumption of conditional independence, which led us to an inordinately high estimate of a posterior probability of disease, is violated. First, we find that the probability of both RG^+ and IVP^+ among patients with the disease is 69.0 per cent compared with

$$P[RG^+|RVD] \cdot P[IVP^+|RVD] = (0.85)(0.78)$$

$$= 0.663,$$

or 66.3 per cent if we assume independence. This is not a large divergence and cannot be the source of our problem. The assumption of conditional independence *given disease* seems reasonable.

Our mistake must involve those patients *without* disease. The probability of both RG^+ and IVP^+ among patients without the disease is 8.0 per cent compared with

$$P[RG^+|\overline{RVD}] \cdot P[IVP^+|\overline{RVD}] = (0.10)(0.11)$$

$$= 0.011,$$

or 1.1 per cent if independence is assumed. This large difference indicates that the joint occurrence of false positives in both tests is far more common than we would suspect if the tests were conditionally independent. In fact, of the 10 per cent of patients without disease who have a false-positive result on the RG, eight of ten also have a false-positive IVP finding. Hence, if we knew that a patient without the disease had a false-positive result on the RG, the probability that the patient would also have a false-positive finding on the IVP would be 0.08/0.10, or 80 per cent. Clearly, false positives in these two tests tend to occur together and not independently.

Observations on the Assumption of Conditional Independence.　Except in extreme cases, data are rarely available on the joint characteristics of tests, and you may have to assume conditional independence as a first approximation. But beware of the obvious exceptions.

The most extreme case, of course, occurs when the tests are redundant; that is, they provide exactly the same information. In such a case one test result is positive only when the other is positive and vice versa. Then either test alone contains all the information of both combined, and to assume independence would be very misleading. In a less extreme situation, one test result is positive only if the other is positive, but the opposite is not true. Or the tests may give identical results only if the disease is absent. In all of these instances, interpreting the test results as if the tests were conditionally independent can lead to serious errors, as we have seen in the example of the IVP and the RG.

Probability Revision in a Prescreened Population.　Another very common source of error should be avoided. Suppose that in the example in this section our population had been prescreened to determine those patients with a positive IVP result. Hence, we might revise our prior probability of disease *for this selected population* using Bayes' formula. We have calculated this revised probability, $P[\text{RVD}|\text{IVP}^+]$, as 0.441. It would then be correct to use 0.441 as our new prior probability for this population. However, if we perform a renogram and get a positive result, what is the new posterior probability of disease? We might be tempted to repeat Bayes' formula as follows:

$$P^*[\text{RVD}|\text{RG}^+] = \frac{P[\text{RG}^+|\text{RVD}] \cdot P^*[\text{RVD}]}{P[\text{RG}^+|\text{RVD}] \cdot P^*[\text{RVD}] + P[\text{RG}^+|\overline{\text{RVD}}] \cdot P^*[\overline{\text{RVD}}]}, \quad (5\text{--}4)$$

where the asterisks indicate that these probabilities apply to the prescreened population with IVP^+. Thus, using the individual characteristics of the RG (Table 5–3), we calculate

$$P^*[\text{RVD}|\text{RG}^+] = \frac{(0.85)\,(0.441)}{(0.85)\,(0.441) + (0.10)\,(0.559)}$$

$$= 0.870.$$

But we know that $P^*[\text{RVD}|\text{RG}^+]$ is simply the probability of disease among patients with a positive IVP finding first and then a positive RG result. Since the order of the tests does not matter, it must be that

$$P^*[\text{RVD}|\text{RG}^+] = P[\text{RVD}|\text{RG}^+, \text{IVP}^+],$$

which we computed earlier to be 0.489. So, we have made a mistake. The mistake is that in using the individual characteristics of the renogram to revise the "post-IVP" probability of disease we have implicitly assumed the IVP and the RG to be conditionally independent. In fact, we can use Table 5–5 to show that

$$P[\text{RG}^+|\text{IVP}^+, \text{RVD}] \neq P[\text{RG}^+|\text{RVD}],$$

and the expression on the left-hand side of the inequality, not on the right-hand side, should have been used in Equation 5–4. From Table 5–5 we compute

$$P[\text{RG}^+|\text{IVP}^+, \text{RVD}] = \frac{0.69}{0.78}$$

$$= 0.884,$$

and

$$P[\text{RG}^+|\text{IVP}^+, \overline{\text{RVD}}] = \frac{0.08}{0.11}$$

$$= 0.727.$$

We might call these the *conditional* (upon IVP^+) true-positive and false-positive rates for the RG. Now, the correct form of Equation 5–4 is given by

$$P[\text{RVD}|\text{RG}^+, \text{IVP}^+] = \frac{P[\text{RG}^+|\text{IVP}^+, \text{RVD}] \cdot P[\text{RVD}|\text{IVP}^+]}{P[\text{RG}^+|\text{IVP}^+, \text{RVD}] \cdot P[\text{RVD}|\text{IVP}^+] + P[\text{RG}^+|\text{IVP}^+, \overline{\text{RVD}}] \cdot P[\overline{\text{RVD}}|\text{IVP}^+]},$$

which is simply Bayes' formula with *everything* conditional upon IVP$^+$. When we substitute the correct probabilities, we find that

$$P[\text{RVD} \mid \text{RG}^+, \text{IVP}^+] = \frac{(0.884)\,(0.441)}{(0.884)\,(0.441) + (0.727)\,(0.559)}$$

$$= 0.489.$$

This result agrees with our earlier result (p. 155), as it must.

The lesson is this: In using a test to revise a probability in a selected population, be sure that you use the characteristics of that test (i.e., the sensitivity and the specificity) conditional upon its use in that selected population and not the characteristics conditional upon its use in the general population. Unless the test is conditionally independent of the screening procedure, the two will give different answers, and only one is correct.

FALSE POSITIVES AND TEST PANELS: THE HAZARDS OF MULTIPLE TESTING

Having developed the analytic techniques required to revise probabilities based on multiple test results, we turn our attention briefly to a common problem of inference in the clinical setting.

Physicians increasingly order panels of tests — 12, 20, or more. Suppose that each of 12 tests in a panel has a false-positive rate of 5 per cent. In other words, the probability that each test result will appear abnormal when, in fact, the patient does not have any disease is 5 per cent. Moreover, suppose that these 12 tests are conditionally independent in patients without disease. What is the probability that at least one of the 12 results will be abnormal in a perfectly healthy patient?

The answer follows from the definition of conditional independence. Denoting the tests by $T_1, T_2, \ldots, T_{12}$, we can compute the probability that all 12 test results will be negative, or normal, in healthy patients:

$$P[T_1^-, T_2^-, \ldots, T_{12}^- \mid \overline{D}] = P[T_1^- \mid \overline{D}] \cdot P[T_2^- \mid \overline{D}] \cdot \ldots \cdot P[T_{12}^- \mid \overline{D}]$$

$$= (0.95)^{12}$$

$$= 0.54.$$

Hence, in a healthy patient there is a 54 per cent chance that all of the test results will be normal. This leaves a probability of 46 per cent that *at least one* test result will be abnormal. This is a sobering thought. Of course, if the tests are not conditionally independent, the probability of a false-positive result would be less than 46 per cent.

In any case, the probability of a positive test result's being due to error increases as the number of tests increases. This fact should be kept in mind when the clinician draws inferences from the results of a large panel of tests.

ERRORS IN THE USE OF MULTIPLE TESTS: CONSERVATISM, LIBERALISM, AND EXCESSIVE DATA COLLECTION

The value of Bayes' formula lies in its ability to improve upon the inferences reached by intuitive thinking. Studies of human decision making suggest that unaided decision makers generally do not combine test information appropriately.[237,260]

When data are processed in a block or when prior probabilities are in the middle range (from 0.3 to 0.7), the most common error is *underestimating* the collective impact of data. When people use intuition alone, they often state probabilities of 0.7 or 0.8; when they use Bayes' theorem to combine the individual probabilities, they arrive at a "correct" posterior probability well above 0.9. Underestimating revised probabilities occurs particularly when the components of the test information are conditionally independent. We might label this tendency *conservatism* in probability revision.

On the other hand, when data are processed in sequence or when prior probabilities are very low (as in the battered child example of Chapter Four), there is a tendency to overpredict, that is, to be more certain than is warranted. Apparently each test result is treated as nearly perfect, independent information. We might call this countervailing tendency *liberalism* in probability revision.

The limitations of physicians as information processors may lead to the collection of redundant data. When clinical tests are not independent, additional tests may provide little additional information. The clinical decision could be made just as well by a formula (e.g., Bayes') that used fewer variables but weighted them properly. For example, one study of the use of a battery of 12 laboratory tests showed that most of the meaningful information could be extracted by a formula for weighting and combining the results of just four of these tests.[280] A lack of conditional independence among the tests accounted for the redundance. Similarly, another study showed that a very satisfactory formula for predicting high-risk pregnancy eliminated the necessity for much of the information obtained by a questionnaire.[182]

A clinician often prefers to seek direct evidence of what could be logically deduced from the data already gathered, and this leads to the collection of more data than would be needed by a more efficient information processing technique. Formal analysis using Bayes' formula may help in this regard.

Moreover, excessive data collection may actually impede the process of clinical inference because the sheer volume of facts can impair the clinician's ability to sort out and focus upon the relevant variables. Decision analysis, or even simply drawing a decision tree, can help to focus attention on the information that is truly relevant to the decision at hand.

From the clinician's viewpoint, however, there may be a number of rationales for repeating a test. We turn to this matter in the next section.

5.4 THE VALUE OF REPEATED TESTS

Having developed the concepts of precision (Section 5.2) and conditional independence (Section 5.3), we are now in a position to use the methods of decision analysis to draw some conclusions about the repetition of tests. We observed in the preceding section that physicians tend to repeat tests more than is optimal. Here, we consider the value of repeated tests.

Sometimes a physician repeats a test in order to observe a change in the value of some clinical variable over time. The measurement of serum levels of cardiac enzymes (SGOT, LDH, CPK) at intervals following hospital admission for suspected myocardial infarction is done for this reason; the changes in these enzyme levels during the period following myocardial infarction are as much a part of the diagnostic data base as the enzyme levels themselves. A physician may also repeat a test to monitor a patient's response to treatment over time. We will not address ourselves to tests that are repeated in order to establish a time-dependent trend in a clinical variable.

A physician sometimes repeats a test because the levels of the variable being measured fluctuate over time and the physician is interested in the long-term level of the variable. Blood pressure measurements are repeated, in part, for this reason. Because a person's blood pressure fluctuates during the course of the day, a physician will often take several measurements at different points in time in order to obtain a valid indication of the central tendency of the blood pressure. This, too, is generally an appropriate reason for repeating a test. Although it is not our primary concern, we will later discuss one caveat in the interpretation of repeated tests of this kind, regression toward the mean (p. 162).

A third reason that a physician may order a test to be repeated is that it may be unreliable, or imprecise. If a measurement is subject to random errors from test to test, the effects of this imprecision can often be mitigated by repetition of the test. If the problem is inaccuracy and not imprecision, repetition will not add information.

How, then, should the physician revise probabilities of disease given the results of repeated measurements? This is the subject of the following section.

PROBABILITY REVISION USING REPEATED TESTS

We introduce this topic, as we have introduced other topics, with a clinical example.

Occult Blood and the Diagnosis of Colon Cancer

One approach to screening for asymptomatic cancer of the colon is the detection of occult blood in the stool. It has been estimated that the true-positive rate for such a test is 91.7 per cent and that the false-positive rate is 36.5 per cent.[180]

The director of a clinic is interested in missing as few cases of colon cancer as possible and estimates that the prevalence of undiagnosed colon cancer in the population under study is 0.5 per cent. Seeking to achieve a high predictive value negative, the director proposes that patients be screened three times using three sequential stool tests. What is the predictive value negative of this sequence of tests, assuming that a result is to be called positive if any of the three test results is positive?

First, consider the predictive value negative of a single test. It is given by

$$P[\overline{D}|T^-] = \frac{P[T^-|\overline{D}] \cdot P[\overline{D}]}{P[T^-|\overline{D}] \cdot P[\overline{D}] + P[T^-|D] \cdot P[D]}$$

$$= \frac{(0.635)(0.995)}{(0.635)(0.995) + (0.083)(0.005)}$$

$$= 0.99934.$$

Fewer than one patient among 1,000 patients with negative results would actually have cancer because

$$P[D \mid T^-] = 1 - P[\overline{D} \mid T^-]$$

$$= 1 - 0.99934$$

$$= 0.00066.$$

Next, consider the predictive value negative of *three* sequential tests. Let us assume — and this is a big assumption — that the errors in the test are due not to its lack of discrimination or accuracy but to its lack of reliability. Suppose that each time the test is run on a patient with cancer, there is an 8.3 per cent chance of an error, but the errors occur *independently* from one test to the next. In terms of the concepts of this chapter, we assume that the second and third stool tests are conditionally independent of the first.

Assuming conditional independence of the three repeated tests, the reduction in the false-negative rate (8.3 per cent on a single test) is calculated as follows:

$$P[T^-, T^-, T^- \mid D] = P[T^- \mid D] \cdot P[T^- \mid D] \cdot P[T^- \mid D]$$

$$= (0.083)(0.083)(0.083)$$

$$= 0.00057.$$

The true-negative rate is also reduced from 63.5 per cent to the following:

$$P[T^-, T^-, T^- \mid \overline{D}] = P[T^- \mid \overline{D}] \cdot P[T^- \mid \overline{D}] \cdot P[T^- \mid \overline{D}]$$

$$= (0.635)(0.635)(0.635)$$

$$= 0.256.$$

The predictive value negative for the three tests is therefore equal to

$$P[\overline{D} \mid T^-, T^-, T^-] = \frac{P[T^-, T^-, T^- \mid \overline{D}] \cdot P[\overline{D}]}{P[T^-, T^-, T^- \mid \overline{D}] \cdot P[\overline{D}] + P[T^-, T^-, T^- \mid D] \cdot P[D]}$$

$$= \frac{(0.256)(0.995)}{(0.256)(0.995) + (0.00057)(0.005)}$$

$$= 0.99999,$$

so that a patient with a negative test result has only a one in 100,000 chance of having cancer. If it is important to detect colon cancer, it appears that repeating the test three times may be of value; the predictive value negative is improved from 0.99934 to 0.99999. (Again, we are not considering at this time the economic implications of any test strategy.)

Now suppose instead that we were dealing with a test whose errors are due not to a lack of reliability but to a lack of accuracy in some patients with cancer. In the extreme, suppose that this new test gives the same result each time; it simply fails to diagnose 8.3 per cent of cases of cancer. For this test, the results of successive repetitions are *not* conditionally independent; instead,

$$P[T^-, T^-, T^- \mid D] = P[T^- \mid D].$$

Hence, the predictive value negative for three tests would be no higher than that for a single test.

Conditions Under Which Repeating a Test May Be of Value

To the extent that test results are imprecise, sequential results show conditional independence. When the probability of disease is revised according to Bayes' formula, both the predictive value positive and the predictive value negative will improve relative to a single test. It is important to realize, however, that the incremental improvement in the expected value of clinical information tends to drop off rapidly with additional test replications, so that it is seldom worthwhile to incorporate more than a few repetitions.

If the errors in a test are due in large part to a lack of accuracy, the improvements in predictive value are more modest. This is because the assumption of conditional independence among repeated tests no longer applies. In the section dealing with the revision of probabilities when tests are conditionally independent (p. 154), we saw that the predictive value is always greatest when multiple tests are conditionally independent; here we point out that this conclusion applies to repetitions of the same test as well as to different tests.

REGRESSION TOWARD THE MEAN

On many occasions a physician must interpret several successive measurements of a clinical variable in a patient. Often the patients selected for repeated measurements are those whose first measurement was abnormally high. When patients are selected for repeated testing on the basis of early measurements and when test-retest variations are due either to a lack of reliability or to random fluctuations in the actual clinical variable, the stage is set for a phenomenon of which all physicians should be aware but which is counterintuitive to many. It is called **regression toward the mean.** We illustrate this phenomenon with an example.

Suppose that the probabilities of the diastolic blood pressures in a population are distributed as shown in Table 5–6. For any given measurement, however, the observed blood pressure may deviate from this value because of actual fluctuations or measurement error. Suppose that there is a 0.2 chance that the measured value will be "low" by one interval of 5 mm Hg, a 0.2 chance that the measured value will be "high" by one interval, and a 0.6 chance that the measured value will be on target.

An initial measurement is taken, and the physician decides to retest patients whose initial readings were 85 mm Hg or above. For what proportion of those patients do you think the second reading will be higher than, be lower than, or be within the original interval? The answer may be surprising, so let us work it out.

Consider a patient whose first measured blood pressure is between 95 and 99 mm Hg. The probability of this occurring in a patient whose true blood pressure is between 95 and 99 mm Hg is (0.6) (0.07); the probability of this occurring as a "high" reading in a patient whose true blood pressure is between 90 and 94 mm Hg is (0.2) (0.09); and the probability of this occurring as a "low" reading in a patient whose true blood pressure is between 100 and 104 mm Hg is (0.2) (0.03). Hence, the overall probability of a first reading between 95 and 99 mm Hg is

$$(0.2) (0.09) + (0.6) (0.07) + (0.2) (0.03) = 0.066.$$

TABLE 5–6 PROBABILITY DISTRIBUTION OF DIASTOLIC BLOOD
PRESSURES (mm Hg) FOR A HYPOTHETICAL POPULATION

DIASTOLIC BLOOD PRESSURE (mm Hg)	PROBABILITY
< 60	0.02
60–64	0.04
65–69	0.09
70–74	0.16
75–79	0.20
80–84	0.16
85–89	0.12
90–94	0.09
95–99	0.07
100–104	0.03
⩾ 105	0.02
Total	1.00

Therefore, given a first reading between 95 and 99 mm Hg, the revised probability that this patient has a true blood pressure between 90 and 94 mm Hg is

$$\frac{(0.2)\,(0.09)}{0.066} = 0.273;$$

the revised probability that the true blood pressure is between 95 and 99 mm Hg is

$$\frac{(0.6)\,(0.07)}{0.066} = 0.636;$$

and the revised probability that the true blood pressure is between 100 and 104 mm Hg is

$$\frac{(0.2)\,(0.03)}{0.066} = 0.091.$$

These revised probabilities for the true blood pressure given a first reading between 95 and 99 mm Hg are shown in Table 5–7. Now, the second reading can be from 85 to 89 mm Hg, from 90 to 94 mm Hg, from 95 to 99 mm Hg, from 100 to 104 mm Hg, or greater than or equal to 105 mm Hg, depending on the true blood pressure. For example, the probability that the second reading is between 95 and 99 mm Hg is equal to

$$(0.2)\,(0.273) + (0.6)\,(0.636) + (0.2)\,(0.091) = 0.454.$$

The probabilities of each possible second reading given a first reading between 95 and 99 mm Hg are shown in the last column of Table 5–7. We observe that the probability of a second reading that is *higher* than the initial reading is 20.0 per cent (0.182 + 0.018), of a second reading that is *equal* to the initial

TABLE 5–7 REVISED PROBABILITY DISTRIBUTIONS OF BLOOD
PRESSURE GIVEN AN INITIAL READING BETWEEN
95 AND 99 mm Hg AND A "TRUE" DISTRIBUTION
GIVEN IN TABLE 5–6

DIASTOLIC BLOOD PRESSURE (mm Hg)	REVISED PROBABILITY OF TRUE BLOOD PRESSURE	PROBABILITY OF SECOND READING
< 85	0	0
85–89	0	0.055
90–94	0.273	0.291
95–99	0.636	0.454
100–104	0.091	0.182
⩾ 105	0	0.018
Total	1.000	1.000

reading is 45.4 per cent, and of a second reading that is *lower* than the initial reading is 34.6 per cent (0.055 + 0.291). The second reading is more likely to be below than it is to be above the first, although it may seem that there should be an equal probability of the measurement rising or falling.

Repeated measurements that are subject to imprecision tend generally to move toward the middle of the distribution. Hence, if we select patients for repeated measurements on the basis of high initial readings, we would expect to observe a downward shift in the measured values. If we select patients on the basis of low initial readings, we would anticipate an upward shift in the measured values. This phenomenon is generally known as **regression toward the mean.**

We observed regression toward the mean in our blood pressure example. The downward trend in blood pressures at successive readings was not due to a downward trend in true blood pressures (these were assumed to be constant) nor to a downward bias in measurement (there was assumed to be no bias). The observed trend is explained entirely by a phenomenon associated with random variations in measured values: regression toward the mean. In interpreting the results of successive tests, we should keep in mind the possibility of regression toward the mean before we infer that a real trend in the clinical variable has been observed.

5.5 SUMMARY OF CHAPTER FIVE

Clinical tests rarely determine the presence or absence of disease without error. The source of error may be natural variation in the test variable among patients with and without disease, or it may be measurement error in the test. The ability of a test to separate patients with different conditions may be referred to as its **discrimination**; the greater the overlap between the distributions of the separator variable under different disease states, the poorer is the discrimination. Measurement error introduces still more uncertainty into the interpretation of test results. **Precision**, or test-retest **reliability**, refers to the ability of a test to achieve consistent measurements without random variations. **Accuracy** refers to the tendency of a test measurement to approximate the true value, irrespective of random variation around that value.

The process of probability revision extends to tests that are subject to measurement error, and probability tree inversion is often the most straightforward method.

The **expected value of clinical information (EVCI)** is the difference between the health outcome with a test and the outcome without the test. It can be estimated by averaging out and folding back a decision tree to the decision point at which the options are to test and not to test. Measurement error in the results of an imperfect test lowers its EVCI. Diagnostic tests that provide imperfect information have positive value whenever (1) the information can result in a change in some probabilities and (2) the change in probabilities can produce a change in the preferred subsequent treatment. To be worthwhile, a diagnostic test must have a positive *net* expected value, that is, a positive value after any risk of the test itself has been accounted for.

The value of multiple tests is greatest when test results are **conditionally independent**; under that circumstance the process of probability revision is simplified. When tests are not conditionally independent, their aggregate value is less than might be anticipated, and probability revision requires assessments of the conditional probabilities of each *combination* of test results given each disease state. When using a test result to revise probabilities for a patient who has been prescreened by a previous test, one should use probabilities of test results that are conditional upon the result of the previous test. The assumption of conditional independence for tests and the use of liberalism and conservatism in revising probabilities using multiple tests are among the factors that lead to excessive testing.

Repeated tests have their greatest value when errors in measurement are conditionally independent from test to test. For a test that is imprecise but reasonably accurate, repeated measurements are likely to be of value. For a test that is precise, repetition is of value only if the clinician is interested in observing a real change in a clinical variable that would lead to a different treatment decision. When interpreting measurements with successive tests, the clinician should be aware that **regression toward the mean** increases the likelihood of drift toward the "normal" range.

EXERCISES FOR CHAPTER FIVE

EXERCISES FOR SECTION 5.2

1. *Liver Biopsy Revisited*
   We previously modified the problem of doing a liver biopsy to determine hepatitis by assuming a prior probability of hepatitis equal to 0.6. The test is 90 per cent sensitive for hepatitis and 95 per cent specific. Verify that the revised probabilities of hepatitis and cirrhosis given the biopsy result are those shown in Figure 5–10.

2. *Open-Lung Biopsy for Pneumocystis Revisited*
   Recall the problem regarding the decision whether to do an open-lung biopsy to determine the presence of *Pneumocystis* (Chapter Three, Exercise 6). Assume that all the data are the same as before, but in this case the biopsy does not yield perfect information.

a. Assume that the open-lung biopsy is 100 per cent sensitive but only 90 per cent specific for *Pneumocystis*. What is the expected value of clinical information for the biopsy?

b. What is the maximum mortality attributable to the lung biopsy that would still make the biopsy preferable to no biopsy?

c. Suppose instead that the lung biopsy were only 80 per cent sensitive and 90 per cent specific for *Pneumocystis*. What would its EVCI be?

EXERCISES FOR SECTION 5.3

3. *Two Diagnostic Tests*

There are two diagnostic tests for disease X with the following characteristics: 80 per cent of people with disease X have a positive result on test A; 70 per cent of people with disease X have a positive result on test B; 10 per cent of people without disease X have a positive result on test A; and 10 per cent of people without disease X have a positive result on test B. Both test results are positive in a patient selected from a population in which the prevalence of disease X is 1 per cent.

a. What is the probability that this patient has disease X if the tests are conditionally independent given the presence or absence of disease?

b. Suppose the tests are not necessarily conditionally independent. What is the minimum probability that this patient has disease X?

4. *Two More Diagnostic Tests*

There is a disease, D, for the diagnosis of which two tests, T_1 and T_2, may be used. The positivity criterion for each has been established, and individuals from a study population are separated according to disease status into a 2×2 table, with the probabilities for each test result shown in Table 5–8. The prevalence of disease D in the general population is 10 per cent.

TABLE 5–8 PROBABILITIES OF RESULTS OF TESTS T_1 AND T_2 IN THE
DIAGNOSIS OF DISEASE D*

TEST RESULT	DISEASE STATUS	
	D	$\bar{D}$
T_1^+	0.3	0.1
T_1^-	0.7	0.9
T_2^+	0.4	0.05
T_2^-	0.6	0.95

*D indicates the presence of disease, and $\bar{D}$, the absence of disease.

a. Calculate the revised probability of disease given a positive result on test T_1.

b. Calculate the revised probability of disease given a positive result on test T_2.

c. Calculate the revised probability of disease, assuming conditional independence given the presence or absence of disease, for the following:
   i. Positive results on tests T_1 and T_2.
   ii. A positive result on test T_1 and a negative result on test T_2.
   iii. A positive result on test T_2 and a negative result on test T_1.
   iv. Negative results on tests T_1 and T_2.

d. Actually, tests T_1 and T_2 are not conditionally independent. In fact, if the result of T_1 is positive, it guarantees that T_2 is positive given the presence of disease, D. The joint characteristics of the tests are shown in Table 5–9.

TABLE 5–9 JOINT PROBABILITIES OF RESULTS OF TESTS T_1 AND T_2
IN THE DIAGNOSIS OF DISEASE D*

TEST RESULTS	D			$\bar{D}$		
	T_1^+	T_1^-	Row Totals	T_1^+	T_1^-	Row Totals
T_2^+	0.3	0.1	0.4	0.005	0.045	0.05
T_2^-	0.0	0.6	0.6	0.095	0.855	0.95
Column totals	0.3	0.7	1.0	0.1	0.9	1.0

*D indicates the presence of disease, and $\bar{D}$, the absence of disease.

What is the probability of disease given
  i.   Positive results on tests T_1 and T_2?
  ii. A positive result on test T_1 and a negative result on test T_2?
  iii. A positive result on test T_2 and a negative result on test T_1?
  iv   Negative results on tests T_1 and T_2?
e. Compare your answers in parts c and d.

Chapter Six

Sources of Probabilities

6.1 SOURCES OF PROBABILITY ASSESSMENTS

Informed clinical decisions depend on probability assessments, such as the prior probability that a patient has a disease, the probability that a treatment will alleviate symptoms, and the probability that a patient will die without treatment. The physician facing such a decision often lacks the information needed for a confident assessment of probabilities. Decision analysis, by structuring a decision problem, makes these gaps in knowledge apparent, but this same information is lacking in less systematic clinical decision making as well. Once the probabilities that require assessment have been identified, the physician must face the task of quantifying them on the probability scale.

Sometimes, objective estimates of probabilities may be derived from the medical literature or from some other data base, such as medical records. These would produce probability estimates based on observed frequencies in a population. Other times, however, such data are not available, and the physician who wishes to quantify the relevant probabilities must rely upon personal experience and judgment. The concept of a probability, then, is no longer simply an observable frequency in a population; it becomes a measure of the decision maker's strength of belief that a particular state of the world is occurring or will occur.

The process of quantifying one's strength of belief in the occurrence of an event, which we call **subjective probability assessment,** is discomforting because the physician is not usually forced to be so explicit about such judgments. The thoughtful physician will recognize, however, that such judgments must, *with or without decision analysis,* underlie any clinical decision. Another type of judgment — the assignment of values to possible clinical outcomes — is the other area in which decision analysis forces sometimes uncomfortable explicitness, and this is the subject of the next chapter.

We begin with a brief discussion of probability assessments derived from the medical literature before turning to the main topic of this chapter, subjective probability assessment. Then we discuss the relation between subjective probabilities and sensitivity analysis and conclude with a brief exposition of methods for combining objective and subjective information.

6.2 PROBABILITY ESTIMATES FROM THE LITERATURE

Sometimes, but not as often as one would like, the probability one is looking for can be inferred from a study that someone else has done or from a series of cases that someone has reported in the literature or recorded in a data bank. This is generally considered the most satisfactory way of assessing a probability, because it involves the use of quantitative evidence.

The estimation may be straightforward. Suppose that we want to know the probability that a particular surgical procedure will result in perioperative death. A report in the literature states that of a series of 1,000 patients who underwent the operation, 23 died in surgery. Thus, an obvious estimate of P[Death] is 23/1,000, or 0.023. This is the proportion of patients who died in this particular sample of 1,000 patients. The larger the sample, the more confident we can be that the observed frequency in the sample is a good estimate of the actual probability in the general population.*

Now there are several caveats in translating a study result into a probability estimate for use in your particular decision problem.

First, the treatments (or diagnostic procedures) may not be entirely comparable to yours. Different personnel, equipment, facilities, or variations in the actual procedure may result in different probabilities. For example, while a study may be based on the experiences with a new surgical procedure, the performance of surgeons may have improved considerably since that time.

Second, the study population may be different in some important respects from your patient. Those patients in the study population may have been older or younger, or in better or worse health. They may have volunteered or have been specially selected for the treatment in question. A randomized study would help to eliminate this latter problem, but not completely: Someone with the characteristics of your patient might have been excluded from the study altogether.

An implication of these caveats is that a probability should not necessarily be adopted from a study or data set just because it is available. A modified assessment for your patient, based in part on your experiences, your knowledge of the patient, and the judgments of experts, may reflect more adequately your feelings about the particular probability for this patient. Let us consider next the meaning — and limitations — of personal, or subjective, probabilities.

---

*Statisticians have developed "theories of estimation" that provide a means of quantifying the degree of confidence one can place in estimates derived from such samples. Discussion of the statistical estimation of an unknown proportion may be found in any good introductory text on statistics. See, for example, Mosteller, Rourke, and Thomas, Chapter Eight.[175]

6.3   SUBJECTIVE PROBABILITY

In Chapter Three we defined *probability* as the frequency of an event in a population. Sometimes, however, it is not possible to assess such a frequency from "hard" data. Even if we are comfortable in assuming that the patient at hand is representative of some well-defined population, we may not have available any data on what proportion of individuals in that population have experienced the event of interest. The procedure in question, for example, may be too new for any reliable studies to have been published. Moreover, it can be argued that each patient and each circumstance is unique. Therefore, while data on other patients might help us to assess each individual situation, a physician must often rely on personal judgment. A probability based on a judgment as to one's strength of belief that an event will occur is called a **subjective probability** (or **personal probability** or **judgmental probability**). We measure such a degree of belief by analogy to known, frequency-based events, but we do not restrict the use of the word "probability" to events for which true, underlying frequencies exist.

A DEFINITION OF SUBJECTIVE PROBABILITY

Leaving the medical world temporarily, suppose that you are asked to estimate the probability that the next president of the United States will be a Republican. One approach might be to look at the record over the past century; if 13 of the last 25 elections had been won by Republicans, you might estimate the probability as 13/25, or 0.52. But this might be viewed as a poor estimate, because times have changed. An alternative approach would be to marshal all the information at your disposal to answer subjectively questions of the following kind:

"Do you think it more or less likely that a Republican will be elected than that a flip of a coin whose sides are equally weighted will come up heads?"

An answer of "more likely" indicates that

$$P^*[\text{Republican}] > 0.5,$$

where the asterisk reminds us that this is a subjective probability. (Once we are accustomed to the notion of subjective probability, we will do away with the asterisk.) An answer of "less likely" means that

$$P^*[\text{Republican}] < 0.5.$$

Suppose that your subjective answer is "less likely," so that P^* is less than 0.5. Then you might proceed by answering the following question:

"Do you think it more or less likely that a Republican will be elected than that the roll of a six-sided die will come up with one or two dots?"

An answer of "more likely" narrows the range further. Now

$$1/3 < P^*[\text{Republican}] < 1/2.$$

We could continue to narrow the range by analogy to "known" probabilities until we settle on a point estimate.

This process will lead to a probability assessment between 0 and 1, as long as the probability assessor is careful to be consistent with the principle of *transitivity*; that is, if event A is thought to be more likely to occur than event B and event B is thought to be more likely to occur than event C, then event A is thought to be more likely to occur than event C. This procedure of probability assessment can be used, for our purposes, as a definition of subjective probability.

Definition. Suppose that a person believes that an event E is just as likely to occur as another event whose probability of occurrence is defined objectively as p^*. Then p^* is this person's **subjective probability** that event E will occur.

In many clinical decision problems, it is not important to reduce the assessment to a point estimate; a range of probability (e.g., $0.3 < p < 0.4$) will suffice. This observation suggests a close relation between sensitivity analysis (or threshold analysis) and subjective probability. We shall return to this relation in Section 6.4.

WHY USE SUBJECTIVE PROBABILITIES IN CLINICAL DECISION ANALYSIS?

When the probabilities used in a clinical decision analysis are based on objective evidence, the clinician may have confidence in using such an analysis to help guide decision making. In effect, the decision analysis provides a structure for the information the clinician wants to take into account in reaching a decision. The analysis incorporates this information and the structural assumptions in a systematic fashion so that conclusions may be drawn.

When all of the required probabilities are not available from objective data, however, and subjective probabilities are used, the decision analysis continues to produce a quantitative conclusion that one strategy is better than another. By the nature of the method, however, the conclusion drawn is no more than a synthesis of the information that enters into the analysis. Therefore, if the probabilities are based on incomplete evidence or unsubstantiated personal judgment, then why bother with a formal analysis? This is a serious question and one that requires a serious answer, because most probabilities that are needed for clinical decision analyses are not available from the medical literature. Here we offer a brief response to this question; we return to this issue in Chapter Ten in the context of arguments for and against decision analysis with subjective probabilities.

First and most important is the observation that clinical decisions must be made with or without decision analysis. Consider the following scenario.

Suppose that you structure a clinical decision analysis for a problem you face but find that one key probability cannot be estimated objectively. You agonize over this situation, but in the end you are unwilling to base your decision on an analysis into which is built a "best guess" at this unknown probability. Since you have to make a decision, you do so based on your best intuitive judgment. In effect, you are discarding the entire analysis because of one weak link, this unknown probability. Now, suppose that you were to use decision analysis, but instead of inserting your "guess" for the unknown probability, you perform a threshold analysis that will indicate over what range of this probability the decision you actually chose would be optimal. You find that the decision you chose would be optimal only if this probability is greater than 0.9. Therefore, in effect, your decision is consistent with an implicit belief that this probability is greater than 0.9. Whatever your beliefs about this unknown probability, you have acted *as if* the probability were greater than 0.9. If, in fact, you are quite confident that the probability, while unknown, is less than 0.5, you have acted inconsistently. Would it not have been better to make a subjective assessment of the probability, if only so that you could take advantage of the rest of the analysis? Then, when you find the result, you can always go back and do a sensitivity analysis with respect to that probability.

The point here is that decisions must be made and are implicitly based on judgments about probabilities of uncertain events. Why not be as explicit as possible about your strength of belief if you are going to act implicitly on that strength of belief in any case?

A related point is that sensitivity analysis and threshold analysis are always available as ways of improving your confidence in the conclusions of a clinical decision analysis. We will return to the role of sensitivity analysis in the context of subjective probabilities shortly.

An important advantage of pursuing the analysis, even with subjective probabilities, is that it permits a more focused discussion of a clinical problem among physicians. We believe that clinical discussions are much more productive when the source of the disagreement over a treatment decision can be isolated than when the discussion ranges unsystematically from issues of treatment efficacy to issues of valued outcomes to issues of treatment options. It is helpful to be able to focus on a subjective probability (or, as we shall see in the next chapter, a utility value) as the source of dispute. The evidence pertaining to this probability can then be marshaled and, if a consensus cannot be reached, at least the parties to the discussion may be able to agree as to the reasons for their disagreement.

Finally, subjective probabilities, as we have defined them, obey all of the laws of objective probabilities, such as the summation principle.[204] The numbers are, therefore, logically and mathematically equivalent to objective probabilities, and one can be unhesitatingly substituted for the other in Bayes' formula.

PROBABILISTICALLY DISTRIBUTED PROBABILITIES

You might be wondering why subjective probabilities should be expressed as point estimates if, in fact, the decision maker feels uncertainty about the probability. Some readers, especially those who have been exposed to statistics, may feel that what is needed is some notion akin to "confidence intervals" surrounding the unknown probability. Suppose that some probability is subjective: It is not known with certainty, as is a frequency-based probability, such as a coin toss. For example, suppose that your best assessment is that p^* equals 0.3, but it could be 0.2, or 0.4, or even 0.0 or 1.0. You just do not know. Can and should this vagueness about the probability be taken into account?

To clarify our thinking about this, let us consider a slightly more structured analogy. Suppose that we are estimating the probability that a coin toss comes up heads. We are told that the coin will be drawn at random from a box containing nine coins, each of which is weighted with a different probability of coming up heads. In particular, suppose that the first coin comes up heads 10 per cent of the time, the second coin comes up heads 20 per cent of the time, and so on up to the ninth coin, which comes up heads 90 per cent of the time. Thus, the probability of heads *might be* 20 per cent, or 40 per cent, or 90 per cent.

The answer is unknown because we do not know in advance which coin will be drawn from the box. But, for all practical purposes, the probability of heads can be easily calculated. It is 10 per cent (with a probability of 1/9), 20 per cent (with a probability of 1/9), and so forth, up to 90 per cent (with a probability of 1/9). Therefore, the probability of heads can be calculated easily by averaging out the probability tree in Figure 6–1. It is equal to

$$(0.1)(1/9) + (0.2)(1/9) + (0.3)(1/9) + \ldots + (0.9)(1/9) = 0.5.$$

It simply does not matter from the viewpoint of the decision maker before the coin was chosen whether there were nine coins whose sides were equally weighted in the box or whether the box held the collection of weighted coins it actually did.

Figure 6–1 *Probability tree for tossing a coin with an unknown probability of showing heads.*

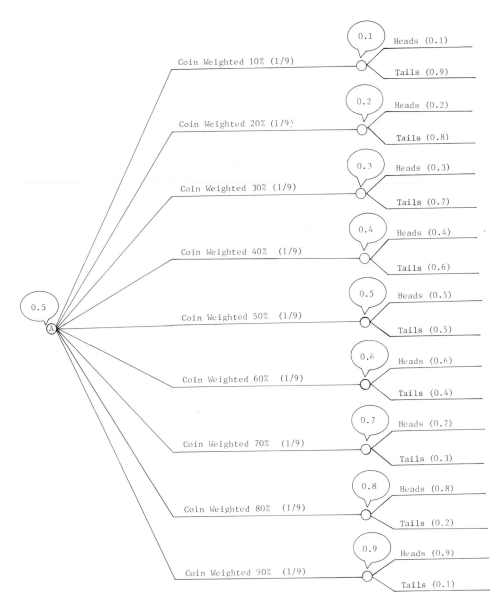

Now suppose we need to use such a probability estimate in a decision analysis. In particular, suppose we are comparing two treatment options. Treatment A gives the patient a "known" survival probability of 40 per cent. Treatment B gives the patient an "unknown" survival probability, where the uncertainty about the unknown probability is analogous to the previous coin example. Assume, somewhat fancifully, that the actual survival probability for treatment B will be determined by a lottery in which, with probabilities of 1/9 each, the treatment will lead to a survival rate of 10 per cent, 20 per cent, 30 per cent, 40 per cent, 50 per cent, 60 per cent, 70 per cent, 80 per cent, or 90 per cent.

In Figure 6–2 the probability assessment for treatment B is broken down into two steps. First, at chance node Ⓐ the likelihood that each survival probability will occur is revealed. Next, the outcome based on the corresponding probability is revealed. The expected chance of survival with treatment B, which is calculated by averaging out, is 0.5. But note that this is the same result we get by collapsing the two stages of probabilities to a single averaged-out probability, namely, the 0.5 we computed previously. The collapsed probability tree is shown at the bottom of Figure 6–2. The choice is treatment B, because a 50 per cent chance at survival is better than a 40 per cent chance at survival.

This finding may be generalized: If we are dealing with "probabilities of probabilities," then it is only the averaged-out, or expected, probability that matters at any given chance node. This means that the "spread" around a subjective probability assessment does not matter;* you can treat that probability as if it were a point estimate without affecting the decision at hand.

There is one important exception to the rule that the spread around a probability estimate does not matter. This arises when it is possible to apply new information to revise the probabilities that any probability will pertain. For example, suppose that you intend to administer treatment B to two successive patients whom you consider identical for the purpose of assessing a response to this treatment. You give treatment B to the first patient, and he dies. For the next patient, then, the probability that the survival rate is 90 per cent is reduced considerably; if the survival rate were 90 per cent, the first patient would most probably have lived. A method for calculating revised probabilities in this situation is given in Section 6.5. For now, remember that when the probability distribution associated with an unknown probability might change during the course of the decision process, it is important to keep track of the distribution around the unknown probability. This situation will infrequently arise for a decision involving an individual patient; for example, if the decision involved the application of an experimental treatment for a chronic condition, an initial treatment could give the physician information as to its efficacy in subsequent applications.

LIMITATIONS OF SUBJECTIVE PROBABILITY ASSESSMENT

There is a line of argument that states that decision analysis based on subjective probabilities should not be used because of limitations in the abilities of people to give valid probability assessments. The argument contends that the process of forcing explicit probability assessments can actually lead to distortions

---

*The translation from objective uncertainty about the true probability, as in our examples, to completely subjective probability is controversial because some theoreticians doubt the validity of averaging out probabilities.[206]

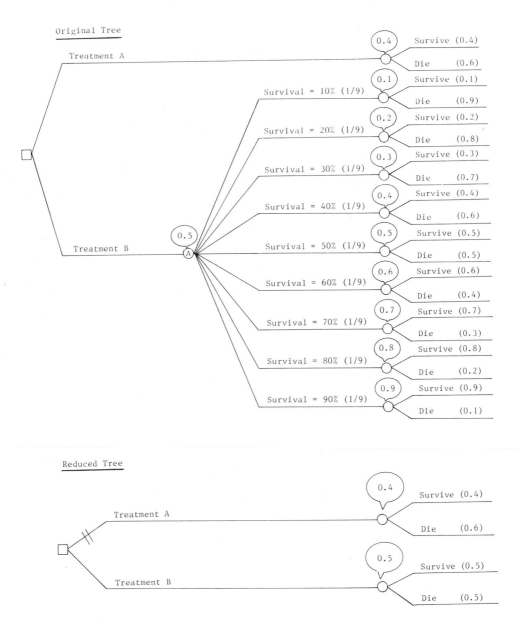

Figure 6–2 *Probabilities of survival following two treatments, one of which has uncertain efficacy.*

of the clinician's best judgments and that the clinician is better off relying on unaided decision making. We offer a rebuttal to this argument in Chapter Ten. There are, however, important limitations to subjective probability assessments. As we review these, we consider the psychological processes used to generate the numbers we call subjective probabilities, the degree of accuracy with which these quantities can be assessed, and the possibility that different means of estimating them make a difference in their accuracy. In the following section, we consider some techniques designed to improve a clinician's skill in probability assessment and to permit several clinicians to pool their opinions in a structured way.

Errors in Probability Assessment

Psychologists have found that subjective probabilities are often biased (i.e., inaccurate) when they are not assessed by direct reference to frequencies of observed events. Tversky and Kahneman[260] have identified three heuristic principles that are commonly employed to generate subjective probability estimates. These are *representativeness, availability,* and *anchoring.* Each may lead to biased judgments under conditions of uncertainty.

The principle of *representativeness* is employed when the probability assessment for an uncertain event is influenced by the degree to which the event is similar in essential properties to a larger class of events. For instance, people generally expect that a sequence of events generated by a random process should fully represent the essential characteristics of that process, even when the sequence is short. For example, in considering tosses of a coin for heads or tails, people expect {heads, tails, heads, tails, tails, heads} to be a more likely sequence than {heads, heads, heads, tails, tails, tails}, since the latter does not appear to be random. In fact, both sequences contain three heads and three tails and are equally likely if the coin is fair and the tosses are independent.

The mistaken belief in the so-called law of averages — that good outcomes are more likely after a string of bad outcomes, and vice versa — is another example of the representativeness principle. As another example, suppose that the clinical picture of a particular case resembles but does not exactly match the typical picture of two alternative diseases, one of which is more common than the other. Because the observed findings of the case fit both larger classes about equally well, many clinicians would judge both alternatives to be equally probable. In so doing, the different prevalences of the two alternatives have been ignored.

Availability is employed when the probability of an event is judged by the ease of recalling instances or occurrences of similar events. Recall can be affected by factors other than frequency and probability. In particular, the meaningfulness of an event can affect how well it is recalled. Thus, one might expect that observations that do not make sense or cannot be explained by theory tend to be forgotten, even though such observations should be committed to memory for purposes of estimating frequencies. More recent events ("I had a patient last week who...") are likely to be better remembered than more distant ones. But recall is also affected by what might be called exoticism: Commonplace events tend to be forgotten but unusual ones are remembered well. Every clinician can remember a case seen just once, with the result that the probability of this rare event is likely to be overstated. Finally, preoccupation with the consequences of a possible disaster may make it seem more likely. In medicine, the probability of a serious illness may be overestimated: A medical student concludes that the problem is cancer when the patient complains of a headache. Perhaps the probability of a malignancy is exaggerated because of the consequences of failing to properly diagnose a case.

In many situations in which a probability assessment is required, people start from an initial value and adjust from that point to derive the final answer. These adjustments are typically insufficient; this is the problem that characterizes the principle of *anchoring.* Conservatism in probability revision (see Sections 4.10 and 5.3) is one manifestation of anchoring. Another typical problem is that people tend to anchor their prior probabilities near the midpoint of 0.5, with the consequence that rare events tend to receive excessively high probability assessments. This tendency aggravates the errors in probability assessment associated with the principle of availability to give greater weight in one's memory to more exotic occurrences. On the other hand, others may tend to anchor near the extremes of 0 and 1. In this case, the physician would assign unduly low probabilities to rare events and be overconfident that the most likely possibility will occur.

Decision analysis relies on assessments of probability, and for most clinical problems these assessments will be subjective probabilities, since the relevant objective data are rarely available. Thus, in light of the preceding cognitive tendencies, the following question arises: How accurate are clinical subjective probabilities, and what difference do errors in these assessments make in the process of clinical decision making? We address this question next.

Accuracy of Clinical Subjective Probabilities

Research on the question of accuracy has yielded mixed results. When evaluating uncertainty, we tend to underestimate our ignorance and to believe that we know more than we do. In a word, we are usually overconfident. Training, however, might reduce this tendency somewhat by making us more aware of our ignorance.

A small number of studies deal with the problem of the validity of subjective probabilities in clinical medicine. One study asked physicians to combine *subjective* likelihood ratios with *objectively* derived prior odds to obtain posterior odds on three diagnostic possibilities.[98] There was little difference between the probabilities assigned to the correct diagnosis by this method and the probabilities derived from objective likelihood ratios and prior odds. Since both sets of assessments used the same initial frequency-based prior odds and differed only in using subjectively assessed or objectively derived likelihood ratios, this study provides some encouragement in the use of subjective probabilities.

Another study found that a computer, using objective probabilities of disease and frequencies of symptoms in alternative diseases, correctly diagnosed the cause of acute abdominal pain more often than clinicians did.[142] When the physicians' subjective assessments of symptom likelihoods were used instead of the observed frequencies, the computer performed no better than the physicians. In this study the clinicians' subjective assessments were wrong in many instances. This finding is especially distressing, since the assessments sought were not of especially rare or unusual diseases with which probability assessors are known to have difficulty. Rather, clinicians were asked to estimate the probabilities of certain symptoms given diseases, a matter about which physicians could reasonably be expected to be knowledgeable and for which the probabilities are not especially small.

Several other studies suggest that physicians can provide reasonably accurate subjective probabilities. One study examined how six urologists used information provided by the intravenous pyelogram (IVP).[253] The investigators found that their estimated probabilities of a normal roentgenogram corresponded well with the actual frequencies of normal results. They concluded that physicians untrained in probability assessment can convey usable information with numerical estimates and that these subjective assessments are fairly accurate.

Another study similarly found that physicians were reasonably accurate in predicting the frequency of neurologic disease in patients examined for that disorder.[70] Also, a Danish study of physicians' abilities to predict the course of duodenal ulcer disease found that the mean estimates of a large number of clinicians conformed very closely to observed experience.[95]

A related question is whether it would be better to seek probability assessments directly or in terms of odds or likelihood ratios. On this issue the evidence is also mixed.[70,81,98,142,253] Perhaps different people use different formats more effectively.

Are subjective probabilities provided by clinicians accurate? This is not a simple question, as the experimental literature is conflicting. There is some evidence that both clinical experience and experience in making probability assessments facilitate accuracy.[80]

TOWARD IMPROVED SUBJECTIVE PROBABILITY ASSESSMENTS

Subjective probabilities may not be perfectly accurate, but often in clinical medicine they are the only ones available and have to be used, either implicitly or explicitly, because a decision must be made. Clinicians can learn to appreciate the human tendencies toward error and thus improve the accuracy of their probability assessments. In addition, methods exist for pooling the opinions of groups of probability assessors in a way that is purported to minimize the effects of individual biases. Here we discuss both the individual and group approaches to improved probability assessment.

The Improvement of Individual Skills in Probability Assessment

What strategies are available to help the clinician improve the accuracy of personal probability assessments? The general strategy of decision analysis is to divide a complex problem into more manageable steps; the same strategy can be used to assess probabilities.

The first step is to describe the uncertain event in question thoroughly in nonquantitative terms and to relate it to other events more familiar to the probability assessor. The second step is to arrange events in order of probability before grappling with precise probability values. This part of the procedure assumes a willingness to say that the probability of event A is less than the probability of event B, even though the assessor would be unwilling to say that either event has a probability of 0.43, 0.03, 0.001, 0.0001, or the like. For example, a clinician might be willing to state that the mortality from a surgical procedure is greater than that from a hernia operation but less than that from coronary artery bypass graft surgery.

After various events have been arranged from most likely to least likely, more specific quantitative measures are gradually introduced. For instance, the assessor may attempt to judge how many times more likely than the least likely event is the most likely; this would yield an estimate of odds that can be used to relate the probabilities of the various possible events and to place upper and lower bounds on them. For example, suppose that the most likely of three possibilities is judged to be ten times as probable as the least likely. Then we can calculate that its probability must be at least 10/21, because (10 + 10 + 1)/21 equals 1.

Finally, each event can be compared with some "standard" external events whose probabilities are known. These reference events include both reference processes, such as drawing a particular number in a lottery or being dealt a certain type of hand at poker, and naturally occurring events, such as the weather and other more familiar medical events. In the previous example in which the mortality from an operative procedure is said to be less than that from coronary artery bypass graft surgery but greater than that for hernia surgery, estimates of the latter two probabilities, if available, could be used to bound the assessment of the probability in question. The numerical expression of subjective probability is no more than a refinement of this type of comparison to a set of reference events.

Serious probability assessors can also improve by learning to *calibrate* themselves. Over a period of time, they may find that of the instances assessed as p equals 0.9, the event occurred 80 per cent of the time, and of the instances assessed as p equal 0.1, the event occurred 23 per cent of the time. Recognizing this experience, an assessor may be guilty of a very common error, which is a special instance of the problem of *anchoring* mentioned earlier. This hypothetical assessor is reluctant to move far from the "anchors" at 0 and 1, with the result that the assessments are too close to the extremes. Noticing this experience, the assessor may then learn to call high probabilities less high and low probabilities less low, thus improving the calibration. (Other assessors may have the opposite problem: They may anchor near 0.5, which results in an underestimation of the probability of likely events and an overestimation of the probability of unlikely events. They will correct this tendency by learning to call high probabilities even higher and low probabilities even lower.)

Probability Assessments by Groups of Experts: The Delphi Method

One approach to obtaining probability assessments is to poll a group of experts. The premise in doing so is that, by interacting with each other, the group members will not be as prone to the biases we have been describing. Formal methods for obtaining group assessments are most likely to be useful in situations in which it is desirable to convince others of the validity of the decision analysis, objective estimates are not available, the personal opinions of a single decision maker will not suffice, and sensitivity analysis indicates that the conclusion is especially sensitive to a particular probability assessment. One method for obtaining the consensus of a panel of experts is called the **Delphi method.**[47] Under this method each member of the group of experts is asked for an assessment of the probability in question, along with the reasons for the assessment. Then, the results of this round of assessments are fed back to the members of the group, but in a way that preserves the anonymity of the assessors. Thus, they might be told that five assessors gave a probability between 0.2 and 0.25, ten assessors gave a probability between 0.25 and 0.30, and so forth. Then another round of assessments is solicited, and the process of feedback is repeated. The process continues until some specified level of consensus is reached or until a certain number of rounds have been conducted, whichever happens first.

The theory behind the Delphi method is that the interaction of opinions will lead toward a consensus and will help eliminate individual biases. It is also held that the anonymity of responses will prevent the participants from reaching an agreement simply because of peer pressure. The method has been applied in studies of medical decisions,[223] and convergence was achieved.

A possible serious drawback of the Delphi method is that the tendency toward consensus may reinforce, and not eliminate, the biases that underlie some of the participants' probability assessments. Moreover, there is no guarantee that an assessment is accurate just because a group of experts can be made to agree to it. Caution should therefore be exercised in interpreting the probability assessments derived from a Delphi procedure. Sensitivity analysis should always be used, just as for individual assessments, and there should be no misconceptions that a Delphi study of expert opinion is a substitute for a well-designed clinical study.

Despite their drawbacks, techniques such as the Delphi method do have a place in clinical decision analysis, although they should be used cautiously. For purposes of a clinician's own decision making, however, group assessment methods are generally impractical, although they can be used in certain hospital and group practice settings as part of a program of clinical rounds.

6.4 SENSITIVITY ANALYSIS AND SUBJECTIVE PROBABILITIES

Any clinical decision analysis that relies on subjective probabilities should be subjected to a sensitivity analysis, or a threshold analysis, with respect to those probabilities. We say this despite our earlier observation that the spread, or vagueness, surrounding a subjective probability assessment should not generally affect the analysis of decisions regarding the clinical care of individual patients. The value of a sensitivity analysis depends on the extent to which the analyst expects the results of analysis to be used by other decision makers or to be applied to decisions affecting many patients now or in the future.

The case for sensitivity analysis when the analysis must be persuasive to others is clear. No responsible clinician should accept unthinkingly the results of an analysis in which the subjective opinions of others compose an important part of the data base. Therefore, in order to allow other decision makers to rely on their own subjective opinions, the analyst should provide a sensitivity analysis to show how the conclusions depend on each subjective probability. If the conclusions can withstand broad variations in these probabilities, then narrower differences in opinion over those probabilities do not matter. If, on the other hand, the results are sensitive to the probabilities, then the users of the analysis may be encouraged to substitute their own subjective judgments; a sensitivity analysis or threshold analysis can facilitate this.

The case for sensitivity analysis when the decision analysis is to be applied to many patients, either by the same or several clinicians, is also clear. Because of individual variations, probabilities that apply to one patient will not apply to the next patient. Therefore, it is helpful to know which probabilities make the most difference and how the conclusions depend on those probabilities. Moreover, when we extend our concern to decisions for future patients, sensitivity analysis can point the way to priorities for clinical research. If there is little (or conflicting) objective information about a key probability, clinical studies to improve our understanding may enable future decisions to be made more confidently — and perhaps, better.

Even when an analysis is used by a single clinician for an individual patient, one advantage of sensitivity analysis is that it may provide peace of mind. Even the most skillful probability assessor may feel a bit uncomfortable acting on the results of a decision analysis that depends heavily on subjective probability assessments. But the fact that you feel uncertain about a particular probability assessment does not alter the fact that a decision has to be made anyway. You can at least gain some confidence in your decision by performing a sensitivity analysis. You would vary the less secure probabilities over the plausible range to see how much difference they make. If they do not make much difference, you need not spend more time searching the literature for more refined information, nor need you worry about your insecurity with the assessments. If small changes in a probability do make a difference, then all you can do is think hard about the assessment, scour the literature, solicit expert opinion, and convince yourself that this probability reflects your strength of belief and any objective evidence that is available. If you do a sensitivity analysis and the result is sensitive to such a probability assessment, you have no choice but to make the best decision you can based on your best assessment. You will feel uneasy about the decision, but, of course, one often feels uneasy about close decisions.

6.5 THE COMBINATION OF SUBJECTIVE AND OBJECTIVE INFORMATION

We observed in the section on probabilistically distributed probabilities that there is one very important circumstance in which the "spread" around a probability assessment does matter, and that is when the opportunity exists to revise that assessment using new information. Consider the example in Figure 6–2 once more. If you choose treatment A, the probability of survival is 0.4. Assuming that this objective probability is based on experience with thousands of patients, new results in a handful of patients would not alter your assessment of 0.4. You could use treatment A 15 times in a row, and every patient could die, and still your assessment of the probability of survival for the next patient would be only minutely less than 0.4. This is because the experience with these 15 patients is vanishingly small compared with the numbers treated in the past.

Suppose, instead, that you choose treatment B, for which you do not *know* the probability of survival. You assess that the survival probability could be 0.1, 0.2, 0.3, and so on up to 0.9, and you think that each probability is equally likely. Hence, for example, your subjective probability of a survival rate of 0.3 is 1/9. For purposes of a single decision, however, we have argued that the probability of survival should be viewed as if it were *known* to be

$$(1/9)(0.1) + (1/9)(0.2) + \ldots + (1/9)(0.8) + (1/9)(0.9),$$

or 0.5.

Let us change the circumstances a bit. Suppose that treatment B is chosen and that a trial is conducted once and leads to death. What is your estimate of the probability of survival the next time treatment B is used? Intuitively, you should see that it is no longer 0.5, because it is now much more likely that the probability of survival is, for example, 0.1 than 0.9. Thus, we expect that the new probability of survival is less than 0.5, but how much less?

We can compute the new probability. Let $P[10 \text{ per cent}]$ represent the *prior* probability that treatment B has a 10 per cent survival rate. We have stated that

$$P[10\%] = 1/9.$$

Similarly, let $P[20 \text{ per cent}]$, $P[30 \text{ per cent}]$, and so on up to $P[90 \text{ per cent}]$ represent the prior probabilities that each of these is the survival rate. Now, let $P[10 \text{ per cent} | \bar{S}]$ represent the *posterior* probability that treatment B has a 10 per cent survival rate, given that the patient did not survive in the first trial.

By Bayes' formula,

$$P[10\%\,|\,\bar{S}] = \frac{P[\bar{S}\,|\,10\%] \cdot P[10\%]}{P[\bar{S}]}$$

$$= \frac{(0.9)\,(1/9)}{0.5}$$

$$= 0.2.$$

(Note that $P[\bar{S}\,|\,10$ per cent] equals 0.9, because the probability of death with a 10 per cent survival rate is 0.9.) Hence, the probability that the probability of survival is 0.1 has risen from 1/9 to 2/10.

It can be calculated similarly that

$$P[20\%\,|\,\bar{S}] = 8/45,$$

$$P[30\%\,|\,\bar{S}] = 7/45,$$

and so on down to

$$P[90\%\,|\,\bar{S}] = 1/45.$$

Thus, the new assessment of the probability of survival, for purposes of the *next* decision, decreases to

$$(0.1)\,(9/45) + (0.2)\,(8/45) + \ldots + (0.9)\,(1/45) = 0.367$$

from a prior value of 0.500. The sample information for the first treatment has caused us to revise our probability assessment from p^* equals 0.5 to p^* equals 0.367.

The same principles apply whether the source of uncertainty surrounding an unknown probability is genuine vagueness or the kind of "objective vagueness" portrayed by the nine coins in Figure 6–1. The former is always the case in clinical decision making. Subjective probabilities can and should be revised when new evidence becomes available. If you are unsure of a probability (it might be 0.1, it might be 0.2, and so on), then the results of a new clinical study should be incorporated into your thinking to revise the subjective probability under consideration.

Indeed, one value of clinical research in decision-analytic terms lies in its ability to provide information that allows us to revise uncertain probability estimates. Clinical research can also provide information that improves our ability to structure a decision problem. The concept of the expected value of clinical information may be applied to the evaluation of clinical research to refine probability assessments as it has been applied to clinical tests to revise the probability of a diagnosis.

This concept of probability revision can be related to the earlier discussion of the use of the medical literature. We claimed that it was reasonable to estimate a probability by using the frequency observed in some study of a sample of patients. It turns out that this simple estimate is approximately the same result you get when you work through the probability revision calculations we demonstrated in the preceding example, *provided* that your subjective prior probability distribution across the range from 0 to 1 is evenly distributed. Such was roughly the case with treatment B. A priori, each of nine possibilities

(0.1, 0.2, ..., 0.9) was considered equally probable, perhaps because we had no basis for thinking that one was more probable than another. Some would describe this situation by saying that we had a "flat" prior distribution with respect to the unknown probability. If the prior distribution is flat, then the posterior (revised) probability is approximately equal to the observed frequency.*

If your prior distribution is not flat because of past experience or expertise, then you probably do not want to adopt the unadjusted observed frequency as your probability assessment. Instead, you want to revise by the method we used with treatment B, except that you will assign different weights to the different probabilities from 0.00 to 1.00. We do not develop this method further in this text but leave the stylized example of treatment B as a suggestive analogue.[204]

6.6 SUMMARY OF CHAPTER SIX

Probability assessments may be derived from the medical literature, clinical experience, personal opinion, or some combination of these. Subjective probabilities are obtained by comparing one's strength of belief that an event will occur with reference events of known probability. Subjective probabilities make explicit the judgments that underlie clinical decisions in any case. An advantage of this explicitness is that it facilitates communication between clinicians who wish to isolate the reasons for disagreements about the choice of treatments.

Subjective probabilities are prone to certain biases, but practice and experience probably can improve one's ability as a subjective probability assessor. A sensitivity analysis may be helpful to deal with many subjective probabilities in the analysis of a decision problem, to make the analysis more persuasive to others, to make the analysis more applicable to many patients, and to increase one's confidence in a difficult decision.

From a decision-analytic point of view, clinical research can provide improved probability assessments for the presence of disease given a clinical presentation and for the effects of treatment.

---

*If the observed frequency is r/n, then the posterior probability, given a flat prior distribution, is equal to $(r + 1)/(n + 2)$. In our example, $r = 0$ and $n = 1$, so that $(r + 1)/(n + 2) = 1/3$. This differs from our computed probability of 0.367 because we have used a discrete approximation to a continuous prior probability distribution in the range from 0 to 1.

Chapter Seven

Utility Analysis: Clinical Decisions Involving Many Possible Outcomes

7.1 INTRODUCTION TO THE PROBLEM OF VALUES

This chapter brings us to the third of the three major elements in the systematic analysis of clinical decision problems. To review, the first is the construction of a decision tree that portrays the temporal sequence of decisions, acquisition of information, and outcomes (Chapter Two). The second includes the assessment of information about uncertainties and the analysis of probabilities (Chapters Three through Six). The final element has to do with assigning values to the possible outcomes of a clinical decision. How, for example, does the physician or patient decide whether to accept some risk of immediate death in order to achieve a reduction in pain or disability? How should survival, quality of life, and other values be considered in evaluating the outcomes of alternative decision strategies? How can all of these competing considerations, or attributes of a clinical outcome, be taken into account?

Value judgments underlie virtually all clinical decisions. We shall argue that these value judgments can and ought to be considered systematically and explicitly, just as the probability assessments are. In decision-analytic terms, value judgments are translated into numbers at the tips of the decision tree, to be averaged out and folded back. In this chapter we will describe a method called **utility analysis** for defining values that reflect a decision maker's degree of preference among possible outcomes in an analytically sound and consistent manner.

Eliciting value judgments is difficult, and there are important problems and limitations with this stage of analysis for clinical decisions. A fundamental concern is whose preferences ought to be considered: the patient's, the physician's, or both? We shall return to this problem at the end of the chapter.

You may wonder why we have proceeded this far into a book on clinical decision making without introducing value trade-offs. We have done so because there is much to gain from clinical decision analysis without quantifying values. Many clinical decision situations can be simplified to problems in which the overriding objective is to maximize some probability, such as that of recovery, or to minimize some probability, such as that of death. For those situations, the methods developed in the first six chapters are sufficient, because the process of averaging out and folding back is well defined. When value trade-offs do arise, much can be gained from structuring the problem with a decision tree and assessing and revising the key probabilities, even without formally assigning values to be averaged out and folded back.

Another reason for delaying the discussion of utility analysis is that it is less developed as a practical set of techniques and, admittedly, more controversial than most of the material presented thus far. Our aim is to present the elements of utility analysis as an approach that some readers will find practical in the analysis of clinical decisions and from which all clinicians can gain insights that will sharpen their thinking about decisions.

One dimension of outcome that we do not consider in this chaper is cost, that is, the cost of health care resources such as a physician's time, hospital beds, and equipment. Part of what makes the problem of cost difficult is that the individual patient often does not bear the cost directly; instead, the cost is shared by members of society through insurance premiums and taxes. Because of the special nature of the problem of including cost as a consideration in clinical decision making, we devote Chapter Eight to this problem. Here, we focus only on the health outcomes to the individual patient — length of life and quality of life — that follow from the detrimental effects of disease and from the risks and benefits of diagnosis and treatment.

EXAMPLES OF CLINICAL DECISIONS
INVOLVING VALUE JUDGMENTS

To begin, consider the following three examples of the kinds of clinical decision problems in which value considerations are paramount. As you read each case, you might wish to try to structure the problem in a decision tree, indicating chance and decision points. You might also want to reflect on the following questions: How do the outcomes at the tips of the trees differ from those in the appendicitis and liver biopsy examples given in Chapter Three? What numbers would you use to average out and fold back?

> *Example: Case 1: Vascular Insufficiency in a Diabetic Patient.* A 68-year-old patient has suffered for years from peripheral vascular disease. Now, after a penetrating foot injury, the patient has developed an infection and possibly gangrene in the left foot. One response would be prompt amputation, but at this stage it is possible that the patient's foot will heal with careful medical care. If surgical amputation is delayed, however, there is a risk that infection and gangrene could spread, necessitating amputation above the knee or even resulting in death. If surgery is performed now, the amputation can be done below the knee, with less resulting disability and deformity than that associated with amputation above the knee. Limb amputation is a relatively safe procedure, but there is always some risk of operative mortality. Given this description of the circumstances and of the decision problem, should surgery below the knee be performed immediately, or should you wait to see if the foot heals?

Example: Case 2: Choice of Operation for Duodenal Ulcer. * As a surgeon you are considering two surgical options for your 50-year-old patient with recurrent duodenal ulcer; vagotomy and partial gastrectomy. Much controversy surrounds the appropriate choice between these two procedures. The main outcomes of concern are further recurrence of the ulcer and early postoperative death. In addition, a small proportion of surgically treated patients may develop a condition called dumping syndrome (faintness, a sensation of warmth, nausea, stomach distention, and diarrhea, which occur about a half hour after eating). Most cases of dumping syndrome are relatively mild, however, and there is little evidence of any differences in the incidence of this condition when vagotomy or gastrectomy has been performed. It is estimated that the perioperative death rate for vagotomy is lower than that for gastrectomy but that the rate of ulcer recurrence is higher. A third option is not to perform surgery and to continue with medical management. What is the best course of action for your patient?

Example: Case 3: Surgical or Medical Management of Coronary Artery Disease. Your 45-year-old male executive patient has suffered recurring chest pain for almost five years. He can usually walk up and down stairs without pain but cannot play tennis as vigorously as he used to because it precipitates chest pain. Sometimes the pain occurs when he is running to his train at the end of the day. The nitroglycerin that you have prescribed for him relieves the pain promptly, but you are nonetheless contemplating coronary artery bypass graft (CABG) surgery for this patient. The outcome of the operation is uncertain: It may or may not alleviate the pain, it may shorten or prolong life, and it may result in early postoperative death. After assessing the evidence, you conclude that surgery will probably improve the prognosis for pain relief, but at the risk of early postoperative death. Should you have your patient catheterized for coronary angiography, and if the results indicate that the patient is a candidate for surgery, recommend the CABG procedure? Or should you continue with medical management to control the symptoms?

DECISION ANALYSIS OF THE EXAMPLES

If you tried to structure these three examples, you surely discovered that the outcomes at the tips of the tree are much more complicated than those in the appendicitis and liver biopsy examples given in Chapter Three. In those examples, all outcomes were described as probabilities of death or survival. Indeed, in terms of ultimate outcome only two possibilities were considered: survival and death. In these examples, as in most actual clinical decisions, there are more than two possible outcomes. For example, in the vascular insufficiency problem, there are at least four possible outcomes: death, cure with loss of limb above the knee, cure with loss of limb below the knee, and cure with the limb intact. To analyze the decision tree, there is no simple numerical scale that can be averaged out and folded back, as we did with the probability of death in the appendicitis and liver biopsy problems. Can these more realistic decision problems with many possible outcomes still be analyzed systematically? We believe that the answer is yes, but to do so requires explicit consideration of preferences. To be explicit about incorporating preferences into the clinical decision analysis, let us assign probabilities and structure the first two of these examples to see where the analysis leads us. We shall return to the third example, coronary artery bypass surgery, later on in the chapter.

---

*This example is based on Cox.[42]

Case 1: Vascular Insufficiency in a Diabetic Patient

A decision tree for whether or not to amputate immediately the limb of the patient with gangrene is shown in Figure 7–1. If the decision is to amputate immediately, then the only uncertainty is whether the patient survives the operation. A probability of 0.99 is assigned to survival. If the patient survives, the outcome is the loss of limb below the knee. An alternative outcome is that the patient does not survive the operation. If, on the other hand, the operation is delayed, the probability that the foot will heal is estimated to be 0.7, with the resulting outcome of total cure. Assuming that continuous monitoring of the leg is not possible, the probability is 0.3 that the disease will spread, necessitating amputation above the knee. The probability of survival, given that the disease has spread and that the amputation may be too late, is estimated to be 0.9. If successful, this operation results in the loss of limb above the knee.

The decision tree in Figure 7–1 is ready for analysis, with one notable omission. There are no simple outcomes (e.g., probabilities of death) at the tips of the tree to permit averaging out and folding back. Instead, at each end point is one of four qualitative and apparently incommensurate outcomes: total cure (C), below-knee amputation (B), above-knee amputation (A), and death (D). If we could somehow assign numerical values to these four outcomes, then we could proceed with the decision analysis as we did for the appendicitis and liver biopsy problems. Now, you can readily rank the four possible outcomes in order of preference (C is preferred to B, B to A, and A to D), but how much do you prefer one outcome to another? What basis is there for choosing any one set of values and for asserting that it is appropriate to choose the strategy with the highest averaged-out "value"? Before answering these questions, let us consider the second case example.

Figure 7–1 A decision tree for the vascular insufficiency example.

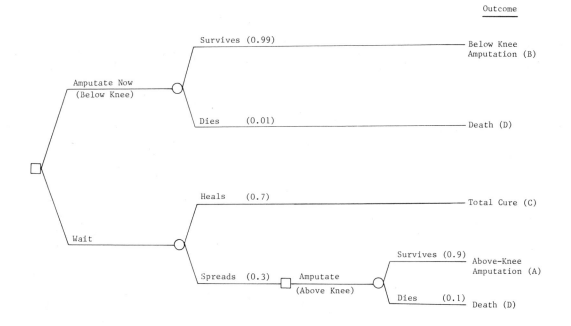

Case 2: Choice of Operation for Duodenal Ulcer

We simplify this problem by ignoring the alimentary complications of surgery, because there is no clear evidence that one operation results in a greater risk of these than the other. Consider the decision tree shown in Figure 7–2. The choice is among gastrectomy, vagotomy, and no surgery. The probability of early postoperative death is estimated to be 4 per cent with gastrectomy, but only 1 per cent with vagotomy. The risk of recurrence, however, is estimated to be 80 per cent without surgery, 10 per cent with vagotomy, but only 2 per cent with gastrectomy. There is a clear trade-off, but not a clear choice. The outcome possibilities are, in order of preference, survival with no recurrence (S, $\overline{R}$), survival with recurrence (S, R), and death ($\overline{S}$). (One might argue that the value placed on recurrence would depend on whether a patient has undergone no surgery, vagotomy, or gastrectomy. This would add several outcomes with intermediate value, and determining the implications for defining and valuing outcomes is left as an exercise at the end of the chapter.) Given this decision tree but no method to assign numbers to the outcomes for purposes of averaging out and folding back, how do you make the choice?

By now we hope that the dilemma is clear. It is necessary not only to enumerate the outcomes that result from each decision and subsequent event but somehow to "value" them. The values that come into play may include competing concerns regarding survival, pain, and disability as well as less tangible concerns, such as anxiety and patient satisfaction. We need an approach that allows the decision maker to incorporate into the decision-making process explicit or implicit statements of preference concerning these values, whether they be the patient's preferences, the family's, or the physician's, or some mixture of these. Analysis based on probabilities alone is not enough; a systematic approach to outcome valuation that is acceptable to the clinical decision maker is needed. Value judgments will be made implicitly in these decisions in any case; these value judgments ought to and can be brought into the decision analysis along with the information on probabilities.

Figure 7–2   A decision tree for the ulcer surgery example.

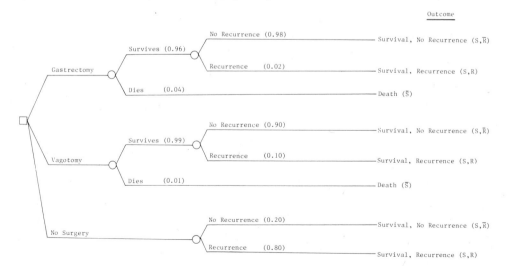

7.2 EXPECTED VALUE*

When we defined the process of averaging out (Chapter Three, Section 3.3), we restricted ourselves to situations in which the outcomes at a chance node were probabilities of some event, such as death, survival, or cure. Recall that when we average out at a chance node, as in Figure 7–3, we simply multiply the outcome at the tip of each branch by the corresponding probability on the branch and add the values across all branches. Hence, the averaged-out value at point Ⓐ in Figure 7–3 is

$$(0.5)\,(0.8) + (0.3)\,(0.6) + (0.2)\,(0.1) = 0.6.$$

We demonstrated in Chapter Three that the process of averaging out, when the outcomes themselves are probabilities of some reference event, is equivalent to the application of elementary laws of joint and conditional probability.

When we presented the concept of averaging out, we introduced the term **expected value.** In the example of Figure 7–3, we would say that the expected value at chance node Ⓐ is 0.6. In this example, of course, the expected value is expressed as a probability.

The concepts of expected value and averaging out can be generalized to situations in which the outcomes at the tips of the tree are not probabilities but some other numbers, such as days of illness or years of life. Thus far, we have justified averaging out only when the numbers being averaged out are probabilities of some reference event. In this chapter we will show how a special kind of numerical scale, called a **utility scale,** can be constructed by the decision maker so that it is as appropriate to apply averaging out to those numbers as to probabilities. First, however, we define the generalized concept of expected value and describe one of its most important applications — life expectancy.

THE DEFINITION OF EXPECTED VALUE

Suppose that we have a probabilistically distributed quantity (PDQ), such as the number of days a patient will remain ill following the onset of upper respiratory symptoms. For example, the patient might have a 20 per cent chance of

---

*This section may be skipped or skimmed by readers already familiar with the concept of expected value.

Figure 7–3 Averaging out when outcomes are probabilities.

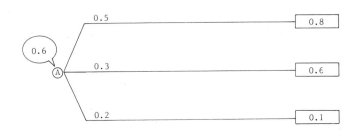

getting well after one day, a 25 per cent chance of getting well after two days, and so forth. We display such a probability distribution at the chance node in Figure 7–4.

The **expected value** of this PDQ is defined in just the same way as we defined it when the PDQ itself was a probability. We take a weighted average of the values of the PDQ (one, two, three, four, or five days in the example) for which the weights are the corresponding probabilities (0.20, 0.25, 0.30, 0.15, and 0.10, respectively, in the example). Thus, the expected value of the number of days of illness is

$$(0.20)\,(1) + (0.25)\,(2) + (0.30)\,(3) + (0.15)\,(4) + (0.10)\,(5) = 2.7.$$

If the PDQ is denoted by the symbol X, then we shall write its expected value as $E[X]$, which is read, "the expected value of X." Thus, if N is the number of days of illness in our example, we have calculated that

$$E[N] = 2.7.$$

The expected value is also called the **mean** of the PDQ.*

Definition. Consider a probabilistically distributed quantity that may have values of V_1, V_2, and so on up to V_n. Suppose that the probability of V_1 is p_1, the probability of V_2 is p_2, and so forth. Then the **expected value**, or **mean**, of this quantity is the weighted average of the possible values, the weights being the corresponding probabilities. Mathematically, the expected value is equal to

$$p_1 V_1 + p_2 V_2 + \ldots + p_n V_n.$$

---

*Statisticians usually refer to a PDQ as a random variable and to its expected value as its mean or expectation.

Figure 7–4   Computing the expected value of a probabilistically distributed quantity.

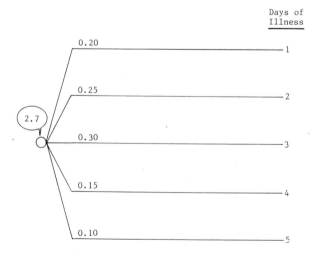

$$2.7 = (0.20)(1) + (0.25)(2) + (0.30)(3) + (0.15)(4) + (0.10)(5)$$

AVERAGES, EXPECTED VALUES, AND
THE LAW OF LARGE NUMBERS

The expected value of a PDQ is closely related to the usual notion of an "average," and the relation is more than coincidental. Suppose that we observe 100 patients like the one in our example and then compute the average number of days of illness. Keep in mind that the average is simply the sum of all the days of illness divided by the number of patients. Now, you know intuitively that if you observe enough patients and the probabilities are correct, the average will tend to be very close to 2.7, which is the expected value of the PDQ. Statisticians call this property the *law of large numbers:* As the number of independent, identical PDQs becomes very large, their average is likely to get very close to the mean of the PDQ. A more familiar example involves a coin-tossing game. If you win one dollar when heads comes up but lose one dollar when tails comes up, your winnings on a single toss define a PDQ with values of one dollar (with a probability of 0.5) or minus one dollar (with a probability of 0.5). The expected value of this PDQ is

$$[(1/2) (\$1)] + [(1/2) (-\$1)] = \$0.$$

The law of large numbers states that in the long run the average winnings per coin toss will be approximately zero.

LIFE EXPECTANCY

The most familiar medical example of an expected value is life expectancy. We can view the number of years in a person's life as a PDQ. Let us denote the event "an individual lives exactly N years" simply by N. Then the probability of living exactly N years is $P[N]$.

Life expectancy is simply the expected value of the number of years of life. For example, if a person has a 0.25 chance of living to age 40, 50, 60, or 70, then that person's life expectancy is

$$40 \cdot P[40] + 50 \cdot P[50] + 60 \cdot P[60] + 70 \cdot P[70]$$

$$= (40) (0.25) + (50) (0.25) + (60) (0.25) + (70) (0.25)$$

$$= 55 \text{ years}.$$

When the number of years of survival is the outcome of concern in a clinical decision problem, one possible approach would be to average out and fold back using life expectancy as the criterion for decision making, just as we have been using the probability of a reference event. We shall discuss the implications of such a criterion later in this chapter.

7.3   A TAXONOMY OF VALUE PROBLEMS

We have seen that the case examples in Section 7.1 present more complicated value problems than the problems we considered in Chapter Three. A taxonomy of problems involving values will illustrate the ways in which some value choices are more complicated than others.

TWO POSSIBLE OUTCOMES

The first and simplest kind of value problem is one in which there are only two possible outcomes. Examples might be such dichotomies as survive or die, cure or no cure, success or failure, patient satisfied or dissatisfied. The appendicitis and liver biopsy problems fall into that category, and in such cases the need for explicit value assessment does not arise. Our criterion for decision making is simply to choose the strategy that gives the highest probability of the better outcome.

MANY POSSIBLE OUTCOMES: THE SINGLE-ATTRIBUTE CASE

The second and more complex type of value problem occurs when there is a spectrum of possible outcomes, ranging on a scale from least preferred through somewhat preferred and very preferred and up to most preferred. One representative of this type of problem is the case of the patient with peripheral vascular disease who faces the possibilities of total cure, amputation below the knee, amputation above the knee, and death. In what follows, we shall show that it is not sufficient merely to rank these outcomes from worst to best. We must accurately portray *how much* worse amputation above the knee is compared with amputation below the knee, and so forth. The introduction of numbers will help us to be precise in this task.

Sometimes, in this second class of problems there is an underlying scale associated with the outcomes, which might naturally serve as the values we are seeking. Thus, for example, if the outcome is adequately described by the number of years of survival, then this continuum of possible outcomes automatically has a set of numerical values — the number of years of survival. We may wish to select the strategy that yields the highest expected value (i.e., the greatest life expectancy). But perhaps we may not. It may be that the patient would prefer nine years of survival over a 50–50 chance between 20 years of survival and immediate death. We may, therefore, wish to modify this underlying scale to account for the possibility that a person may be **risk averse** (a term we shall define rigorously later on). Thus, when an underlying scale of outcomes presents itself, we may or may not wish to use it as the scale for averaging out and folding back.

MANY POSSIBLE OUTCOMES:
THE MULTIPLE-ATTRIBUTE CASE

In the third and most complex class of value problems there are two or more dimensions or values. In the coronary artery bypass surgery decision, for example, each possible outcome has two components. One of them has to do with survival, and the other has to do with pain. The simplest approach to determining a scale for these two dimensions of outcome would be to divide them into discrete possibilities and to consider immediate death, short survival, and long survival on the survival scale, and lots of pain, a little pain, and no pain on the pain scale. As in the previous example, we then would have the task of assigning some relative values to all possible combinations. The worst outcome would be immediate death; the next worst would be a short survival period with lots of pain; the best would be a long survival period with no pain. In order to rank the outcome combinations, we must decide how to make trade-offs between the competing values associated with the two dimensions, or **attributes**, of the outcome. For example, we must assess whether lots of pain with a long period of survival is better or worse than a little pain with a short period of survival. Moreover, we need to know how to assign values on a scale from death to a long survival time with no pain. This chapter shows how numbers can be assigned to such valued outcomes so that (1) they reflect the true preferences of you or your patient and (2) they are appropriate for averaging out and folding back.

7.4 THE CASE OF TWO POSSIBLE OUTCOMES:
A GLANCE BACK AT THE LIVER BIOPSY PROBLEM

Consider the example of the patient with chronic progressive liver failure for whom a liver biopsy is being considered. In this problem, which we analyzed in Section 3.6, the possible outcomes are survival and death. In that analysis, we explicitly assigned no numerical values to these two outcomes; rather, we looked for the strategy that had the highest probability of the favorable outcome, namely, a two-year survival. When we averaged out and folded back the decision tree, we were doing no more than calculating the expected probability of survival down each branch. In doing so, we observed that the expected value of a probability is just another probability: A 0.5 chance at a 0.75 chance at some outcome is just the same as a 0.375 (i.e., (0.5) (0.75)) chance of that outcome. That is why we had no hesitation about multiplying those probabilities together and using their expected values to trim off branches and arrive at an optimal decision strategy. We had only to rank the two possible outcomes and then to maximize the probability of the better one.

AVERAGING OUT PERCENTAGES

Instead of approaching the problem that way, let us assign explicit numerical values to the outcomes of survival and death. Since death is an undesirable outcome, let us arbitrarily assign to it the value of 0. We want to apply a higher value to survival, so, to simplify arithmetic, let us set survival equal to 100. Now, with these numerical values at the tips of the tree, let us carry out the averaging-out-and-folding-back process as shown in Figure 7–5. Notice that as we average out just one step back from the tips of the tree, the numbers we obtain are precisely the percentages of survival that we had at the tips of the tree in our original formulation (Chapter Three, Figure 3–14). Therefore, the expected value of this quantity is identical to the percentage of survival, and maximizing this expected value is equivalent to maximizing the probability of survival. This is because at each step in the averaging-out-and-folding-back process the numbers are the same.

AVERAGING OUT WITH DIFFERENT NUMERICAL SCALES

Now let us see what happens if we shift our numerical scale and assign a value of 0 to survival and of −100 to death. Figure 7–6 shows the result of this averaging-out-and-folding-back process. As can be seen, the result is that the optimal strategy does not change. Moreover, because of the particular scale

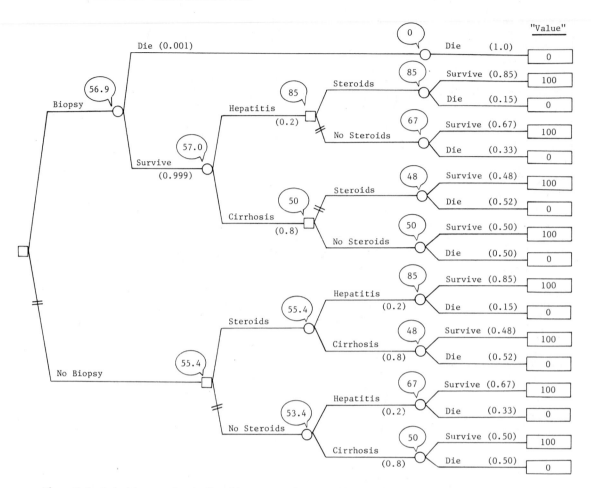

Figure 7–5 *A decision tree for the liver biopsy example. (An arbitrary value of 0 has been assigned to death and a value of 100 to survival.)*

selected here, the expected values (in boxes) represent precisely the negatives of the death rates per 100 (and the death rates equal 100 minus the survival rates in Figure 7–5).

It is beginning to seem as though it does not matter what numerical values we assign to the outcomes of survival and death. Try averaging out and folding back the decision tree of Figure 7–5 with the value 1 for survival and 0 for death. What happens to the numbers and to the optimal strategy? Then you might want to try the value 7.5 for survival and 3.1 for death. Do you see what is happening?

After trying different values, you should be convinced that no matter what numerical value, x, we assign to the outcome of survival and what lesser numerical value, y, we assign to the outcome of death, when we average out and fold back, the optimal decision remains the same. This is no accident. When the final outcome is dichotomous, as it is in this example, any numbers assigned to the two outcomes give the same answer, as long as the preferred outcome is given the higher value. The actual numbers we might assign have no mysterious value attached to them, and we need not be concerned about the apparent arbitrariness with which they were chosen. They were merely useful aids to numerical accounting in our calculations for the expected probability of survival (Figure 7–5) or the expected probability of death (Figure 7–6). To assign a value of

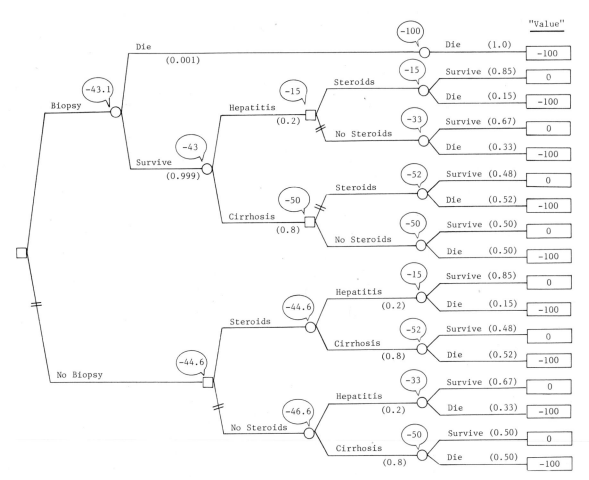

Figure 7–6 A decision tree for the liver biopsy example. (An arbitrary value of –100 has been assigned to death and a value of 0 to survival.)

–100 to death does not imply, in any sense, that death represents a loss of 100 units of anything. It is just a number to compare with the corresponding higher number for survival. The precise values of these numbers make no difference at all when there are only two possible outcomes because, in effect, we are doing no more than maximizing the expected probability of achieving the better of two outcomes.

By convention, we will usually assign the value of 1 to the better of the two outcomes and 0 to the worst. Then, a numerical assignment at an intermediate node on the tree (arrived at by averaging out and folding back) represents the *probability* of eventually arriving at the better outcome from the vantage point of that node. This is illustrated for the liver biopsy example in Figure 7–7. Thus, for example, with no biopsy and a choice of steroids, the probability of survival is 0.554.

7.5 THE CASE OF THREE OR MORE POSSIBLE OUTCOMES: UTILITY ANALYSIS

Encouraged by the simplicity of the liver biopsy problem, let us return to the vascular insufficiency problem (Figure 7–1). Recall that there are four

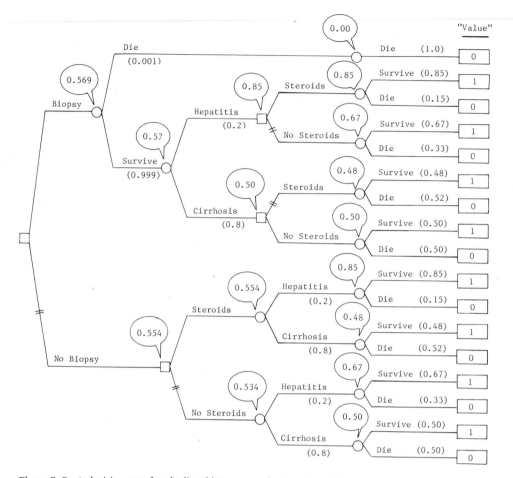

Figure 7-7 *A decision tree for the liver biopsy example. (A value of 0 has been assigned to death and a value of 1 to survival. All averaged-out values represent probabilities of survival.)*

possible outcomes: total cure (C), below-knee amputation (B), above-knee amputation (A), and death (D). This problem differs from the liver biopsy problem in one crucial respect: It no longer makes sense to seek the strategy that maximizes or minimizes the probability of any one of the outcomes. It no longer makes sense simply to choose the strategy that gives the lowest probability of death, because that strategy also has a high probability of severe disability. What we want is the strategy that properly balances the risks of death and disability. Hence, if we are going to assign values, we had better do so in a way that reflects an assessment of the relative severity of the four possible outcomes.

How shall we go about assigning relative values to the outcomes of total cure, amputation above the knee, amputation below the knee, and death? One approach would be simply to rank these outcomes in order of their preference and assign the numbers 1 through 4 to them. We might be tempted to try this because of our experience with the dichotomous outcome problem in which the absolute values made no difference.

Let us apply two arbitrary weighting schemes and see whether or not they affect our choice of strategies. For the decision tree of Figure 7–1, suppose you were to assign arbitrary numerical values to the outcomes as follows — C equals 4, B equals 3, A equals 2, and D equals 1 — and average out and fold back to find the optimal decision. Now suppose you were to assign these values — C equals 1,000, B equals 999, A equals 998, and D equals 0 — and average out and fold back again. Does your preferred strategy change? You might wish to try these calculations as an exercise.

It turns out that the numerical values assigned to the outcomes do make a difference. This is generally expected to be the case whenever there are more than two possible outcomes. (In this example, the value assigned to death, relative to the other outcomes, makes a big difference.) Since our attempt to use an arbitrary numerical scale has failed to provide consistent answers, we must seek a less arbitrary scale that somehow expresses the patient's or the physician's subjective intensity of preference among the possible outcomes.

DIRECT SCALING METHODS

One approach to ranking preferences would be to ask the patient to locate the four outcomes on a linear scale, or "ladder." For example, examine the scale in Figure 7–8. The value 1.00 on the scale represents functioning with both legs, and 0.00 represents death.

Now, pretend that you are the patient. Mark an x on the scale at the relative value you would place on the state following amputation below the knee with

Figure 7–8 *A scale of values for the vascular insufficiency example.*

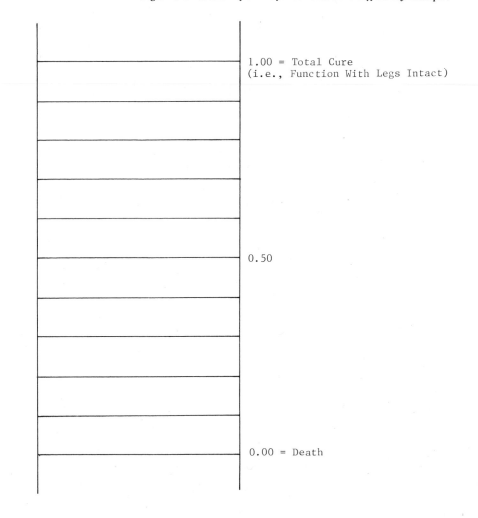

1.00 = Total Cure
(i.e., Function With Legs Intact)

0.50

0.00 = Death

the best functioning compatible with that condition. Similarly, mark a y at the value you would assign to the state following amputation above the knee with the best functioning compatible with that condition. The location of x and y on the scale should show how close or far these states are from perfect functioning (1.00) or death (0.00) and how near or far they are from each other. Write the exact number on the scale to correspond with the position you have assigned to x and y.

If you are like most people, you had some difficulty in making these judgments. People we have asked usually locate amputation below the knee at around 0.9 and amputation above the knee at approximately 0.8. That is, most people respond to a ladder approach like this by spacing the relative values fairly widely on the scale. Faced with the whole scale, people refrain from bunching their intermediate values near one end (e.g., 0.99 and 0.98).

Let us carry out the averaging-out-and-folding-back process, using the values of 1.0, 0.9, 0.8, and 0.0. The analysis is shown in Figure 7–9. We see that the "wait" strategy has the higher expected value, a conclusion that may seem to violate your true feelings about the decision. It is very possible that, in a sense we shall make precise in the next section, the assessments of values (0.9 and 0.8) do not reflect your true preferences about these outcomes.

The problem with this scaling approach is that the numbers involved have no concrete interpretation. There is no justification for using expected value based on them (i.e., averaging out) in comparing decision alternatives. Decision analysts have developed a technique for assigning values to such outcomes that is designed explicitly so that the averaging-out-and-folding-back process will lead to decisions that are consistent with your true feelings. We present this technique next.

UTILITY SCALES

In the liver biopsy example (Figure 7–5), we found that we were able to reduce the analysis to one of selecting the alternative that maximized the proba-

Figure 7–9 Analysis of the vascular insufficiency example, using values of 0.8 for amputation above the knee and of 0.9 for amputation below the knee.

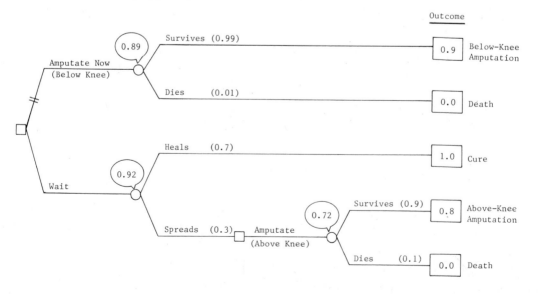

bility of the preferred of two outcomes. If we could convert our vascular insufficiency problem to such a dichotomous case, we should be able to use the same averaging-out approach. This conversion must involve an explicit assessment of preferences.

A Hypothetical Dialogue

Suppose that a patient indicates a descending order of preference, from best to worst, of total cure (C), amputation below the knee (B), amputation above the knee (A), and death (D). The patient's physician, who understands decision analysis, wants to elicit from the patient how much of a risk of death the patient is willing to take in order to avoid each level of disability. What follows is a dialogue between the patient and the physician. This is not, of course, the best way to approach all patients. Later, we will discuss ways in which thoughtful physicians can approach the same kinds of value problems.

The dialogue follows:

Physician: You know that we are facing a tough decision about whether to proceed now with surgery on your leg.
Patient: Yes, you've been pretty good about explaining just what I'm up against, and I appreciate that.
Physician: It would be helpful to me in advising you if you could give me a better idea of your feelings about the possibilities ahead. This will require us to play a kind of betting game with each other, but it's a game with a serious purpose. Are you willing to try?
Patient: Well, I'm not sure I know just what you mean, but if you think it will help, I'm willing to try.
Physician: O.K. I want you to imagine that you are standing this very moment in front of two doors, through one of which you *must* go. If you go through the door on the left, you must play Russian roulette with a gun having ten chambers, one of which is loaded with a bullet. This means that you have a 10 per cent chance of dying. But you have a 90 per cent chance of surviving with complete functioning of your legs as they are now. Now, if you go through the door on the right, there is no risk at all of death. But you will, without risk, undergo amputation above the knee. So here is your choice. Are you willing to run a 10 per cent chance of death by going through the door on the left in order to avoid the disability of amputation above the knee?
Patient: I don't have any problem with that choice at all. An above-the-knee amputation is bad, but it is not so bad that I would risk a 10 per cent chance of dying.
Physician: Well, then, what if the gun had a million chambers and only one bullet loaded? That would mean that choosing the door on the left carried a risk of death of one in a million in order to avoid the disability of amputation above the knee. Which door would you choose then?
Patient: Well, in that case, the door on the left. One in a million is a risk I certainly would accept in order to avoid the disability of the above-the-knee amputation.
Physician: So you're willing to take a risk of one in a million. How about a risk of one in a thousand?
Patient: Yes, I'd take a risk of one in a thousand.
Physician: How about a risk of one in a hundred?
Patient: Well, if I had a 99 per cent chance of coming out alive and intact, yes, I think I would take that risk.
Physician: But a risk of 10 per cent is too high. Right?

Patient: Right. I think 10 per cent is too high, but I see what you are driving at.

Physician: It seems that somewhere between 1 per cent and 10 per cent there must be a point where you would be just as willing to go through the door on the right and have your leg amputated without risk as to go through the door on the left and take a chance of staying as you are but also run the risk of dying.

Patient: I guess so. I guess I would have a hard time choosing between the doors if the risk of death were around 5 per cent.

Physician: Well, then, when the chance of surviving the Russian roulette is 95 per cent, the left door is equivalent to the right door.

Patient: Yes, that seems right.

Physician: What about amputation below the knee? At what risk of death would you be indifferent between a below-the-knee amputation and a game of Russian roulette in which you might emerge as you are but also might die?

Patient: Well, let's see. Amputation below the knee causes less disability than amputation above the knee, so I wouldn't be willing to run such a high risk of death to escape it. I guess I would rather have a below-the-knee amputation than run a 5 per cent risk of death by choosing that left door. On the other hand, if the risk of death were only one in a thousand, I would take that chance rather than the amputation. I suppose that a 2 per cent risk would make it very difficult for me to choose between them. But I really have trouble thinking about these numbers. It could be 1 per cent or 3 per cent.

Physician: That's all right. It may not make that much difference what the exact number is. For now, though, shall we say that when the chance of surviving the Russian roulette is 98 per cent, the left door is equivalent to the right door?

Patient: O.K.

The physician in this dialogue has elicited from the patient a statement that the outcome of above-the-knee amputation (A) is valued the same as a gamble consisting of a 95 per cent chance of total cure (C) and a 5 per cent chance of death (D). We shall say that the patient is "indifferent" between the two branches at the decision node at the top of Figure 7–10.

To simplify our notation, we will denote the gamble consisting of a 95 per cent chance of C and a 5 per cent chance of D as

$$<(0.95), C); (0.05, D)>.$$

We shall also use the symbol "$\sim$" to denote indifference (i.e., no preference) between two outcomes or gambles; it is read "is indifferent to." Hence, for our hypothetical patient, we write

$$A \sim <(0.95, C); (0.05, D)>, \tag{7-1}$$

which means simply that the two branches at the decision node at the top of Figure 7–10 are equally (un)desirable. We use this notation to express this same choice at the bottom of Figure 7–10.

The patient in the dialogue also told the physician that amputation below the knee (B) is the equivalent of a gamble consisting of a 98 per cent chance of total cure (C) and a 2 per cent chance of death. Hence, we write

$$B \sim <(0.98, C); (0.02, D)>. \tag{7-2}$$

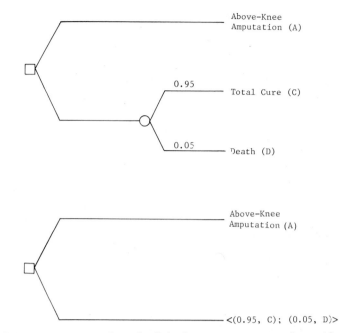

Figure 7–10 Two representations of a choice between an outcome and a gamble.

An Analysis of the Vascular Insufficiency Example

Now refer back to Figure 7–1. Suppose the patient's stated preferences are those expressed previously in Equations 7–1 and 7–2. That is, the patient is indifferent between the certain loss of limb above the knee and a gamble giving a 0.95 chance of survival with the limb intact and a complementary 0.05 chance of death. The patient is also indifferent between the certain loss of limb below the knee and a gamble giving a 0.98 chance of survival with the limb intact and a complementary 0.02 chance of death.

We can take advantage of this new information to eliminate the two intermediate outcomes from the decision tree in Figure 7–1, thereby reducing the problem to the two-outcome type with which we are already familiar. First, we eliminate outcome A from the decision tree by *substituting* the equivalently valued gamble <(0.95, C); (0.05, D)> for A where it occurs in Figure 7–1. This substitution has been made at chance node Ⓐ in Figure 7–11. Next, we eliminate outcome B by *substituting* the gamble <(0.98, C); (0.02, D)> for B where it occurs in Figure 7–1. This substitution has been made at chance node Ⓑ in Figure 7–11. The result of this substitution is a decision tree with only two outcomes, as we had for the liver biopsy example in Figure 7–5. Now, all we have to do is choose the strategy with the higher expected probability of the preferred outcome, total cure (C). The result of this averaging-out-and-folding-back procedure, given the preferences elicited, is that the better choice is to amputate, since the probability of cure is 0.970 compared with 0.956 if surgery is delayed.

You may wonder how much meaning to attach to these numbers if they are based on estimates with which the patient feels uneasy. One way of responding to this concern is to perform a **sensitivity analysis** or **threshold analysis** with respect to these estimates. Another way of responding is to use a method we

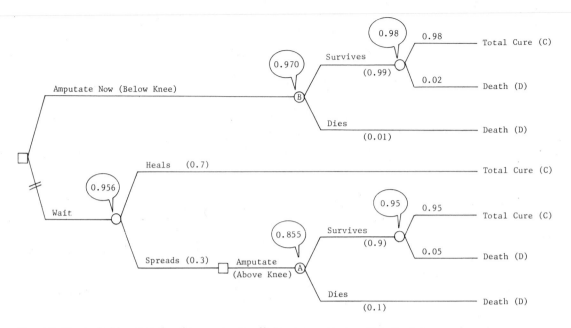

Figure 7–11 *A decision tree for the vascular insufficiency example in which the intermediate outcomes have been eliminated by substitutions.*

shall call **consistency checking.** We shall return to these methods and to this example after generalizing the procedure we have just defined.

Basic Reference Gambles

The procedure employed in converting Figure 7–1 to Figure 7–11 can be generalized. First, choose the best and worst outcomes. (This may itself be a value judgment; for example, is total paralysis worse than death?) Then, for each outcome, X, ask a hypothetical question that will elicit a probability p_X that creates indifference between the outcome X and the gamble giving a chance of p_X at the best outcome and a chance of $1-p_X$ at the worst outcome. We call this probability, p_X, the **break-even probability** for the outcome X. Next, substitute these hypothetical gambles with their break-even probabilities for the outcomes at the tips of the decision tree. Note that the break-even probabilities for the best and worst outcomes must be 1.0 and 0.0, respectively. The gambles between the best and worst outcomes are sometimes called **basic reference gambles** or **basic reference lotteries.**

Once basic reference gambles with an appropriate break-even probability have been substituted for each intermediate outcome, it is straightforward to average out and fold back, as in Figure 7–11. The task has been reduced to the familiar one of finding the strategy with the highest probability of the favorable outcome.

Utilities

The dialogue illustrated a way to assign numbers expressing the patient's relative preferences for the four outcomes in the example. Let us indicate these on the ladder in Figure 7–12. First, we place the most preferred outcome at the upper end of the scale and assign to it a value of 1. Next, we place the least preferred outcome at the lower end of the scale and assign to it a value of 0.

In between, we would like to know where to place each intermediate out-

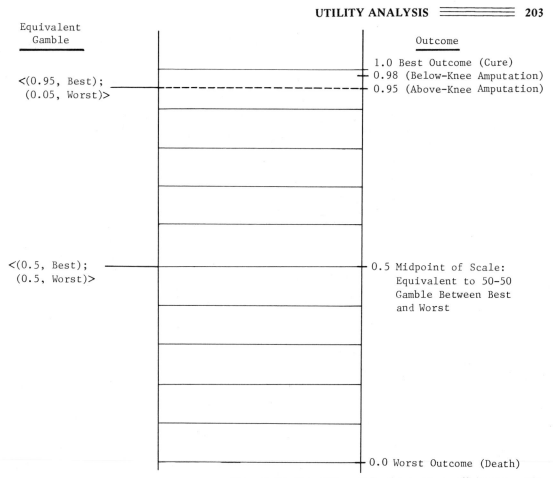

Equivalent
Gamble

Outcome

<(0.95, Best);
(0.05, Worst)>

1.0 Best Outcome (Cure)
0.98 (Below-Knee Amputation)
0.95 (Above-Knee Amputation)

<(0.5, Best);
(0.5, Worst)>

0.5 Midpoint of Scale:
Equivalent to 50-50
Gamble Between Best
and Worst

0.0 Worst Outcome (Death)

Figure 7–12   The utility scale for the vascular insufficiency example.

come. For example, should an intermediate outcome be placed closer to the
most preferred or the least preferred outcome? What does it mean to be "closer"?
We respond by defining the midpoint of the scale as equivalent to a gamble
giving a 50 per cent chance at the best outcome and a 50 per cent chance at
the worst outcome. If the intermediate outcome in question is preferred to this
even gamble (as is the case for both intermediate outcomes in our example),
then place it closer to the top of the ladder than to the bottom.

The patient in the dialogue placed the outcome "amputation above the
knee" much closer to the best outcome, "cure," than to the worst outcome,
"death." In fact, it was placed at a point 95 per cent of the distance to the top
of the scale, as shown in Figure 7–12. We have given this point a precise meaning:
It is equivalent to a gamble giving a 0.95 chance at the best outcome and a 0.05
chance at the worst.

Generally, if a person places an outcome, X, at the value p on this scale,
this indicates that the person is indifferent between this outcome and a gamble
giving a chance of p at the best outcome (whose value is 1) and a chance of
$1-p$ at the worst outcome (whose value is 0). We call such a scale a **utility scale,**
and we call these values **utilities.**

Definition. Suppose that the best and worst outcomes in a decision problem
have been identified, and that outcome X is valued equivalently to a gamble
giving a chance of p at the best and a chance of $1-p$ at the worst. Then p is the
utility of outcome X on a **utility scale** of 0 to 1.

In complicated decision problems, it would be tedious indeed to actually go through the exercise of substituting these basic reference gambles and the associated break-even probabilities at each tip of the tree. Fortunately, all we really have to do is keep track of the values of the break-even probabilities or utilities themselves and treat those as the quantities to be used for averaging out and folding back.

Thus, for the particular set of expressed preferences in the example, the utility of total cure (C) is 1.00, the utility of an outcome of below-the-knee amputation (B) is 0.98, the utility of an outcome of above-the-knee amputation (A) is 0.95, and the utility of death (D) is 0.00. We may abbreviate these by writing $u(C)$ equals 1.00, $u(B)$ equals 0.98, $u(A)$ equals 0.95, and $u(D)$ equals 0.00. We read "$u(B)$," for example, as the "utility of B."

Now, the value of the utility scale lies in the fact that we can use these numbers in the averaging-out process. The reason is that *choosing the decision strategy that gives the highest expected value of utility is equivalent to substituting basic reference gambles for each outcome and then averaging out and folding back.* The key is that utilities, as we have defined them, are really just probabilities (in a basic reference gamble), and we know that it is appropriate to average out probabilities.

In the present example of Figure 7–1, given the statements of preference previously elicited, we could proceed directly to the formulation in Figure 7–13, which is the equivalent of that in Figure 7–11. The numbers at the tips of the tree are the utilities for the outcomes. Compare Figures 7–11 and 7–13 to be sure that you understand that they are equivalent.

The utility approach may seem more difficult than direct scaling methods. But the utility scale based on break-even probabilities is the only numerical scale for which expected value (i.e., averaging out) is meaningful.

Consistency Checks

The process by which preferences are elicited using basic reference lotteries based on the best and worst outcomes is often referred to as **utility assessment,**

Figure 7–13 Decision analysis for the vascular insufficiency example, with utilities assigned.

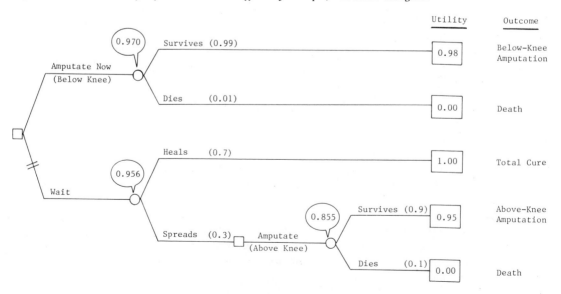

since the result is a set of utilities, or a numerical scale upon which to average out and fold back. The utility assessment procedure is, in practice, very difficult and may involve dialogues of the kind we illustrated earlier. The dialogue in our example resulted in convergence to $u(A)$ equals 0.95 and $u(B)$ equals 0.98. But surely these numbers are very difficult to think about clearly, particularly when they are all very close to 1, as they usually are when death is in the basic reference lottery. (This is because survival with almost any disability is far better than death for most people.)

To facilitate the utility assessment process and to provide a double check for consistency, it is often useful to construct a different basic reference lottery using one of the intermediate outcomes as one of the extremes. For example, consider a lottery between total cure and loss of limb above the knee. We might have started by asking what probability of total cure would make the gamble equivalent to amputation below the knee. In other words, what value of p results in the following indifference?

$$B \sim <(p, C); (1 - p, A)>?$$

This may be easier to think about than Russian roulette games involving life and death. Suppose a patient is indifferent at a value of p equals 0.6. Then we write

$$B \sim <(0.6, C); (0.4, A)>. \tag{7-3}$$

This enables us to place the outcome of below-the-knee amputation on the scale between the outcomes of total cure and above-the-knee amputation, but it does not enable us to place all three in relation to death. That requires a second assessment. For that purpose, we use the assessment with which the patient felt more comfortable in the dialogue, namely, that above-the-knee amputation is considered as desirable as a 95 per cent chance of total cure and a 5 per cent chance of death:

$$A \sim <(0.95, C); (0.05, D)>. \tag{7-4}$$

These two assessments in Equations 7–3 and 7–4 are sufficient to derive all of the utilities. We set $u(C)$ equal to 1 and $u(D)$ equal to 0, because these are the best and worst outcomes, respectively. Also, $u(A)$ equals 0.95 according to Equation 7–4. To find $u(B)$ we need to do some averaging out, as illustrated in Figure 7–14. The first step represents the patient's expressed preference (Equation 7- 3). The second step involves substituting for the outcome of above-the-knee amputation the equivalent gamble involving total cure and death (Equation 7- 4). The third step is simply based on averaging out the probability tree in the second step, where

$$0.6 + (0.4) (0.95) = 0.98.$$

Hence, the below-the-knee amputation outcome is considered indifferent to a gamble giving a 98 per cent chance of total cure and a 2 per cent chance of death. We can then proceed to use $u(B)$ equals 0.98 in the analysis of the decision tree.

The derived utility value for below-the-knee amputation happens to agree with the original assessment from the Russian roulette dialogue. If all three

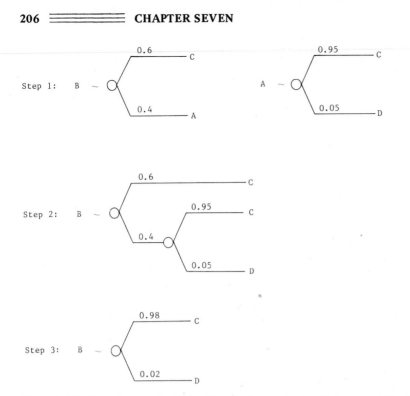

Figure 7-14 *A consistency check of utilities in the vascular insufficiency example. (C indicates cure; B, below-the-knee amputation; A, above-the-knee amputation; and D, death.)*

assessments in Equations 7–2, 7–3 and 7–4 are independently obtained and are **consistent** (in the sense that two of the assessments logically imply the third), then one can have more confidence in their validity. If, on the other hand, the patient insists that u(B) equals 0.99 despite the analysis in Figure 7–14, then there is an inconsistency.

As with probabilities, people usually feel uneasy when dealing with utilities very close to 1 or 0. The patient in the dialogue expressed this uneasiness with regard to the assessment of 0.98 for the outcome of below-the-knee amputation. As a rule, it is best to follow the course exemplified by the assessments in Equations 7–3 and 7–4: "Stretch out" one end of the utility scale as much as possible by creating basic reference gambles with intermediate outcomes treated as "worst" outcomes.

If inconsistencies persist or if the physician and patient continue to feel uneasy about the utility assessments, then a sensitivity analysis or threshold analysis is indicated. In fact, we recommend that sensitivity or threshold analysis be used as a matter of course in any clinical decision analysis, especially where utilities are prominently involved. We illustrate this process in the next section.

A Threshold Analysis Involving Utilities

In the vascular insufficiency example we may feel uncomfortable directly assessing break-even probabilities in gambles involving death. It may be that the only assessment with which we are comfortable is the placement of the outcome of below-the-knee amputation on the scale between the outcomes of total cure and above-the-knee amputation, as expressed by Equation 7–3. Where does this leave us?

Fortunately, we can proceed with a **threshold analysis** with respect to the utility of above-the-knee amputation. That is, we can seek to determine the range of utilities over which the amputation strategy is preferable. Continue to assume that Equation 7–3 still holds for amputation below the knee; then, for what utilities of amputation above the knee would the strategy to amputate now be preferred? Let $u(A)$ equal u, as represented in the first step of Figure 7–15. Then, as shown in steps 2 and 3 of Figure 7–15, we can derive the utility of amputation below the knee:

$$u(B) = 0.6 + (0.4)\,(u).$$

Now, substitute these utilities for $u(A)$ and $u(B)$ into Figure 7–1, and average out and fold back. We find that the expected value of the "amputate now" branch is

$$(0.99)\,[0.6 + (0.4)\,(u)] + (0.01)\,(0),$$

or

$$(0.99)\,(0.6) + (0.99)\,(0.4)\,(u),$$

and that the expected value of the "wait" branch is

$$(0.7)\,(1) + (0.3)\,[(0.9)\,(u) + (0.1)\,(0)]$$

or

$$0.7 + (0.3)\,(0.9)\,(u).$$

Figure 7–15 *The calculation of utilities for threshold analysis in the vascular insufficiency example. (C indicates cure; B, below-the-knee amputation; A, above-the-knee amputation; and D, death.)*

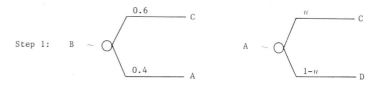

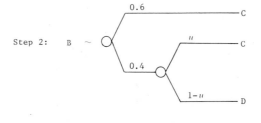

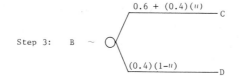

We complete the threshold analysis by calculating which values of u make the amputation strategy preferable. Specifically, amputation is preferred (i.e., has the higher expected utility) if

$$(0.99)(0.6) + (0.99)(0.4)(u) > 0.7 + (0.3)(0.9)(u). \qquad (7\text{--}5)$$

Solving Inequality 7–5 for the unknown utility, we find that amputation is preferred so long as

$$u > 0.84.$$

Let us interpret this finding. It says that, as long as above-the-knee amputation is preferred to a gamble giving a 0.84 chance of cure and a 0.16 chance of death, amputation is the preferred strategy. Now, our patient would seem to have no trouble with this comparison: The patient clearly prefers the outcome of above-the-knee amputation to this gamble. Unease about setting the value at 0.95 rather than at 0.94 or 0.96 does not seem to matter. This assumes, however, that the patient is reasonably comfortable with making the outcome of below-the-knee amputation equivalent to a 0.6 chance of cure and a 0.4 chance of above-the-knee amputation. If the patient were to reassess that break-even probability to be 0.5, for example, then the new threshold analysis for $u(A)$ would be

$$(0.99)(0.5) + (0.99)(0.5)u > 0.7 + (0.3)(0.9)u$$

or

$$u > 0.91.$$

Hence, *if* the patient considers below-the-knee amputation no better than a 50–50 gamble between above-the-knee amputation and cure *and* the patient considers above-the-knee amputation less desirable than a 0.91 chance of total cure and a 0.09 chance of death, then the optimal decision would be to wait.

Notice that it should be easier to think about whether the outcome of below-the-knee amputation is closer to 0.6 or 0.5 on the reduced scale between total cure and above-the-knee amputation then to agonize over whether the utility of below-the-knee amputation is 0.98 or 0.99 or even 0.999. The decision maker must be clever enough to ask the utility questions that are easiest to contemplate and rely on threshold or sensitivity analysis to gain confidence in the conclusions of the analysis.

Transformations of the Utility Scale

The utility scale upon which we can base our averaging out and folding back is anything but arbitrary. It has a very precise meaning in terms of basic reference gambles and is a well-defined shorthand for converting an unmanageable multiple-outcome decision tree into a manageable dichotomous one. This shorthand was illustrated by the equivalence between the analyses represented in Figures 7–11 and 7–13.

We have seen that it is not permissible to change the utility values arbitrarily, as could be done in the dichotomous case. Those intermediate utility values have real quantitative importance. What you can do, however, is change the units of measurement on the scale. Instead of anchoring the best and worst outcomes at 1 and 0, respectively, you may want to relabel the scale so that the best outcome is perhaps 100, and the worst is 0. Or possibly you might want one of the intermediate outcomes to be 0, in which case the worst outcome would have a negative value.

Why change the units? For one reason, you might be interested in using a natural scale, such as years of life expectancy, as a utility scale. Such a scale does not range from 0 to 1, but would permit you to use expected longevity as a criterion for decision making. Another reason for changing the units of the scale is to coincide with the utility assessment procedure. In the vascular insufficiency example, given the method on which we settled for assessing utilities, it would have been convenient to place $u(A)$ equal to 0 and $u(C)$ equal to 1. Then, according to Equation 7-3, $u(B)$ equals 0.6. On that scale, of course, $u(D)$ would be negative.

You can think of this kind of scale transformation as analogous to a change from Celsius to Fahrenheit on the temperature scale. On the Celsius scale the boiling point of water is 100 degrees and the freezing point is 0 degrees. On the Fahrenheit scale these bench marks are relabeled 212 degrees and 32 degrees, respectively. To go from Celsius (C) to Fahrenheit (F), you multiply by 1.8 and add 32; that is,

$$F = 1.8C + 32.$$

Notice that this linear transformation, which is simply a change of scale, involves multiplying the original value by a positive constant (1.8) and adding another constant (32).

Similarly, you can assign different values to a utility scale by multiplying by a positive constant and adding another constant. Thus, if we want to change the units of measure for our utilities for the vascular insufficiency example, we could multiply them all by 100 and subtract 95. This would result in $u(C)$ equals 5, $u(B)$ equals 3, $u(A)$ equals 0, and $u(D)$ equals −95. Using these values in the decision tree of Figure 7–13 would give the same optimal strategy as that of the original utilities; this had to be the case, since we did no more than to change the units of measurement.*

This does not mean that the scale is arbitrary but only that a proportional stretching or shifting of the units of the scale does not change the optimal decision rules. Thus, the scale of 100, 98, 95 and 0 for C, B, A, and D, respectively, is equivalent to 50, 49, 47.5, and 0 but *not* to 50, 40, 30, and 0. You can fix the utility value for the best and worst outcomes, as in the dichotomous case, but beyond that the scale is determined by preferences as expressed in terms of the basic reference gamble.

Maximizing Expected Utility and Minimizing Expected Disutility

Up to this point we have defined utility scales as ranging from 0 (or some

---

*In general, if $u(X)$ is the utility scale for the outcomes denoted by X, then

$$u^*(X) = a \circ u(X) + b$$

is an equivalent utility scale (provided that a is greater than 0, to preserve the rank order of outcomes). Statistically speaking, the reason is that the expected value of a quantity, $E[X]$, has the property that $E[aX + b] = aE[X] + b$.

low value) for the worst outcome up to 1 (or some higher value) for the best outcome. Thus, more utility is better, and we want to get the highest possible expected value. Sometimes, however, it is more convenient to define a *disutility scale* rather than a *utility scale,* with the highest values being the least desirable. For example, in the appendicitis example of Chapter Three, 1 might be the *disutility* of death and 0 the disutility of survival. In that case we would select the strategy with the *lowest* expected disutility. If the value 1,000 represented death and 0 represented survival, then the expected disutility would be equivalent to the death rate per 1,000 patients, as we observed in Chapter Three. One can always convert a disutility scale to a utility scale, or vice versa, by multiplying all values by -1; care must be taken, however, to keep track of whether one is maximizing (for utilities) or minimizing (for disutilities).

UTILITIES BASED ON NATURAL UNDERLYING SCALES

Consider a decision problem in which the only outcome of concern is the length of survival, that being measured in years, or another decision problem in which the only outcome of concern is the number of days spent disabled (e.g., out of work, in bed). In both of these cases we might be tempted to use the underlying scale as the utility scale. Thus, if the number of years of life were the utility scale, we might choose the strategy that gives the greatest life expectancy.

Let us pursue the implications of using a numerical scale, such as the number of years of life, as the utility scale. Suppose that in a given situation the maximum possible longevity to which a probability other than 0 is attached is 50 years. This is the best outcome. The worst outcome is immediate death, or zero years. What is the utility of 25 years? In our precise terms, what must the value of p_{25} be so that the gamble

$$<(p_{25}, 50 \text{ Years}); (1 - p_{25}, 0 \text{ Years})>$$

is considered equally as desirable as the certainty of 25 years of life? The answer for any particular individual need not be 0.5. Indeed, an individual may prefer a certainty of 20 years to an even gamble between zero and 50 years.

The Certainty Equivalent of a Gamble

Suppose an individual is indifferent between a certainty of 15 years and the gamble

$$<(0.5, 50 \text{ Years}); (0.5, 0 \text{ Years})>.$$

Then, 15 years is said to be the **certainty equivalent** of the gamble.

Definition. Consider a gamble in which each possible outcome is expressed on some numerical scale (not necessarily a utility scale). The **certainty equivalent** of the gamble is the outcome along the scale such that the decision maker is indifferent between (1) that certain outcome and (2) the gamble.

Risk Aversion

The certainty equivalent need not be the same as the expected value, which is 25 years for the lottery in question. If the certainty equivalent is less than the expected value, the individual is said to be **risk averse** with respect to longevity.

The degree of **risk aversion** with respect to longevity is a matter of personal preferences. It may depend on one's age, family responsibilities, and many other factors. For example, an individual with young children may be very risk averse in order to ensure sufficient time to provide for their future, while a young single person may be less risk averse. In addition, people may assign greater value to the more proximate years of life than to the more distant years; this preference would appear as a source of risk aversion.

In terms of the utility scale, a risk-averse individual would assign utilities according to a schedule such as the concave curve in Figure 7–16. Thus, in our example 15 years would be assigned a utility of 0.5, indicating an indifference probability of 0.5 in the basic reference gamble.

An individual whose utility assessments lie along the straight line in Figure 7- 16 is said to be **risk neutral.** For such an individual, utility is proportional to longevity, and therefore expected utility is proportional to expected longevity (i.e., life expectancy). Since we can multiply the utility scale by any constant without changing its properties, we can multiply by 50 in this case, so that utility equals longevity. For such an individual, excluding concern with the quality of life or other considerations, the quantities at the tips of the tree are life years, and the averaging-out-and-folding-back process is equivalent to computing and maximizing life expectancy. The important caveat, however, is that a patient may be risk averse, and in such a case life expectancy would not be a decision criterion consistent with preferences.

Figure 7–16 *Utilities on the longevity scale: risk-averse and risk-neutral individuals.*

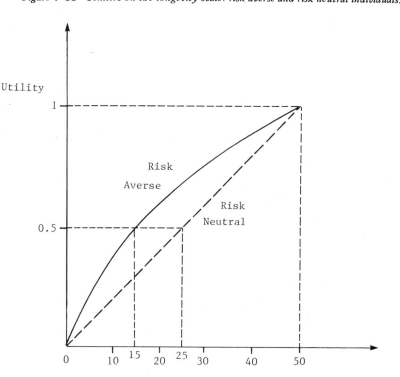

MULTIPLE-OUTCOME PROBLEMS IN WHICH
UTILITY JUDGMENTS CAN BE AVOIDED:
THE PRINCIPLE OF PROBABILISTIC DOMINANCE*

Threatened Stroke in a Very Ill Patient

A hospitalized 68-year-old man with diabetes mellitus, hypertension, and cardiovascular disease develops weakness, unusual sensations, and difficulty speaking, but these symptoms resolve within 15 minutes. A neurological consultant believes that the patient is very likely to develop a cerebrovascular accident, or stroke. If nothing is done, the consultant estimates that the risk of stroke is 90 per cent and that, if stroke occurs, it is equally as likely to be major (paralysis and prolonged disability) as it is to be minor (less severely disabling).

One possibility is to treat the patient with anticoagulant medication. This carries some risk because of bleeding and is assessed to have a 2 per cent chance of causing death in this already ill patient. If the patient develops no fatal complications, the risk of stroke would be reduced to 75 per cent; if a stroke does occur, it would be less likely to be major (a probability of 0.4) than minor (a probability of 0.6). Another intervention that entails greater risk would be to perform surgery on the arteries leading to the brain. The neurosurgeons assess the risk of death from surgery for this patient to be 20 per cent. But if the patient survives surgery, he will have only a 70 per cent risk of stroke and, if a stroke occurs, only a 0.3 chance that it will be major. Both the risks of stroke and of major stroke are lower with surgery than with medical treatment with anticoagulants.

Even without considering the risks of performing an angiogram, which would be necessary prior to surgery, you think that surgery ought to be ruled out for this very ill patient. But the improved prospects for avoiding a stroke after successful surgery make you want to consider further that possibility before dismissing it altogether. It is possible, in fact, to justify your inclination to rule out surgery without relying on utility judgments, even though there are more than two possible outcomes.

A decision tree for this problem is shown in Figure 7–17. The four possible outcomes are no stroke (N), minor stroke (Mi), major stroke (Ma), and death (D). (Each of the outcomes of minor and major stroke stand for a range of possible consequences, including, for major stroke, death at the time of the stroke. Death consequent to the treatment options is distinct from these future possibilities and is included in the decision tree.)

Consider Table 7–1, which shows the path probabilities associated with each possible outcome for each decision option. When the medical option is compared with the surgical option, it appears that one would need to know utility values in order to be able to decide which option is better. After all, although medical treatment gives a higher probability of the best outcome (N) and a lower probability of the worst outcome (D), the comparison for the middle two outcomes seems to be ambiguous. If a major stroke is bad enough (i.e., has a utility close enough to 0), then perhaps surgery would be preferred. But further examination indicates that such is not the case.

First, note that the medication option gives a lower probability of death

---

*This section is not essential to what follows and may be skipped without loss of continuity.

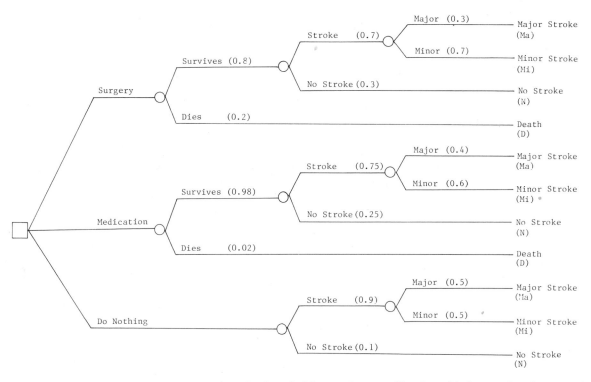

Figure 7–17 *A decision tree for a very ill patient with threatened stroke.*

TABLE 7-1   PATH PROBABILITIES OF ALTERNATIVE DECISION
OPTIONS FOR THE VERY ILL PATIENT WITH
THREATENED STROKE

OUTCOME	DECISION OPTION		
	Surgery	Medication	Do Nothing
No Stroke (N)	0.24	0.25	0.10
Minor Stroke (Mi)	.39	.44	.45
Major Stroke (Ma)	.17	.29	.45
Death (D)	.20	.02	.00
Total	1.00	1.00	1.00
Major Stroke or Death (Ma or D)	0.37	0.31	0.45
Minor Stroke or Major Stroke or Death (Mi or Ma or D)	.76	.75	.90

than surgery does. Next, determine which of these two options gives the lower
probability of major stroke *or worse* (i.e., major stroke or death). Again, medication is better (0.31 versus 0.37). So even if a major stroke were as bad as
death, the medication option would be better than surgery. Finally, determine
which option gives the lower probability of a minor stroke *or worse* (i.e., Mi,
Ma, or D). Again, medication is superior (0.75 versus 0.76). Regardless of where
we draw the line between outcomes, medication is preferred over surgery, no
matter what utilities we might assign to the four outcomes. This is an example
of the principle of **probabilistic dominance.**

Probabilistic Dominance

Definition. One strategy is said to have **probabilistic dominance** over a second strategy when (1) for each possible outcome the probability of achieving this outcome or any worse outcome is no greater for the first strategy than for the second, and (2) for at least one possible outcome, the probability of achieving this outcome or any worse outcome is lower for the first strategy than for the second.

The general principle is as follows. Suppose there are four possible outcomes, which are, in decreasing order of preference, W, X, Y, and Z. Let the path probabilities of these outcomes be w, x, y, and z, respectively. The rank order implies that it is desirable to shift probabilities from the less preferred to the more preferred outcomes. Hence, for example, the modified gamble,

$$<(w, W); (x + 0.01, X); (y - 0.01, Y); (z, Z)>$$

is preferred to the original gamble,

$$<(w, W); (x, X); (y, Y); (z, Z)>,$$

because X is preferred to Y. Suppose now that there is an alternative strategy that yields a different set of path probabilities — w', x', y', and z', respectively, for the four outcomes. The principle of probabilistic dominance says that the former strategy is preferred to the latter if

$$z \leq z', \qquad (7\text{--}6a)$$

$$y + z \leq y' + z', \qquad (7\text{--}6b)$$

and

$$x + y + z \leq x' + y' + z'. \qquad (7\text{--}6c)$$

In our example, z equals 0.02, z' equals 0.20, y equals 0.29, y' equals 0.17, x equals 0.44, and x' equals 0.39, so that all of the required inequalities hold.

When these conditions are not all met, then a swing in utilities can reverse the decision, and probabilistic dominance does not apply. The latter is illustrated by the comparison between the medication option and the option to do nothing in the example. The probability of death is lower if we do nothing (0.00 versus 0.02), but the probability of major stroke *or worse* (Ma or D) is lower with medical treatment (0.31 versus 0.45). Therefore, the choice depends on the utilities assigned to the outcomes. If a major stroke has a utility near the utility of death, then medication will be preferred. For example, let $u(N)$ equal 1, $u(Mi)$ equal 0.95, $u(Ma)$ equal 0.90, and $u(D)$ equal 0. Then the expected utility with medication is

$$0.25 + (0.44)(0.95) + (0.29)(0.9) = 0.929,$$

and the expected utility of taking no action is

$$0.1 + (0.45)(0.95) + (0.45)(0.9) = 0.933.$$

Taking no action is preferred. If, however, $u(Ma)$ equals 0.5 and the other utilities remain the same, then the expected utility with medication is

$$0.25 + (0.44)(0.95) + (0.29)(0.5) = 0.813,$$

and the expected utility of taking no action is

$$0.1 + (0.45)(0.95) + (0.45)(0.5) = 0.753.$$

Medication is now preferred. This shift in preferences cannot happen if probabilistic dominance holds.

When probabilistic dominance holds, it can simplify the decision problem considerably, since the only required value judgment is the ranking of outcomes. Unfortunately, probabilistic dominance rarely holds.

Often, even when probabilistic dominance does not hold, the decision is not sensitive to utilities over some range of values. We saw this in the vascular insufficiency example. It is advisable to do a sensitivity analysis or threshold analysis to see how variations in utilities might affect a decision. In the example of the threatened stroke just discussed, the utility of stroke has to be unrealistically high in order to make no action appear superior to medication. If the choice does not change over a wide range of plausible utility values, then you can feel more comfortable about the decision. If the choice is sensitive, you may want to give the utility assessment extra thought or try to probe the patient's values more deeply.

7.6 OUTCOMES WITH MULTIPLE ATTRIBUTES: TRADE-OFFS BETWEEN LONGEVITY AND QUALITY OF LIFE

Case 3: Surgical or Medical Management of Coronary Artery Disease

The third example presented at the outset of this chapter — the choice between coronary artery bypass graft surgery and medical management for a patient with coronary heart disease — involves two dimensions of outcome. These are, to simplify considerably, (1) longevity and (2) the degree of relief from chest pain (angina pectoris). Each of these dimensions has associated with it a continuum of possible outcomes (for example, the number of years of life saved or lost, the degree of pain relief). To allow us to use decision analysis to guide this complex decision, we need to be able to describe these outcomes in a way that can be managed in a decision tree, converted to a utility scale, and then averaged out and folded back to suggest a preferred course of action.

A simple decision tree that might be used is shown in Figure 7–18. Here the patient is being considered for angiography, an x-ray procedure used to discover the nature and operability of the disease (e.g., the number of coronary arteries involved, their operability, and the level of cardiac function). The description of the patient includes personal characteristics (e.g., a 45-year-old male), medical characteristics (e.g., severe angina pectoris with no history of myocardial infarction), and personal preferences with respect to longevity and relief from chest pain. The latter, which may be strongly affected by the amount of physical activity the patient enjoys or requires, will undoubtedly have to

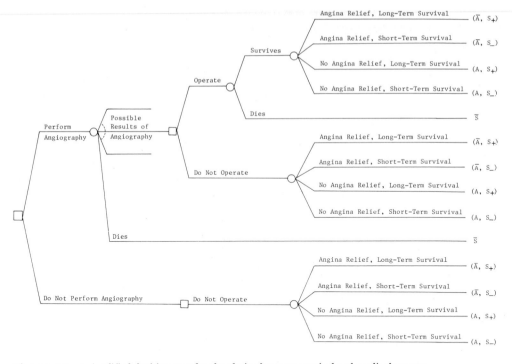

Figure 7–18 *A simplified decision tree for the choice between surgical and medical management of coronary heart disease. (Long-term survival is defined arbitrarily as survival of greater than or equal to ten years. Short-term survival is defined arbitrarily as survival of less than ten years but beyond the perioperative period.)*

enter into the assessment of utilities corresponding to the outcomes at the tips of the tree.

Notice that in Figure 7–18 we have taken the dimension of angina relief and dichotomized it into two values: $\overline{A}$, which denotes that the angina has been relieved, and A, which denotes that the angina has not been relieved. We define relief arbitrarily as an improvement for at least ten years or half of the life span, whichever is less. The dimension of survival is also simplified by creating three possible states: long-term survival (e.g., at least ten years), short-term survival (e.g., less than ten years), and perioperative death. These outcomes are denoted by S_+, S_-, and $\overline{S}$, respectively, at the appropriate tips of the decision tree. By dividing one dimension into two outcomes and the other dimension into three outcomes, we have created a situation in which there is only a small number of combinations of outcome. The best is represented by $(\overline{A}, S_+)$, which stands for angina relief with a long survival time; the worst is represented by perioperative death, $\overline{S}$. There are three intermediate outcomes between these two extremes — $(\overline{A}, S_-)$, (A, S_+), and (A, S_-) — and there are, therefore, five utility values to be assessed. In principle, this could be done by the method of the basic reference gamble.

Situations may arise in which such simplifications of the two dimensions are too gross, and a more refined analysis is necessary. For example, one might want to know how to value 14 years of survival with angina relief for ten of those years, no relief for two years, and a more severe level of angina for the last two years. How would one approach such a problem?

One approach is to use a utility scale in which each year of life is weighted by an index (ranging from 0 to 1) that reflects the quality of life in that year.

Thus, ten years of life with severe angina might have a value of five "quality-adjusted" life years if severe angina represents a quality level of 0.5. If we use such a scale, the averaging-out-and-folding-back process corresponds to choosing the option with the highest quality-adjusted life expectancy. The validity of such a scale as a *utility* scale depends on several implicit assumptions, which are described in the remainder of this section.

RANKING MULTI-ATTRIBUTED OUTCOMES

In the coronary bypass example, each possible outcome is described in terms of two dimensions: longevity and quality of each year of life. How can we rank the possible outcomes?

The Principle of Value Dominance

We say that one outcome **value dominates** a second outcome when the first is preferable in both or all dimensions. (Note that this kind of *value* dominance is different from *probabilistic* dominance, which was described earlier [p. 212]). For example, the outcome of 40 years of life with no angina dominates the outcome of 30 years of life with mild angina. But not many outcomes can be ranked according to the **value dominance** principle. Which is preferred: 40 years with mild angina or 30 years with no angina? Several approaches to ranking such incommensurable outcomes are possible; we offer one that is gaining acceptance among researchers in this field. (The interested reader may wish to consult the bibliography for additional readings on the use of health-status indexes and quality-adjusted life years in the evaluation of medical decisions and health programs.)

Quality-Adjusted Life Years

One approach is to attempt to place the various health states, or quality levels, on a scale of 0 to 1. Perfect health would be assigned the value 1.0, and a state nearly as bad as death would be assigned a value near 0.0. Thus, severe angina might be valued at 0.7 and mild angina at 0.9. A life span of 20 years, including 15 healthy years, three years with mild angina, and two years with severe angina, might then be assigned a score of

$$(15)(1.0) + (3)(0.9) + (2)(0.7) = 19.1$$

quality-adjusted life years. This score is the number of years of full health that would be valued equivalently to the number of years of survival that are expected, including any morbidity during those years. Outcomes can be ranked in order of preference according to the number of **quality-adjusted life years.**

But what is the origin of these weights, or health index values? What do they have to do with personal preferences, which surely must enter into the ranking of possible outcomes? Two ways of deriving these weights are the **basic reference gamble method** and the **proportional trade-off method.**

In the **basic reference gamble method** the object is to choose the value of the probability p_S, such that the decision maker is indifferent between life in health state S and the gamble giving a chance of p_S full health and a chance of $1-p_S$ of death; that is,

$$S \sim \,<(p_S, \text{Full Health}); (1 - p_S, \text{Death})>.$$

Alternatively, in the **proportional trade-off method** the decision maker answers the following question: "Suppose you are faced with a year in health state S. Taking into account your age, pain and suffering, immobility, and lost earnings, what fraction, p_S, of a fully healthy year of life would you be willing to accept in exchange for the state S for the full year?" The answer, p_S, would then be the weight by which a year in health state S would be valued. The weights derived by either method would lead to a measure of quality-adjusted life years of each possible outcome, and this measure could then be used to rank the outcomes.

With some qualifications, quality-adjusted life years can be used as a utility scale in the precise sense we defined it in Section 7.5. In the next section, we will discuss the assumptions that permit quality-adjusted life years to be treated as a utility scale.

QUALITY-ADJUSTED LIFE YEARS AS A UTILITY SCALE*

A scale of quality-adjusted life years may be a helpful way to structure preferences systematically to compare possible outcomes. In the context of decision analysis and utilities as we have defined them, however, is it appropriate to average out and fold back with quality-adjusted life years, thus, in effect, choosing the strategy with the greatest quality-adjusted life expectancy? We were very careful to define utilities earlier in terms of basic reference gambles and their substitution to yield equivalent decision trees with dichotomous outcomes. Is the number of quality-adjusted life years, as defined by either the proportional trade-off method or the basic reference gamble method, a legitimate utility scale in this very precise sense?

The answer is a qualified yes, but only if a set of very specific characteristics of the individual's preferences apply. These are utility independence, the property of "constant proportional trade-off," and risk neutrality with respect to life years.† Each of these characteristics will be discussed shortly.

You can decide for yourself whether it seems reasonable to expect these conditions to apply or, indeed, whether they come close to describing your own feelings. Even if they seem right for you, this does not mean that they apply to every individual or to every decision-making situation. If they do not apply, then the criterion of quality-adjusted life expectancy must be modified. Later we describe a modification for the case in which you want to be risk averse with respect to longevity (p. 220).

Utility independence means that one's ranking of gambles on one attribute (e.g., life years) does not depend on the level or amount of the other attribute (e.g., health status). For example, if the gamble

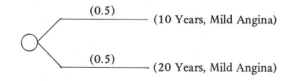

___

*This section is somewhat technical and may be skipped without loss of continuity.
†The mathematically oriented reader interested in a formal proof that these conditions are sufficient may refer to Pliskin et al.[199]

has a certainty equivalent of 14 years with mild angina, then utility independence requires that the gamble

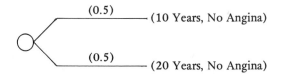

(0.5) — (10 Years, No Angina)

(0.5) — (20 Years, No Angina)

has a certainty equivalent of 14 years with no angina. Moreover, utility independence requires that the utility scale for quality of life, or health status, is the same for any underlying length of life. Thus, if the gamble

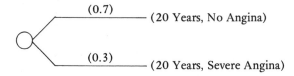

(0.7) — (20 Years, No Angina)

(0.3) — (20 Years, Severe Angina)

has a certainty equivalent of 20 years with *mild* angina, then utility independence requires that the gamble

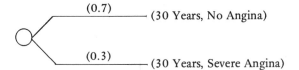

(0.7) — (30 Years, No Angina)

(0.3) — (30 Years, Severe Angina)

has a certainty equivalent of 30 years with *mild* angina. Utility independence means, in short, that utility scales for length of life and quality of life can be specified *independently* rather than *conditionally* upon the level of the other attribute.

Utility independence should not be confused with probabilistic independence as defined in Chapter Three; the probabilities leading to outcomes in an actual decision problem have no bearing on the assessment of utilities, and the two concepts should be kept separate.

The second property required in order for quality-adjusted life years to be a proper utility scale is called the *proportional trade-off property*. This states that one would be willing to give up some fraction of one's life years in order to improve the quality of those years from one level to a preferred level, and that the fraction depends only on the two quality levels and not on the length of life at the outset. Thus, for example, suppose that you are told you have 40 years of life remaining and that you would be willing to give up eight of those years in order to obtain relief from your severe angina pectoris. Then, you are told that you have only 30 years of life remaining. Would you give up six of those years for relief of your angina? If so, and if you would similarly give up one fifth of your life years for such an improvement in quality of life for any underlying length of life, then your preferences satisfy the constant proportional trade-off property.

Risk neutrality with respect to life years was defined earlier and applies to an individual whose utility values are directly proportional to longevity.

One or more of these three assumptions — utility independence, constant proportional trade-off, and risk neutrality — may not reflect your preferences or those of your patient. If not, then it would be, strictly speaking, incorrect to use quality-adjusted life expectancy as a utility scale. On the other hand, these properties may be close enough to your preferences so that it is worth going through the exercise of the analysis to gain the insight it may yield.

ALTERNATIVES TO QUALITY-ADJUSTED LIFE EXPECTANCY

If a decision maker does not want to use quality-adjusted life expectancy as a utility scale but still wants to use a full decision analysis, then we suggest two practical alternatives for carrying out a decision analysis in which both survival and quality of life are considered.

One method, which is always proper, is to revert back to the original definition of a utility scale and to assess each possible outcome in terms of a basic reference gamble between the best and worst outcomes. To make this practical, the number of outcomes considered would, of course, have to be rather small, as in Figure 7–18. The formulation of a decision problem in this way may not be mathematically elegant, but it may yield sufficient insights to obviate the need for a more elaborate analysis.

If the decision maker is unwilling to use quality-adjusted life years as a utility scale because of risk aversion with respect to longevity (e.g., the decision maker prefers a certain 18 years to a 50–50 gamble between 30 years and 10 years), then it is possible to construct a utility scale that accommodates these preferences. One way to do this is to use a concave function of quality-adjusted life years, such as the logarithm or square root, as the utility scale. For example, the curve in Figure 7–16, with quality-adjusted life years on the horizontal axis, would represent a utility scale that would satisfy a risk-averse decision maker.

7.7   UTILITY ASSESSMENT IN CLINICAL SETTINGS

Utility assessment is a means of quantifying a decision maker's preferences in a logically coherent manner so that those preferences can be used to ascertain a preferred clinical strategy. It is a necessary ingredient if decision trees and probability assessments are to be used to their full advantage in realistic decisions involving more than two possible outcomes. Although utility assessment entails some practical limitations and clearly cannot be carried out for all decisions concerning all patients, it raises fundamental issues that every clinician should consider.

LIMITATIONS OF UTILITY ASSESSMENT

The practical limitations of utility assessment in the clinical setting are of four types: (1) variability in an individual's preferences, depending on circumstances; (2) ignorance of the true character of alternative outcomes; (3) lack of familiarity with lotteries and reluctance to think in such terms; and (4) bias introduced by the physician-analyst.

The first problem is that utility estimates obtained under one condition may not apply when conditions are altered. Most serious are changes in preference that may be induced by pain or distress. Some people may feel exactly the same way about possible outcomes regardless of whether they are ill or perceive themselves to be in a life-threatening situation, but others may express very different preferences at such times. There is no completely satisfactory answer to the problem of variable preferences by an individual at different times and under different circumstances.

Second, utilities are expressions of preference among outcome states that the decision maker usually has not personally experienced. If a decision maker has a very wrong notion of what it would mean personally to experience any given outcome, then utility assessments may be correspondingly distorted. This raises the question as to whether the patient or the physician is the more valid source of utility assessments; we return to this question in the next section.

Third, some persons may react negatively to the whole concept of "gambling," and this may inhibit utility assessment. If an individual is willing but unaccustomed to thinking in terms of gambles, it may be difficult to translate felt preferences into utility terms. Chance events are so much a part of our daily lives, however, that this problem may not be encountered too often. The more practice one has with utility assessment, the more readily one can comfortably translate preferences into a utility scale.

One final risk with utility assessment is that the physician-analyst may consciously or unconsciously bias the person whose preferences are being elicited. Patients are especially likely to sense the physician's preferences and be influenced by them.

WHOSE PREFERENCES?

These limitations bring us to a central question: Whose preferences ought to be the basis for clinical decisions, those of the patient or those of the physician? Throughout we have talked about the preferences of the physician or the patient, but there is no reason to expect their values and utility assessments to be the same. Of course, the physician, who has expert knowledge, is the one who must assess probabilities, but who is the appropriate judge of utilities?

In principle, it is tempting to say that of course it is the patient's preferences that matter; after all, it is the patient who is facing the gambles on life and health. On the other hand, can the patient really understand the possible outcomes as well as the physician can? The physician regularly sees patients with many conditions that this patient has never experienced. Who is in the best position to judge the trade-offs between death owing to surgery and a favorable effect on the quality of life, as may be the case in CABG surgery, or between amputation above the knee and below the knee, as in the case of our patient with gangrene?

There may be additional practical considerations that dictate reliance on the physician's utilities or at least the physician's attributions of the patient's preferences. For example, the physician may not want to arouse the patient's concern over a hypothetical outcome that is extremely unlikely. Depending on the patient's mental state, rational assessments may be impossible. The physician may feel that it is improper to be so explicit about a subject as sensitive as trade-offs between life and disability. The patient may not want to participate in such judgments and may be more comfortable placing complete faith in the judgment of the physician.

SOME PRACTICAL INSIGHTS FOR THE CLINICIAN

Despite these limitations and the practical problems of eliciting utility assessments from patients, the clinician can still gain some useful insights for clinical decision making in several ways.

First, family physicians who know patients for many years can be in a better position to estimate their patients' preferences. In fact, an important role of the primary practitioner in referring a patient to a specialist may be to provide this information about the patient's preferences.

Second, research can be done to analyze decisions for classes of patients as opposed to decisions for individual patients. Suppose that you as a clinician had access to an article in which decisions for 30 patients confronting leg amputation were subjected to formal analysis. If these 30 patients expressed a range of possible utility structures, you might at least be able to place bounds on the preferences of your patient and decide on the optimal strategy without making explicit estimates of the patient's unique utilities.

Perhaps the most important insight to be gained by following the logic of decision analysis and confronting the need for utility assessments is that the optimal decision for one patient need not be the same as that for another patient, even if they are identical in terms of history, symptoms, signs, and disease. Their preferences may differ considerably, and this may mean the difference between one treatment and another. The optimal course for the skilled laborer whose angina pectoris precludes physical work might be coronary surgery, while the optimal course for the physically identical but sedentary office clerk might not.

There should be no expectation that everyone will agree on utility assessments. Unlike probability assessments, for which consensus is desirable and for which an underlying "truth" exists by which they may be judged, utility assessments by their nature have no external validity. If the individual patient or physician believes them and understands their implications up to the limits of past and current experiences, then those utility assessments are "correct," and no new scientific evidence of the sort underlying probabilities can alter them.

7.8 SUMMARY OF CHAPTER SEVEN

The decision maker needs to consider explicitly the strength of preferences among possible outcomes whenever more than two final outcomes are possible. Several methods can be used, but only one yields a numerical scale that is appropriate for averaging out and folding back. The method is called **utility assessment,** and the numerical scale is called a **utility scale.**

In utility assessment, the first step is to rank all outcomes from best to worst. Each intermediate outcome is then judged to be equivalent in value to a gamble between the best outcome and the worst outcome. If the outcome is X and the **break-even probability** is p_X, then

$$X \sim <(p_X, \text{Best}); (1 - p_X, \text{Worst})>.$$

The number p_X, whose value is between 0 and 1, is called the **utility** of X, or $u(X)$.

Utilities are then substituted for outcomes at the tips of decision trees. When averaged out and folded back, these trees will yield the decision strategy once the **basic reference gambles,** with their appropriate break-even probabilities, have been substituted for all intermediate outcomes.

Other methods to elicit preferences among outcomes, which are usually variations of direct scaling methods, have been used. These approaches lack a sound interpretation in decision-analytic terms and may lead to inconsistencies in decision making.

Utility scales can be transformed into different units of measurement (other than a scale ranging from 0 to 1) without changing their essential properties. Such a transformation is analogous to converting from Celsius to Fahrenheit on the temperature scale. Conversion of the units of measure makes possible the use of life years, or quality-adjusted life years, as a utility scale.

Utility judgments may be unnecessary in rare instances in which one alternative strategy **probabilistically dominates** others. To test for probabilistic dominance, all outcomes are ranked from best to worst and the probability of achieving each outcome by following each decision option is noted. One option dominates a second if its cumulative probability of reaching a given or worse outcome is always less than the second option's cumulative probability of reaching the same outcomes. When probabilistic dominance does not hold, it may be useful to do a **sensitivity analysis** or **threshold analysis** to see how variations in utilities might affect the decision strategy.

In more complicated clinical problems, outcomes may include many possible levels along two or more attributes, such as longevity and quality of life. In these situations it may be possible to reduce the problem to a single utility scale, given that certain assumptions are satisfied. Quality-adjusted life years may be used as a utility scale, so long as the individual is risk neutral with respect to life years, attaches value to the quality of life independently of the length of life and vice versa, and is willing to trade a constant proportion of longevity to achieve a given improvement in the quality of life regardless of the number of years of life remaining.

A fundamental question raised by utility assessment is, "Whose values are to be represented, the patient's or the physician's?" It would seem desirable for physicians to assess the probabilities of events and for patients to assess their own utilities. A number of practical problems may arise in trying to use a patient's own utilities, including the patient's mental state, ignorance of the true meaning of possible outcomes, and a spoken or unspoken desire to have the physician take responsibility for all decisions. Therefore, a physician might try to infer the patient's utilities from personal attributes or other insights into the patient's personality and to apply these on behalf of the patient. Again, sensitivity analysis will be valuable.

Unlike probabilities, for which an underlying truth exists and consensus may be desirable, there is no way to externally validate utility assessments and no reason to expect one person's utilities to be the same as another's.

EXERCISES FOR CHAPTER SEVEN

EXERCISES FOR SECTION 7.2

In Chapter Three, Section 3.4, we evaluated the problem of deciding on surgery for patients with possible appendicitis in terms of mortality. This is only one, albeit very important, possible outcome measure. We might also analyze the impact of alternative decision strategies on the expected costs of care.

Assume that the cost of six hours of observation in the emergency unit is $60. The average hospital cost for surgery and care of patients with perforated appendices is $3,000. The average cost for surgery and care of patients with inflamed or nondiseased appendices is about $1,500. If you based your decision of whether to operate on expected mortality, as shown in Figure 3–10, what would be the expected financial costs of observing patients for six hours before deciding whether to operate?

2. *Life Expectancy on Kidney Dialysis*

For a cohort of patients beginning a kidney dialysis program, the probabilities of surviving each year are given in Table 7–2. What is the life expectancy of this cohort at the time they begin dialysis? (Assume that each patient lives until the end of the year in which death occurs.)

TABLE 7–2 SURVIVAL PROBABILITIES FOR A COHORT OF
PATIENTS BEGINNING KIDNEY DIALYSIS

END OF YEAR	PROBABILITY OF SURVIVAL
0	1.00
1	0.80
2	0.72
3	0.64
4	0.56
5	0.49
6	0.42
7	0.36
8	0.30
9	0.25
10	0.21
11	0.17
12	0.13
13	0.10
14	0.08
15	0.06
16	0.05
17	0.04
18	0.03
19	0.02
20	0.01
21	0.01
22	0.01
23	0.00

EXERCISES FOR SECTION 7.3

3. *Threshold Analyses for the Amputation Example*
a. In the amputation example of Figure 7–1, suppose $u(A)$ equals 0.95, $u(C)$ equals 1.0, and $u(D)$ equals 0.0. For what range of $u(B)$ would delaying surgery be the preferred course of action? Interpret the meaning of $u(B)$.

b. In the same example, suppose $u(B)$ equals 0.99, $u(C)$ equals 1.0, and $u(D)$ equals 0.0. For what range of $u(A)$ would delaying surgery be the preferred course of action?

c. Suppose that, in the same example, a given patient has the following utilities: $u(C)$ equals 1.0, $u(B)$ equals 0.99, $u(A)$ equals 0.95, and $u(D)$ equals 0.0. Would this patient prefer to lose his leg below the knee for certain or to take a chance consisting of a 0.75 probability of total cure and a 0.25 probability of loss of the leg above the knee (with no possibility of death)?

4. *Surgery for Duodenal Ulcer*
Refer to Figure 7–2 for the structure of the choice between surgical procedures for duodenal ulcer.

a. Describe how you, as the analyst, would get a patient or a physician to assign utilities to the several outcomes. Write a dialogue that illustrates your approach.

b. Assume, as we have, that the outcome of recurrence has the same value whether it follows gastrectomy, vagotomy, or no surgery. Assess your *own* utilities and determine your preferred course of action.

c. Dr. Bard Parker agrees with the probability assessments given in the decision tree (Figure 7–2) but still prefers gastrectomy. What must be true of his utilities? (Continue to assume the same utility for recurrence regardless of the choice of operation.)

d. A medical intern also accepts the probabilities but prefers no surgery at all. What must be true of the intern's utilities?

5. *A Longshoreman with Claudication*
One of your patients, a 52-year-old longshoreman, is unable to work because of the development of severe pain in his right leg whenever he undertakes his usual level of job-related exertion. Your diagnosis is claudication. One option is to insert an arterial graft to improve circulation, but there are several risks. First, although it is a relatively safe procedure, the surgery does carry with it a risk of operative mortality. Second, the graft may fail, resulting in the necessity of amputating the leg. (The amputation itself would then carry its own risk of death.) And, of course, the graft surgery may simply fail to relieve the symptoms. Without surgery the patient would have to live with the pain, most likely for the rest of his life.
You assess the following probabilities. Without surgery there is a certainty of continued symptoms (S). With surgery there is an 80 per cent chance of relief (R), a 12 per cent chance of no change in symptoms, a 6 per cent chance of graft failure with the need to amputate, and a 2 per cent chance of operative death (D). Assume that operative mortality from amputation is 4 per cent and that the outcome following a successful amputation is the loss of limb above the knee (A).

a. Draw a decision tree for this problem.

b. Identify the four possible outcomes and impute utilities to them that might reasonably reflect this patient's preferences. Using these utilities, determine the optimal decision.

c. Suppose that a utility of 0.9 for amputation (A) and of 0.95 for continued symptoms (S) leads you to conclude that the preferred decision is to operate. The next month, a 55-year-old executive and devoted golfer comes to you with similar symptoms. He finds himself unable to play golf because of the development of severe pain in the calves of his legs whenever he walks more than 200 yards. The decision problem is the same as for the longshoreman, and you assess the same probabilities of outcome. Explain, using the utilities in the decision tree, why it might be best not to operate on this patient.

d. Do a sensitivity analysis to determine over what range of utilities surgery is indicated for a patient with symptoms of claudication under the assumptions given.

EXERCISE FOR SECTION 7.6

6. *Kidney Dialysis and Transplantation*
   Assume that a patient undergoing dialysis faces a remaining life expectancy of 10 years. The same patient, given a kidney transplant, would have a 20 per cent chance of dying during surgery. If the patient survives the operation, he faces a 40 per cent chance of losing the transplanted kidney within one year. If he survives the operation and loses the kidney, he undergoes dialysis, and his total life expectancy (including the first year) is 10 years; if he survives the operation and keeps the kidney, his life expectancy is 12.5 years. Assume that if the patient is to lose the transplanted kidney, he will do so within the first year.

   The health status of a patient during the remaining years of life may fall into one of four quality levels:[197]

T_1. The patient is carrying a successful transplant. He is working full time and has returned to his prior level of activity.

T_2. The patient is carrying a successful transplant. He has multiple physical or emotional problems or both. There are limitations on his activity.

D_1. The patient is undergoing dialysis. He is working full time and has returned to near his prior level of activity.

D_2. The patient is undergoing dialysis. He has multiple physical or emotional problems or both. There are limitations on his activity.

A patient carrying a transplant has a 60 per cent chance of having a health status of quality T_1 and a 40 per cent chance of having a health status of quality T_2; a patient undergoing dialysis has a 50 per cent chance of having a health status of quality D_1 and a 50 per cent chance of having a health status of quality D_2.

A physician estimates that a typical patient would be indifferent between

i. ten years of life with quality T_2 and six years of life with quality T_1;

ii. eight years of life with quality D_2 and four years of life with quality D_1; and

iii. ten years of life with quality D_1 and eight years of life with quality T_1.

In answering the following questions, define one year of quality-adjusted life as a year spent at quality level T_1, and assume that the proportional trade-off assumption holds.

a. What is the quality-adjusted life expectancy for a patient undergoing dialysis?

b. What is the quality-adjusted life expectancy for a patient who survives a transplant operation and accepts the kidney?

c. What is the quality-adjusted life expectancy for a patient who survives a transplant operation?

d. What is the quality-adjusted life expectancy for a patient given a transplant?

e. Compare your answer for part a to that for part d, and interpret the result.

f. The most difficult value trade-off is the comparison between the quality of life with dialysis and the quality of life with a transplant. This trade-off is described by statement iii. Perform a threshold analysis indicating how the trade-off in statement iii would have to change in order to change the decision that gives the higher quality-adjusted life expectancy. (Assume that the trade-offs in i and ii still apply.)

Chapter Eight

Clinical Decisions and Limited Resources

8.1 LIMITED RESOURCES FOR MEDICAL CARE

Medical care entails benefits, risks, and costs. Until this chapter our approach has involved weighing benefits against risks for individuals and groups of patients and choosing the actions that provide the greatest expected net benefit. Now we extend our analysis to consider expressly the economic costs of health care.

As with all economic goods and services, the provision of medical care consumes resources. Hospital beds and equipment, medications, medical devices, and the time of physicians, nurses, and other health workers all contribute to medical care. The consumption of these resources constitutes the economic costs of medical care.

Sometimes the term *cost* refers to any negative effect of an action. For example, one might say that a drug's side effects are costs of gaining its benefits. But we shall be careful (and have been careful throughout this book) to use *costs* only in the specific economic sense of resources consumed.

Real resource consumption is different from the transfer of resources from one party to another: The distribution of costs is an important but separate issue from their realization. If the government sends a check to a pharmacist as reimbursement for a Medicaid prescription, this in itself does not constitute a resource cost, because the resource pool is in no way depleted. A cost occurs because the drug is produced and consumed, regardless of whether the patient, the pharmacist, the manufacturer, or the government actually pays for it.

Definition. Costs of medical services are the economic resources (such as equipment, supplies, professional and nonprofessional labor, and the use of buildings) consumed in the provision of those services.

Resources available for medical care are limited in supply. This means that whenever resources are used for one activity, they are not available for other activities. An hour of a physician's time spent with one patient is unavailable for another patient. A hospital bed occupied by one patient cannot be used that day for another patient. Society can add to the resources devoted to health care by training more doctors, for example, or producing more hospital beds, but even in the longer term, resources available for health care will be finite. Any medical decision that entails the use of resources implicitly excludes those resources from alternative possible uses.

Health resources are consumed in order to produce health benefits. Given the limited availability of resources, we are led naturally to ask questions about their most efficient use: "Is this particular expenditure of health resources worthwhile, given the alternative uses to which they might be put?"

Our aim in this chapter is to introduce the conceptual and analytic issues surrounding decisions that involve the allocation of health resources. We will begin by considering different perspectives on health costs and benefits, an exercise that raises dilemmas for doctors, patients, and society. Then we will introduce the principles underlying the efficient allocation of limited resources and discuss the measurement of resource costs and health benefits. We will describe cost-effectiveness and benefit-cost analysis, two methods for analyzing alternative allocations of limited resources. By the end of the chapter, you should comprehend the rationale underlying such analyses, be able to assess them critically, and understand the potential for different conclusions about preferred medical actions and programs when resource costs are ignored and when they are included.

8.2 PERSPECTIVES ON HEALTH CARE: WHO PAYS AND WHO GAINS

So long as we have been concerned with the balance between risks and benefits of different medical decisions (and not with their resource costs), we have encountered no unresolvable conflicts of interest among different decision makers. To be sure, in thinking systematically about individual patient decisions we were concerned about differences between the patient and the physician as decision makers. These differences did not arise from different vested interests, but rather from the lack of complementary information: The physician does not know the values of the individual patient, and the patient does not have the medical knowledge of the physician.

Introducing concern about health resources brings additional perspectives into play, including various health care institutions, insurers, and government. Above all, economic concerns bring into play the perspective of "society," or the aggregate of all patients present and future. All decision makers have their own views of resource costs, because health expenditures affect each differently. Indeed, what is considered an expense by one may be a saving or financial gain for others.

For our purposes, the most salient potential conflict arises between individual patient interests and societal interests. Analyses of resource allocation decisions are normally undertaken from the societal perspective. When such analyses suggest health care choices different from those that would be chosen by individual patients, this presents a dilemma for physicians and other medical decision makers. Further analysis can clarify but not resolve such conflicts in values and perspectives.

PATIENTS INDIVIDUALLY

At the time they receive medical care, individual patients are concerned with costs only to the extent that the individual is responsible for payment. The great majority of Americans have insurance for hospital care, and a growing number have nonhospital health insurance as well. The insured individual pays only when there are deductibles, coinsurance, and limits on coverage, which are sometimes a small fraction of the total costs. The individual use of services may ultimately result in higher insurance premiums for the insured group, but the large number of insured people dilutes the personal impact of an individual's expenses. For example, suppose that a patient incurs a $10,000 expense and that there are 100,000 people in the insured group. The personal burden for this added cost is $10,000 divided by 100,000 subscribers, or $0.10. Thus, at the time health services are contemplated, the insured individual has little disincentive to use health care resources and can act as if they were practically unlimited, or costless.

PATIENTS COLLECTIVELY, OR SOCIETY

On the surface it appears contradictory to assert that the collective interests of all patients can differ from their individual interests. After all, the collective interests should simply be the sum of individual interests. Indeed, earlier in this book we stressed the substitutability of population-based frequencies for probabilities applied to an individual. Why should the relation between populations and individuals be any different when resources are at stake?

The interests of society do differ from the sum of individual interests because health resources are limited, the potential demand for health services exceeds the available resource supply, and health benefits (such as longer life) attained by one individual are not directly transferable to others.

Acting in their own interest as patients, individuals would seek any health service that promises an expected positive benefit. Let us posit two patients, A and B, who stand to benefit personally from utilizing, respectively, treatment I and treatment II, each of which would consume $100 worth of health services. Let us further assume that the expected benefit is not the same for each: Patient A stands to gain one year of life from treatment I, while patient B stands to gain one and a half years from treatment II. Now we would obviously like to provide services to both patients. But suppose we are down to our last $100 worth of services (and the required treatments are not divisible). Given a choice, either patient would opt to receive the needed services (unless knowledge of the other's need led the patient to act altruistically). But if an independent judge could decide, which patient should receive the services?

The "fairness" of choosing to treat one patient over the other in this imaginary example might be rationalized by recourse to a principle of social justice called the original position.[208] Suppose that neither A nor B is yet in need of treatment but that both know they have the same chances of later requiring either of the two treatments. If they had to choose only one treatment to be made available, they would both agree, in this original position, that the treatment offering one and a half years of life (II) should be chosen. They could agree on this if the choice were made before they knew who would require which treatment. Once it is known that patient B is the one who stands to benefit, the original agreement would turn to the advantage of B, but from the perspective of the original position it might just as well have benefited A.

If the judge wants to make a decision based on the original position argument and in this way do the most social good with the last bit of health resources, the resources would go to patient B. That decision would yield an additional half year of human life expectancy (one and a half years for B compared with one year for A). In the interests of equity, the judge might wish that it were possible to assign three quarters of a year of life expectancy from patient B to patient A, but that is not in the nature of health benefits: They go to one patient *or* to the other and cannot be transferred.

In the imaginary example just described, the socially preferred decision is contrary to the best interests of patient A. In real-world decisions to allocate health resources, the limit on total resources may be less tangible and the availability and effects of alternative uses of resources may be less apparent. Surely some resources are now wasted on ineffective or harmful practices, and if they were redirected, individuals as well as society would benefit. Even so, the resources devoted to health care are finite, if enormous, and a constraint on their total prohibits every individual from obtaining every health service that promises an expected positive benefit.

If society wishes to advance the objective of attaining the greatest collective benefit from available resources, the members of society will want to allocate resources according to their effectiveness in alternative applications. This desire motivates the effort to conduct cost-effectiveness and benefit-cost analyses in order to inform these social resource allocation decisions. Beyond analysis, the obstacles to socially optimal resource allocation include finding an acceptable rationing device and, even more difficult, finding an acceptable institutional structure within which to implement it.

PHYSICIANS

Traditionally, the physician is dedicated to the interests of the individual patient and undertakes to do everything possible to benefit the patient without much concern for cost. A physician takes one patient at a time and is not concerned with the fact that, from a societal point of view, resources spent for one patient are resources that are not available to someone else. As patients obtain more insurance, the physician (as well as the individual) is even less inclined to consider cost. And, of course, resources spent on physician services benefit the doctor directly.

At times, physicians do readily make choices among patients when the trade-offs are immediate, pressing, and tangible. If the coronary care unit is full and a patient arrives in the emergency room with a suspected myocardial infarction, that patient's needs must be weighed against the needs of others already in the unit. If two hospitalized patients suffer acute renal failure and only one dialysis machine is available, it is not a matter of "my patient" versus a distant, faceless statistic; instead, it is a choice among real, identified candidates for treatment.

A physician who tries to be sensitive to societal resource consumption as well as to individual patient needs is caught in an uncomfortable dilemma. Individually, we want *our* physicians to act in our interests to the best of their abilities. Collectively, members of society may not want physicians to act solely in the interests of the patient at hand if the aggregate of such behavior works to the detriment of all. This is the crux of the dilemma physicians face in the divergence of interests between patients individually and patients collectively. In countries with national health plans, resources may be explicitly allocated to areas of medical need and restricted from other areas. By virtue of their professional training and in their own interest, physicians are reluctant to limit the use of resources in treating patients unless they are pressed by the exigencies of forced rationing.

This is not to say that the physician necessarily acts in ways that are perfectly consonant with the interests of individual patients. For example, patient waiting time is a cost to the patient but not to the physician and is not typically a prime concern of the doctor. Physicians may also find it possible to conserve their own time (and generate greater revenue) by heavier reliance on laboratory tests, at perhaps some inconvenience to the individual and resource cost to society.

HOSPITALS

Hospitals have many objectives, including high quality patient care, community service, institutional prestige, employee satisfaction, and financial stability. Only a minority of hospitals (for example, approximately 10 per cent of general hospitals in the United States) are in business to make a profit, but all hospitals must be concerned with their own revenues and expenditures. Those revenues and expenditures reflect the consumption of health resources.

Each hospital, in pursuing its own best fiscal interest, may not use society's health resources in the most efficient manner. For example, when a hospital's bed occupancy rate declines, administrators may encourage staff physicians to admit more patients. Without a patient in the bed, no patient or insurer can be billed for days of care, but the hospital still must pay substantial fixed costs associated with an empty bed. From society's viewpoint, an empty bed costs less than an occupied bed, and the admission of patients for marginally valid reasons represents a resource loss to society but a revenue gain for the hospital. As a second example, a small or medium-sized hospital may find it financially advantageous as well as convenient to perform nearly all of its own laboratory determinations. Yet a small or medium-sized laboratory tends to consume more resources per test than larger, more efficient laboratories. This is due mainly to economies that can be gained from highly automated equipment given sufficiently large testing volumes. More societal resources may be consumed by smaller, separate laboratories, but that arrangement helps assure that each hospital's revenues will exceed its costs.

The exact financial incentives acting on a hospital will depend on the mix of payers it bills, particular arrangements with different third-party payers, and any rate regulations under which it operates. Various hospitals thus face very different economic pressures, but their range and variety are not our main concerns here. What does concern us is that hospitals, as individual, fiscally responsible institutions, may tend to employ society's health resources in less than the most efficient way. An analysis of costs and benefits according to a hospital's point of view might thus look very different from an analysis according to society's view.

GOVERNMENT AGENCIES

In discussing various perspectives on costs and benefits, we have stressed the differences and potential conflicts between individual interests and societal interests. One rationale for government intervention in the health care system is the promotion of the allocation of resources in the collective interest of the population of patients and potential patients. Just as physicians may be viewed as agents for individual patients, so government agencies that plan and regulate the distribution of medical services may be viewed as agents for society. In the same way that physicians often act in their own interests, however, government agencies develop bureaucratic and organizational objectives that may not be consonant with the broader public interest. Aside from particular health agencies, the larger government decision-making apparatus has an enormous effect on the resources to be allocated to medical care by virtue of choices among health, education, defense, and other societal needs.

Patients individually and collectively, physicians, hospitals, and government agencies have distinctive views of health costs and benefits. Other decision makers, such as insurers, prepaid group practices, and nonhospital institutional providers, also have their own perspectives. Our purpose in presenting the various viewpoints is not to conclude that some are right and others are wrong but to assert the differences and the importance of bearing them in mind when trying to analyze decisions in which resources count. The policy analyst may prefer a societal perspective, but policy recommendations derived from such analysis would still have to be adopted and implemented by such agencies, institutions, and individuals as those discussed.

8.3 THE EFFICIENT ALLOCATION OF LIMITED RESOURCES

The analytic methods we present in this chapter are premised on a desire to use available resources to gain the most benefit. In this section we will present the principles underlying the efficient allocation of resources and compare two approaches, cost-effectiveness and benefit-cost analysis. These methods presume fixed resources and require knowledge of the differential benefit from alternative uses of those resources. The analyses need not be done in monetary terms, as any scarce medical resource might be the object of analysis, and our first example addresses the allocation of physician time without reference to money. The second example includes both physician time and other resources and demonstrates concretely how concern for costs can alter decisions of patient care.

THE ALLOCATION OF PHYSICIANS' TIME

Physicians in clinical practice know they cannot spend as much time with every patient as might be ideal. A busy physician who is concerned with the health of all patients has to pick and choose how much time to allocate to each patient problem. Time that is spent treating one problem is time that is not spent treating another.

Let us say that the physician's objective is to maximize the overall health benefits to patients, given a limit, for example, of 50 working hours per week. Let us also suppose that the physician has estimated the impact of care on each patient in terms of the expected number of days of disability prevented. Each patient consumes a certain amount of the limited time available. Hypothetical information of this kind is given in Table 8–1.

TABLE 8–1 HYPOTHETICAL HEALTH BENEFITS AND TIME
REQUIREMENTS FOR PATIENT PROBLEMS

PATIENT PROBLEM	EXPECTED HEALTH BENEFIT (B) (DAYS OF DISABILITY PREVENTED)	TIME REQUIRED (T) (HOURS)	TIME-EFFECTIVENESS RATIO (B/T)
A	5	10	0.5
B	1	5	0.2
C	2	40	0.05
D	0.1	1	0.1
E	0	2	0
F	4	10	0.4
G	4	2	2.0
H	10	1	10.0
I	50	20	2.5
J	10	10	1.0
K	5	1	5.0
L	9	3	3.0
M	1	5	0.2
N	1.5	3	0.5

In order to maximize total benefit, the physician should allocate time to patient problems according to the amount of benefits provided per unit of time required, or "time-effectiveness." Thus, in the table the most time-effective use is the allocation of the physician's time to patient problem H, which results in an expected benefit of ten days of disability prevented but consumes only one hour of physician time. The next most time-effective use is the allocation of the physician's time to problem K, which has a time-effectiveness ratio of 5.0. The best decision rule for the physician to follow in meeting the objective is to establish priorities according to this ratio and to treat problems in decreasing order of priority (in descending order of the time-effectiveness ratio) until the available time is exhausted.

In the example given in Table 8–1, the rank order is H, K, L, I, G, J, a tie for A and N, F, a tie for B and M, D, C, and E. Since H, K, L, I, G, J, A, and N occupy the available 50 hours, the remainder are not treated. Note that problem C would gain more benefit than N but that the high time requirement for C renders it a time-ineffective undertaking. Note also that problem E would never be undertaken because the expected benefit from treatment is nil. To be sure, the physician can expand the hours to see more patients, but at some point the line will be drawn, and in general the line must be drawn well above the point at which benefit falls to zero. This would be especially so if patient satisfaction and reassurance were counted among the benefits.

Other examples of this sort of allocation that physicians regularly perform include triage in an emergency room and the allocation of intensive care unit beds. The same principles of ranking in terms of resource-effectiveness and choosing according to the order of greatest efficiency would apply.

TIME AND MONEY: SURGERY FOR PANCREATIC CANCER VERSUS SCREENING FOR COLON CANCER

This second example compares alternative uses of medical resources and takes into account their costs in terms of dollars. The clinical situations are intentionally simplified to make the comparison more clear.

First, we will consider the decision to perform palliative surgery for patients with adenocarcinoma of the pancreas. In this severely ill population, we will assume the operative mortality to be 58 per cent and the mean duration of life for patients surviving surgery to be 134 days.[65] Although the operation is palliative, assume for the sake of discussion that the objective is to maximize the expected number of days of life saved. What is not known is the expected number of days of survival resulting from nonsurgical care. We want to calculate, then, the duration of survival resulting from nonsurgical treatment that would shift the decision in favor of or opposition to surgery.

One approach to this calculation is to find the expected number of days of survival without surgery (call this number X) that makes us indifferent between surgery and no surgery. Then, any length of survival less than X makes surgery preferable, while any length of survival greater than X makes the nonsurgical alternative preferable.

A decision tree for this problem is shown in Figure 8–1. To find the indifference point, average out the two main branches, set the two expected values on either side of an algebraic equation, and solve for X. Thus,

$$(1.00) (X) = (0.58) (0) + (0.42) (134),$$

or

$$X = 56.28.$$

Therefore, if the expected survival time without surgery is greater than 56.28 days, no surgery is the preferred choice. If the expected survival time without surgery is less than 56.28 days, then surgery is preferable. This conclusion does

Figure 8–1 A simplified decision tree for the patient with pancreatic cancer.

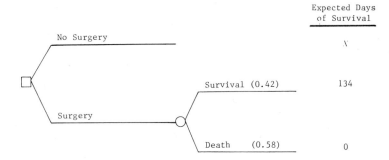

not consider outcomes other than the length of survival (e.g., the quality of the days of survival) and implicitly assumes that they either are of no concern or would be equal under both decisions. The analysis also assumes that the decision maker is risk neutral with respect to the number of days of survival (see Chapter Seven).

This analysis is based only on the health outcome to the individual patient; thus far we have not considered the cost of the resources used. If the resources are limited, then those spent on surgery for this patient cannot be spent on care for another patient with another present or potential health problem. Viewed this way, the choice is for the surgeon to perform an operation in this situation or to release the time and resources for the treatment of other patients. In short, we want to consider the population of patients that this physician might treat and the **opportunity cost** of the physician's time and other resources.

Definition. The **opportunity cost** of a resource is the value of benefits forgone by failing to apply the resource to the most productive alternative use.

Assume that the next best use of the physician's time and resources would be in the outpatient department performing sigmoidoscopies on asymptomatic patients between the ages of 50 and 80 to screen for cancer of the colon. Suppose that this alternative results in the detection of one case of colon cancer for every 2,000 sigmoidoscopies performed at a cost of $25 per examination and that the detection of such a cancer will, on the average, save four years of that patient's life. The cost per year of life saved is then

$$(\$25) \, (2,000)/4 = \$12,500.$$

(Surgical costs for removal of the colon cancer found are not included, because we assume surgery will occur sooner or later whether this cancer is found early or not. In general, a cost analysis need include only costs that vary depending upon the decision.)

With the availability of this alternative use of resources, the decision rule for patients with carcinoma of the pancreas should be adjusted in light of the comparative costs and benefits of surgical treatment for those patients.

Assume that the cost of surgical care is $6,000 if the patient dies during surgery and $20,000 if the patient survives and that the resource cost of managing the condition without surgery is $10,000, including a physician's time and supporting services. Given these costs, how short must survival time without surgery be so that surgery for pancreatic cancer is preferred? When we worked out this example without regard for opportunity costs, we wanted to operate as long as the expected survival time was longer for surgical than for nonsurgical management. Now, however, we want to operate only as long as the cost per year of life saved by performing surgery is less than the cost per year of life saved by screening for colon cancer.

Figure 8–2 shows a decision tree to solve for the longest survival time without surgery (Y) such that surgery would still be preferred. We want to calculate the value of Y for which the cost per year of life saved is just $12,500, the same as the cost per year of life saved by sigmoidoscopy. Now, the expected dollar cost with surgery is

$$(0.58) \, (\$6,000) + (0.42) \, (\$20,000) =$$

$$\$3,480 + \$8,400 = \$11,880.$$

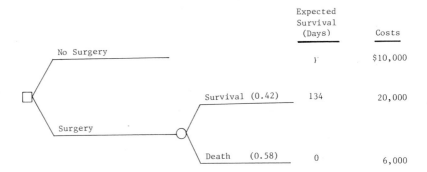

Figure 8–2 A simplified decision tree for the patient with pancreatic cancer, in which the cost of resources is taken into account.

The expected survival time with surgery is

$$(0.58)(0) + (0.42)(134) = 56.28 \text{ days}.$$

The expected cost and survival time without surgery are, respectively, $10,000 and Y. Hence, the cost per year of life saved when surgery is performed compared with that when surgery is not performed is

$$\frac{\text{the difference in costs between surgery and no surgery}}{\text{the difference in survival time between surgery and no surgery}}$$

$$= \frac{\$11,880 - \$10,000}{(56.28 - Y)/365} .$$

At the indifference value of Y, this ratio, the cost per year of life saved, is equal to that of the next best use of resources, which is $12,500. Solving the equation,

$$\frac{\$11,880 - \$10,000}{(56.28 - Y)/365} = \$12,500,$$

we obtain Y equals 1.384 days. Hence, if survival time without surgery is more than 1.384 days, then surgery should not be performed and the physician should spend time in the outpatient department looking for colon cancer. If survival time without surgery is less than 1.384 days, then surgery should be performed.

As Y increases from 1.384 days to 56.28 days, the cost per year of life saved by surgery increases from $12,500 to infinity. This is because a survival time of more than 56.28 days resulting from nonsurgical treatment would make surgery undesirable even if it were absolutely free. The relationship can be graphed as shown in Figure 8–3.

Thus, we find that the indifference point between surgery and no surgery when the physician considers alternative uses of time and resources is very different from the indifference point when the alternatives are ignored. For one patient alone the physician could spend an unlimited amount of time per unit of benefit; when the alternatives are considered, the physician will spend only up to that amount of time at which resources otherwise used could yield more benefits.

This analysis, we repeat, oversimplifies the clinical problem. For one thing,

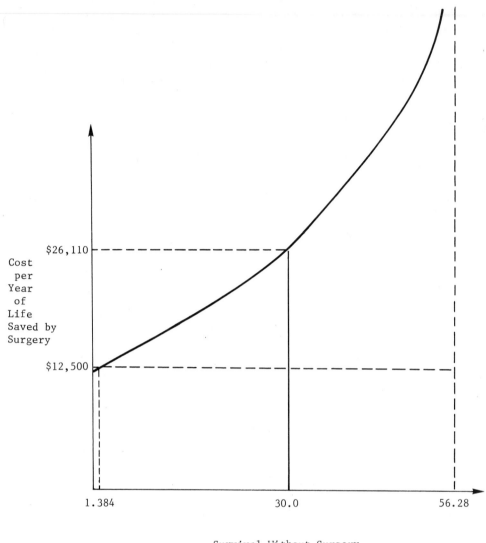

Figure 8–3 *The cost per year of life saved by surgery as a function of survival time without surgery.*

it does not consider differences in the quality of life. One might wish to weigh differently a day of life at home with symptomatic relief and a day in the hospital without relief. The survival time associated with surgical mortality is indicated as zero, whereas, in fact, it may be hours or several days. The analysis gives equal weight to survival for the first day after surgery as for the one hundredth day past surgery. Some of these issues can be dealt with by utility analysis (e.g., valuation in terms of quality-adjusted years of life, as described in Chapter Seven) and by the use of discounting, as described later in this chapter (p. 248).

COST-EFFECTIVENESS AND BENEFIT-COST ANALYSIS

Cost-effectiveness analysis and benefit-cost (or cost-benefit) analysis are two related but distinct approaches to the assessment of health practices. Benefit-cost analysis is intended to compare investments in different programs and proceeds to value all outcomes, including mortality and morbidity, in the same economic (usually, monetary) terms. Cost-effectiveness analysis is intended to determine the most efficient or productive use of limited resources, and it does not require that a monetary value of life and health be assessed. The two approaches are frequently confused, and many analyses that technically measure cost-effectiveness are labeled "cost-benefit analyses."

Cost-Effectiveness Analysis

The underlying premise of **cost-effectiveness analysis** in health problems is that, for any given level of resources available, the decision maker wishes to maximize the aggregate health benefits conferred to the population of concern. (This was assumed in the examples presented earlier.) Alternatively, a given health benefit goal may be set, the objective being to minimize the cost of achieving it. In either formulation the analytic methodology is the same. First, health benefits and health resource costs must each be expressed in terms of some unit of measurement. Health resource costs are usually measured in monetary terms but might equivalently be expressed in units of hospital days or hours of physician time. Health effectiveness (or health benefit) is expressed in terms of some unit of output, such as the number of cases of cancer detected, or in terms of a measure of ultimate outcome, such as the number of lives or years of life saved. The use of quality-adjusted years of life has the advantage of incorporating changes in survival and morbidity in a single measure that reflects trade-offs between them.

The cost-effectiveness measure is the ratio of costs to benefits and is expressed, for example, as the cost per year of life saved or the cost per quality-adjusted year of life saved. Alternative programs or services are ranked from the lowest value of this cost-per-effect ratio to the highest, and then they are selected starting with the highest ranked program or service until available resources are exhausted. The point on the priority list at which the available resources are exhausted, or at which one is no longer willing to pay the price for the benefits achieved, becomes the cutoff level of permissible cost per unit of effectiveness. For example, the level of blood pressure at which antihypertensive treatment is recommended might be based on the corresponding cost-effectiveness cutoff level.[272] The application of this procedure ensures that the maximum possible expected health benefits will be realized, subject to whatever resource constraint is in effect. A limitation of this approach, however, is that comparisons cannot be made between programs or activities with diffferent outputs.

Benefit-Cost Analysis

The **benefit-cost** approach measures all units of output in monetary terms and thereby allows the comparison of programs and activities with widely differing outputs. Presumably, Congress and the President must decide on the amount to be spent on health, education, defense, energy, transportation, and other areas. Implicitly, they must compare very different outcomes. Benefit-cost analysis attempts to make explicit the comparisons across such diverse programs.

Applying benefit-cost analysis to health practices requires converting years of life saved into a monetary value, as will be discussed in Section 8.5. Once benefits and costs have been expressed in monetary terms, net benefits are derived as the difference between the two: If these are positive, the argument goes, the program or practice should be undertaken; if they are negative, it should not.

The major disadvantage of the benefit-cost framework is the requirement that human lives and the quality of life be valued in monetary units. Many decision makers find this difficult or unethical and do not trust analyses that depend upon such valuations. Cost-effectiveness analysis, on the other hand, requires only that health outcomes be expressed in commensurate units (e.g., years of life or quality-adjusted years of life). An advantage of the benefit-cost framework is that costs can be subtracted from benefits, which leads to a positive or negative number (or zero) for each program or practice evaluated. Therefore, benefit-cost analysis does not require knowledge of a cost-effectiveness cutoff level to decide whether a particular practice should be undertaken.

Finally, a limitation of both approaches is that the benefits and costs to different individuals must be aggregated. If the equitable distribution of benefits and costs among individuals or groups is of concern, a single cost-effectiveness measure or benefit-cost calculation will not suffice.

In the remainder of this chapter we will discuss in some detail the measurement of resource costs and health benefits and provide additional examples of analysis in which resources are treated as limited.

8.4   THE MEASUREMENT OF RESOURCE COST

Resources used for one patient are unavailable for use elsewhere. It is this consumption of resources for a patient that constitutes the cost of care. In economic terms, resource costs are valued by their opportunity cost. Although this is a good idea in theory, opportunity costs are not often easy to estimate. In this section we will discuss the meaning and practical measurement of health resource costs.

THE COMPONENTS OF RESOURCE COST

Resource costs for a health service or practice may be considered to have two major components: (1) production costs and (2) induced costs (and savings).

The production costs include direct costs, such as the services of professional and paraprofessional personnel, equipment, and materials, as well as indirect or overhead costs, such as maintenance, electricity, and administration. **Direct costs** are those that are wholly attributable to the service in question. **Indirect costs** are based on costs that are shared by many services concurrently; the indirect costs for one service are the portion of the shared costs attributed to that service.

Induced costs and savings are resource expenditures that are added or averted on account of the initial service or procedure. These induced effects are manifest through changes in the subsequent evaluation and treatment of a patient following the initial service. For example, there may be savings in medical care owing to the prevention of subsequent morbidity that would have required evaluation and treatment. If a procedure has side effects, there may be costs in treating such iatrogenic conditions. Finally, if treatment results in prolonged life because a condition has been cured or early disease has been avoided, then the cost of treating later disease that would not otherwise have arisen must be considered.

For example, a patient who survives a heart attack may subsequently develop cancer. This is not to say that the net effect is negative but simply that the cost of treating the cancer must be counted as a cost, while the benefit of prolonged life is counted on the health benefit side.

The components of health resource costs are summarized in Table 8–2. Note that these costs do not include adverse health effects, such as premature death. Such adverse consequences are not health care resource costs. Instead, they are counted as debits against net health effects, that is, as negative benefits. We will discuss the valuation of benefits in Section 8.5.

TABLE 8-2 COMPONENTS OF HEALTH RESOURCE COSTS

Production Costs
  Direct
    Equipment acquisition and improvement
    Professional and nonprofessional labor
    Materials
  Indirect (Overhead)
    Rent/building depreciation
    Space preparation and upkeep
    Utilities
    Support services
    Other administrative services
Induced Costs (and Savings)
  Tests added or averted
  Treatments added or averted

Costs Versus Charges

The price or charge set by a hospital or other provider of a medical service is often taken as the cost of that service. A hospital bill has the advantages of being readily available and frequently itemized. The problem here is that resource cost and charge may not coincide; this is especially true for some hospital services. Some hospitals make a "profit" (a price greater than the cost) on routine surgery, private rooms, and laboratory and x-ray tests, and lose money (a price less than the cost) on emergency room services, open-heart surgery, and teaching. The analyst should be wary of the unthinking adoption of charges as surrogates for resource costs. An alternative to using charges, the accounting approach to estimating production costs, is described and illustrated in the section on production costs (p. 242).

Incremental Versus Average Costs

In contemplating additional health resource expenditures, we want to decide whether the additional expense is worthwhile. To make this judgment, we should focus on the **incremental cost** (also called the **marginal cost**) of providing additional services. This may be quite different from the **average cost** for the total output.

Definition. The **average cost** of a unit of output (for example, one day in a hospital for one patient) is the total cost of the total number, N, of units of output, divided by N. The **incremental cost** of the Nth unit of output is the total cost of N units of output minus the total cost of $N - 1$ units of output.

Table 8–3 illustrates the difference between the average and the incremental cost for two producers of five units of output. You may wish to think of these units of output as laboratory tests. Producer A has a higher initial production cost and requires $30 worth of resources to produce the first unit, while producer B consumes only $20 worth of resources to produce the first unit. If we want to gain an additional unit of output once both A and B have produced their first units, it would be cheaper to invest in producer A than in producer B. The incremental cost for the second unit produced by A is $1 less than B's incremental cost ($5 versus $6), and A is therefore preferred even though B's average cost for two units ($13) is lower than A's ($17.50). According to similar reasoning based on incremental costs, B would be preferred for investment in the third, fourth, and fifth units of output.

TABLE 8-3   COMPARISON OF AVERAGE AND INCREMENTAL
COSTS FOR TWO PRODUCERS OF FIVE UNITS OF OUTPUT
(e.g., LABORATORY TESTS)

UNITS OF OUTPUT	PRODUCER A			PRODUCER B		
	Total Cost	Average Cost	Incremental Cost	Total Cost	Average Cost	Incremental Cost
1	$30	$30	$30	$20	$20	$20
2	35	17.50	5	26	13	6
3	40	13.33	5	30	10	4
4	45	11.25	5	32	8	2
5	50	10	5	34	6.80	2

Notice that the analysis of which producer has lower costs (i.e., produces more efficiently) depends both on our starting point and on the number of additional units to be produced. If we start at the level of zero and want two units of output, B is cheaper than A (B's average cost is lower). If we start at one unit, A can produce a second unit more cheaply than B can (A's incremental cost is lower). In general, once an expenditure has already been made, it is a "sunk cost," and we should not consider it in comparing alternative expenditures from that point forward.

The discrepancy between the average and the incremental cost will depend on the extent to which the capacity is fixed and is being utilized. For example, if the fixed capacity is less than fully utilized, the incremental cost of a procedure may be much less than its average cost. Thus, the addition of an extra serum sample to a run on an automated chemistry analyzer consumes fewer incremental resources than the average cost per tested serum. At the other extreme, decisions that affect the purchase of new equipment or the building of new facilities entail incremental costs that would include the cost of acquiring the new capacity.

Production Costs

The components of production costs (Table 8–2) include both fixed and variable elements. **Fixed costs,** such as those for equipment, are relatively invariant and are measured per unit of time (usually annual) rather than per unit of volume. **Variable costs** (such as disposable materials) vary directly with the volume of services. An intermediate type of cost, sometimes called **semivariable**, includes both a fixed and a variable component. These costs, including some maintenance costs, do increase with volume, but less than proportionately. The incremental and average costs of a new service, then, depend both on the volume of output at which the analysis begins as well as on the projected increase in volume.

We will turn now to methods for measuring the cost of a particular service. The cost typically includes fixed, variable, and semivariable components. The cost of a service is the sum of the costs for the equipment, labor, supplies, and overhead attributed to that service.

Equipment, Buildings, and Depreciation. New buildings and equipment have useful lives that extend over many years, perhaps 40 years for a building and 10 years for a piece of equipment. Expenditures for relatively long-lasting resources are capital investments. The cost of using a building or equipment may be represented as an annual expense by the method of depreciation.

Definition. Depreciation is a method for spreading the cost of a piece of capital, such as new buildings or equipment, over its useful lifetime.

The simplest method of depreciation is to divide the purchase cost (less any residual value at the end of useful life) by the number of years of useful life. This gives the yearly cost of using the capital investment. If a new hospital is built for $20 million and is fully depreciated over 40 years, its cost could be calculated as follows:

$$\frac{\$20,000,000}{40 \text{ years}} = \$500,000 \text{ per year.}$$

This is called **straight-line depreciation.**

There are a variety of other formulas that can be used to spread these capital costs over time. One is called **amortization.** The amortized annual cost is that amount that would have to be paid during each year of the useful life of the capital investment in order to repay the principal plus interest on a loan (e.g., mortgage) whose principal is the purchase price. In fact, since borrowing is often the means of financing construction and capital equipment, this procedure may well approximate the actual timing of expenditure. If the interest rate is i per cent per annum, the term (or useful life) is N years, and the purchase price is P, then the amortized annual cost (i.e., the annual mortgage payment), C, is given by the formula

$$C = P \cdot \frac{i}{100} \cdot \frac{(1 + i/100)^{N-1}}{(1 + i/100)^N - 1}.$$

From the viewpoint of societal resource cost, the amortized value is more correct than the straight-line value. This is because money tied up in equipment cannot be used productively elsewhere to yield the normal rate of return during the accounting period. Therefore, the imputed annual cost should reflect not only the principal (i.e., the purchase price) but also the forgone interest.

Depreciation is measured as an annual cost, while what we want to measure is the cost of services. Some portion of the capital devoted to producing a service should be counted as part of that service's direct or indirect cost. The accuracy of any estimate of the capital cost per unit of service depends on the accuracy of the estimate of the number of units of service produced in a given time period.

Labor. Typically, a variety of workers, including physicians, contribute to the provision of a medical service. Physicians' fees for services may reflect the doctors' opportunity costs, that is, the amounts they could earn by other activities. However, different physicians charge different amounts for the same procedure, and the appropriate basis for setting fees is controversial. For salaried physicians, services could be valued according to the time spent and their salary per hour plus fringe benefits. For others, the fees that are charged are the most reasonable measures of the cost of professional time.

The wages of employees contribute to the cost of a service in proportion to the working time devoted to the service. Estimating these costs requires the definition of units of a service (such as a laboratory procedure, an ambulatory visit, a day in a hospital bed, and so on), the determination of work time (as a fraction of the total time) devoted to the service, and the salary per unit of time. Then the labor cost for each worker is calculated as follows:

$$\frac{salary\ (\$)}{unit\ of\ time} \cdot \frac{time}{unit\ of\ service} = \frac{worker\ cost\ (\$)}{unit\ of\ service}.$$

The total labor cost would, of course, be the sum of similar calculations for all workers contributing to the service.

Materials. The cost of materials is a variable cost that can be included in a straightforward manner in estimating the cost of a service.

Indirect or Overhead Costs. The production of medical services entails a number of overhead expenses that are necessary for the delivery of services. These indirect costs include such items as building depreciation or rent, building maintenance, utilities, administration costs, and support services (such as purchasing and billing). There are standard accounting procedures for allocating overhead costs to individual services. Often, overhead is distributed among services in proportion to their direct costs, but this may overstate the incremental costs because a portion of this overhead is fixed (such as building depreciation) and incurred regardless of the volume of services. Other portions of overhead (such as electricity) may vary to some degree with the volume.

Care must be taken to avoid counting costs twice, as may occur, for example, if a component of overhead is included in the costs for two different services. An individual analyst may carefully avoid this error in calculating the costs of different services. However, if estimates of costs obtained in separate studies are added to obtain a total, there may be a greater risk of double-counting.

Joint Products. Many hospitals have the joint goals of patient care, teaching, and research. These constitute joint products of many hospital activities. The resources that go into producing one product may simultaneously contribute to a second or third. For example, a nurse providing care for one patient may also be teaching others or learning lessons that will be helpful for future patients. The same record room that provides information about previous hospitalization, which is necessary for the care of patients, may also provide data for clinical research. If all direct and indirect costs are allocated to patient care activities, then patient care bears the burden of some teaching and research costs.

Some teaching and research costs, such as classroom hours and research time, may be distinguishable; to a large degree, however, patient care, teaching, and research are intertwined. One approach to this problem, which is not fully satisfactory, is to attempt to estimate the resource costs of a procedure if no teaching or research were involved, for example, by attributing some fraction of personnel time and overhead to research and some to teaching.[183, 244] In the end, the allocation of costs for joint products is an arbitrary decision.

An Example of Production Cost Analysis: The Barium Enema. Now that we have introduced the major components of resource cost (summarized in Table 8–2) in the production of health services, we can present an illustrative example. In this analysis of costs for a barium enema performed in a hospital, the figures are approximate and do not necessarily reflect current prices. The example does not attempt to distinguish teaching from research components. Nor does this first example include consideration of induced costs or savings (such as the effect on the duration of hospitalization or the use of other tests).

The barium enema is a diagnostic x-ray examination of the colon. The component parts of the cost and the basis used to estimate the cost per examination are summarized in Table 8–4 and are discussed in the following sections.

TABLE 8-4 COMPONENTS OF COST AND BASIS FOR ESTIMATING PRODUCTION COSTS FOR A BARIUM ENEMA

COMPONENT		BASIS FOR ESTIMATING COST OF COMPONENT
Direct		Total of equipment, labor, and materials
Equipment		Depreciated cost divided by frequency of use
Labor	Physician's time	Professional fee
	Other personnel's time	Hours times wages per hour
Materials	X-ray film	Cost per procedure
	Other supplies	Cost per procedure
Indirect (Overhead)		Fraction of other hospital costs allocated to this procedure

EQUIPMENT. The costs of equipment allocated to a procedure depend not only on the purchase price of the equipment but also on the length of time over which it is depreciated or amortized, the method used to compute that depreciation, and the number of procedures for which the equipment is used.

We shall assume the x-ray machine used here has a useful life of ten years and a purchase price of $50,000. If we take an interest rate of 8 per cent, the *amortized* cost would be

$$C = (\$50,000)(0.08)\left(\frac{(1.08)^9}{(1.08)^{10} - 1}\right)$$

$$= \$4,000\left(\frac{2.00}{1.16}\right)$$

$$= \$6,903.$$

This result is the resource cost of using this x-ray equipment for a year. Since the equipment is used for different types of procedures, which vary in the time required, it might be possible to derive a weighted procedure index that would allocate cost to different procedures according to their frequency and duration. In this example, however, we will spread the costs uniformly over all procedures. If the machine is used for 1,000 procedures per year, the average cost per procedure is

$$\$6,903/1,000 \cong \$6.90.$$

LABOR: THE PHYSICIAN'S AND OTHER PERSONNEL'S TIME. The radiologist's fee for a barium enema may reflect the physician's opportunity cost for time devoted to the conduct and interpretation of the examination. The allocated costs for salaried radiologists could be based on the fraction of working time devoted to the examination, as subsequently described for other personnel. In this example we shall use a physician cost of $40 for the barium enema.

In addition to the physician, a radiologic technician contributes time to the performance of the examination.

Assume that the technician spends 30 minutes per barium enema and helps with four of these per day. Suppose that the technician also does 30 chest x-ray films a day, each of which takes ten minutes. Thus, the total working time is

$$4 \cdot 30 \text{ minutes} = 120 \text{ minutes}$$
$$+ 30 \cdot 10 \text{ minutes} = \underline{300 \text{ minutes}}$$
$$= 420 \text{ minutes.}$$

Since the total eight-hour work day consists of

$$8 \cdot 60 \text{ minutes} = 480 \text{ minutes,}$$

there is a difference of

$$480 \text{ minutes} - 420 \text{ minutes} = 60 \text{ minutes.}$$

This difference, as yet unaccounted for, may include lunch, coffee break, and idle time. This unaccounted for time is sometimes allocated to the various units of work in the same proportions as the time directly spent on the different tasks. In our example, let Z represent the amount of this unaccounted for time allocated to the barium enemas. Then, by this accounting device, we have

$$\frac{120}{420} = \frac{Z}{60},$$

or

$$Z = 17.14 \text{ minutes.}$$

The remainder of unaccounted for time (60 minutes − 17.14 minutes = 42.86 minutes) would be allocated to the chest x rays. The total time attributed to barium enemas would thus be

$$120 \text{ minutes} + 17.14 \text{ minutes,}$$

or 137.14 minutes. The time per barium enema, then, would be this amount divided by four (the number of barium enemas per day), or 34.3 minutes. If the technician's salary is $5 per hour plus 15 per cent fringe benefits (retirement plan, health insurance, and so on), then the personnel cost per barium enema is

$$[\$5 + (\$5)(0.15)]\left(\frac{34.3}{60}\right) = \$3.29 \text{ per barium enema.}$$

Certain additional personnel, such as the people who transport patients as well as other aides, might be included here or, as we shall, as part of the administrative overhead costs.

MATERIALS: X-RAY FILM AND OTHER SUPPLIES. For our barium enema example, materials consist of x-ray film and other supplies (including, of course, the barium) that are used to conduct the examination. In this example we will take the cost of film to amount to $10 per examination and of all other supplies to be $12 per examination.

INDIRECT OR OVERHEAD COSTS. The overhead costs attributed to the barium enema derive in part from administrative and other costs in the radiology department and in part from overhead costs related to the buildings and administrative functions of the entire hospital. The fraction of hospital overhead assigned to a single revenue-generating department may depend on that department's space and number of personnel. Normally, the total overhead allocated to radiology would be divided equally among all procedures, although one could allocate these costs according to a weighted index such as that mentioned in our discussion of equipment costs.

If the indirect costs assigned to radiology from general hospital overhead amount to $200,000 for the year and the radiology department itself has an additional $100,000 in overhead expense, then the total overhead would be $300,000 per year. If the department performs 50,000 procedures per year, then the indirect cost per procedure is

$$\frac{\$300,000}{50,000} = \$6.$$

The total production costs for a barium enema are summarized in Table 8–5. Bear in mind that the final figure of $78.19, derived as we have here, overstates the incremental cost of one additional study (since some fixed costs were

TABLE 8-5 SUMMARY OF PRODUCTION COSTS FOR A BARIUM ENEMA

COMPONENT	COST
Equipment	$ 6.90
Physician's time	40.00
Technician's time	3.29
X-ray film	10.00
Supplies (other than film)	12.00
Overhead	6.00
Total	$78.19

included in the allocation) and does not include any induced costs or savings from resulting changes in the use of resources for other tests and treatments. Especially in the case of a diagnostic procedure, these induced effects may be a large fraction of the total resource costs consumed as a result of the procedure. For example, an analysis of the cost-effectiveness of screening for pheochromocytoma found approximately 45 per cent of net costs to be due to induced effects following the initial test.[269]

DISCOUNTING AND PRESENT VALUE

Resource costs accrue over time, and alternative programs that involve the same total investment over time may differ in the annual distributions of those investments. For example, Table 8–6 shows three programs that each consume $100,000 worth of resources over five years, but program A entails uniform investment each year, B requires more resources in the early years, and C is weighted more heavily in the later years. If these programs produce identical benefits, should we be indifferent among them?

TABLE 8-6 RESOURCE COSTS FOR THREE HYPOTHETICAL PROGRAMS OVER FIVE YEARS

YEAR	RESOURCE COST INVESTMENT		
	Program A	Program B	Program C
0 (this year)	$ 20,000	$ 40,000	$ 5,000
1	20,000	30,000	15,000
2	20,000	10,000	15,000
3	20,000	10,000	25,000
4	20,000	10,000	40,000
Totals	$100,000	$100,000	$100,000

Most analysts believe that future costs should be weighted less heavily than present ones. In this section we discuss the reasons for such time-related preferences and describe a method, called **discounting**, to quantify the magnitude of this preference. Discounting enables us to compare future costs (and benefits) with present costs (and benefits).

Inflation in the monetary price of goods and services is by itself *not* a reason for discounting future costs. In estimating costs, it is usually best to express all costs in real, that is, inflation-adjusted, monetary terms. Such inflation-adjusted costs represent real *resource* costs at the time they are incurred. After adjustments have been made for inflation, it is still important to discount future costs.

One reason for discounting future costs is that a dollar that is not spent today can be invested productively to yield a larger number of real dollars in the future. You can take the dollar to the bank and deposit it in a savings account that pays, for example, 7 per cent interest. A year from now you will get $1.07. A dollar's worth of resources in the national economy, if not spent this year, can be put to productive use to yield $1.07 worth of goods and services next year.

A second reason for discounting is that you may prefer to have the goods and services a dollar can buy now rather than to wait a year. In addition, there are risks associated with delay. The bank that holds your money, or the munici-pality that has issued your bond, may fail. You demand a premium in the form of interest if you must postpone consumption.

Definition. **Discounting** is a process for computing how much a dollar, payable one or more years from now, is worth today. The **present value,** or value today, of a future dollar depends on how many years in the future it is obtained and on the annual rate at which it is discounted, or its **discount rate.**

One dollar invested at an interest rate of 7 per cent will bring $1.07 a year from now. We can compute the present value of a dollar obtained one year from now using a 7 per cent discount rate as follows.

Suppose P is the amount of money that, if invested, will yield one dollar one year from now. Then,

$$P \circ 1.07 = \$1.00,$$

or

$$P = \$0.935.$$

At a 7 per cent discount rate, then, the *present value* of $1.00 next year is 93.5 cents.

In the same way, one can calculate the value of a dollar spent or received two years from now.

$1.00 two years from now

$= \$1.00/1.07 = \$0.93$ one year from now

$= \$0.93/1.07 = \$0.87$ today.

Hence, $1.00 two years from now at a 7 per cent discount rate is worth $0.87 today.

The general formula for present value is

$$P = \frac{S}{(1 + r)^N},$$

where P is the present value; S is the amount of future worth (in the preceding example, S is one dollar); r is the discount rate (interest rate or rate of return); and N is the number of periods (in the preceding example, N equals two years).

So the present value of $500 ten years from now at an 8 per cent discount rate is

$$P = \frac{\$500}{(1 + 0.08)^{10}} \cong \$232.$$

Tables giving present values for a future value of S of one dollar over a number of years and at various discount rates are available*; many pocket calculators also provide for the calculation of compound interest and present value.

---

*See, for example, the *Standard Mathematical Tables* published annually by the Chemical Rubber Company, Cleveland, Ohio.

If we are comparing the costs of alternative programs, such as those presented in Table 8–6 in which costs accumulate over time, we would want first to compute the present value of the cost for each program. We may wish to express these costs as annual costs rather than as present values, especially if we are comparing annual costs with annual benefits. In that case we would *amortize* the present value of each program's costs at the discount rate. The time period for amortization would depend on the time period over which this investment produces additional benefits.

Although it is unquestioned among economists that resource costs should be discounted, the rate at which they should be discounted is controversial. In large part differences of opinion stem from variations among interest rates observed in our economy, which in turn reflect the differences between the productive potential of the investment (in machinery and other capital stock) and the preferences of individuals for present versus future consumption of goods and services. Some economists favor inflation-adjusted discount rates as high as 15 per cent. The rate used by the United States Office of Management and Budget is 10 per cent, which is subject to much criticism. Other economists favor rates as low as zero (or negative) per cent. The consensus, however, lies between 4 and six per cent. The further we move into the future, the greater the uncertainty concerning future uses of health resources that will be available. In any cost-effectiveness or benefit-cost analysis, a range of discount rates, perhaps from 0 per cent to 10 per cent, should be tested to see how big a difference may be produced in the results. This is another example of sensitivity analysis.

8.5 THE MEASUREMENT OF HEALTH BENEFITS

The meaning and measurement of health benefits are more controversial than the measurement of costs to provide medical services. Resources expended on health care are intended to produce health benefits, but the immediate effects of medical intervention (e.g., positive test results or cases correctly diagnosed) are intermediate along the way to ultimate health benefits for an individual. These ultimate health benefits may take many forms: prolonged life, improved function and activity, relief from pain and anxiety, greater capacity for work and earnings, and reduced medical care expenses.

The health benefits derived from a clinical practice obviously depend on the nature of the patient's illness (if any) and on the chosen intervention(s). In addition, the benefits obtained will vary from setting to setting, depending upon (among other things) the expertise and experience of practitioners in different places. Some analysts distinguish the "efficacy" of a procedure from its "effectiveness," reserving the former for health benefits derived under ideal conditions of practice and using the latter to mean the average level of benefits obtained.[185] What is important here is not semantics but the recognition that the probabilities of various outcomes and hence the measured benefits will vary with the patient's background (age, sex, and so on) and clinical status, the nature of available treatments, the specific conditions of administration, and the capabilities of the physicians and others caring for the patient.

Some analysts, particularly those attempting benefit-cost analysis, stress the measurement of health benefits in monetary terms. Since life and health themselves are not traded in any marketplace, the effort here is to assign a "market price" to extended or improved life. Such monetary approaches tend to provoke serious philosophical objections, but a great deal of useful analysis can be accomplished without assigning monetary values to benefits. Unlike benefit-cost analysis, cost-effectiveness analysis de-emphasizes the monetary equivalents of health benefits and aims for a combined measure of the length and quality of life that would allow the comparison of alternative health expenditures. In this section we will review briefly the several approaches to valuing health benefits.

MEASUREMENT IN MONETARY TERMS

Lost Earnings

One approach to assessing the value of a human life is to estimate the present value of projected future earnings, taking into account such factors as the age, sex, and education of the individual. This "human capital" approach measures the value of a productive year of life in terms of an individual's annual earnings.[38,210] Some of those who have taken this approach use the *net* present value of earnings (obtained by subtracting the individual's anticipated consumption from anticipated earnings). This, in effect, values only an individual's contribution to the rest of society. Others advocate using the *gross* present value of earnings (which includes the individual's consumption) so that the individual also counts as a valued member of society. The rationale for human capital approaches to valuing life is that society stands to lose the potential consumption of goods and services in proportion to the lost productivity of its members.

The increase in earnings that is due to prolonged life or decreased morbidity is sometimes described as one of the "indirect benefits" of a health program or service. Indirect benefits are distinguished from the "direct benefits," or savings in future health resource consumption as a result of improved health and "intangible benefits," or any improvements in function and well-being that are not directly translated into reduced health expenditures or into increased earnings.[200]

In many instances, intangible benefits (such as reduced pain or relief from anxiety or grief) are very prominent health benefits. Yet these would be excluded from a lost earnings approach. More fundamentally, a human capital measure can violate our intuitive sense of the relative value of human life. For example, according to the present value of their future earnings, very young children have little "value," because it will be 20 years before their average income is substantial. After retirement age the present value dwindles to a neglible amount. Also, men earn more than women, and college graduates earn more than high school dropouts. In some cases even the proper monetary value for work is unclear; should a housewife be valued by the income of the job she forgoes in the marketplace or by the cost of hiring a housekeeper? These numerous difficulties make lost earnings a questionable yardstick for health benefits.

Willingness To Pay

An alternative monetary approach to valuing the extension of life and an improved quality of life is the calculation of the amount an individual is willing to pay for a particular reduction in the risk of death or of illness.[220]

This willingness-to-pay measure takes into account subjective (intangible) values associated with health and life that are not denoted by wages alone. When the values from a population are aggregated, willingness to pay provides a measure of the societal value attached to a given health benefit.

Willingness to pay is favored by some economists, but it has several important limitations as a measure. First, measured willingness to pay varies according to the initial probability of death and the extent of the promised reduction in the probability of death or illness. However, these variations are not linear, and so one cannot extrapolate empirical findings from one range of probabilities to another.[270] Furthermore, the approach may give undue weight to the affluent, since the willingness to pay would increase with wealth. At a practical level, it may be difficult to contemplate how much one would pay to achieve a small change in a low probability of disease or disability.

MEASUREMENT IN HEALTH TERMS

Both philosophic and practical objections arise whenever health outcomes are translated into monetary terms. Such measures, as we have seen in the previous section, may be incomplete and misleading; however, their monetary value makes them directly commensurable with the resource costs of alternative investments, a necessary feature for benefit-cost analysis. In the less demanding cost-effectiveness format, benefits may be measured solely in health terms. In some situations a single, straightforward benefit measure may suffice. More often, however, it is desirable to develop a weighted health outcome measure that combines longevity and morbidity.

Single Health Benefit Measures

Health status is multidimensional, but in any particular instance we may be interested in only a particular health measure and the most efficient means of achieving it. For example, which of two treatment programs will produce the larger number of cures per dollar expended? Which of two diagnostic strategies is more efficient for purposes of detecting disease in a given population? In these two examples the number of cures and the number of cases detected serve as measures of health benefit. They are neither complete nor final outcome indicators, but for purposes of the specific questions asked they will serve nicely. Such limited measures may make practical objects of study, and there is nothing wrong in using them as long as their limitations are recognized. The detection of a case does not necessarily lead to improved treatment (e.g., optimal treatment may already be in effect or the patient may not comply), and better treatment does not ensure a cure.

A single measure for mortality might be expressed in terms of lives saved (or lost). An alternative is to compute the number of years of life that are added by the particular intervention. With this measure the age at death (and not merely the fact of death) is important. In contrast to the lost earnings approach, the cure of childhood disease would be valued relatively highly in terms of years of life saved. Both measures for the lost earnings and the years of life saved place relatively less value on intervention for the elderly. Some would feel that neither measure does justice to their sense of the value of human life at every age.

**Combined Health Benefit Measures: Trade-Offs Between
Longevity and Morbidity**

Alternative health programs are likely to differ in their effects on the length of life and the quality of life. For example, as compared with medication a surgical intervention may offer, on the average, decreased morbidity but a greater risk of mortality. Evaluating the cost-effectiveness of these alternative approaches requires a common unit of measured benefit that properly reflects the trade-off between longevity and the quality of life. The problem is the same as that we faced in Chapter Seven in which decisions with multiple outcomes led us to utility assessment. Here again we use a utility scale to value the quality of life in any one year and then add all years of life to achieve a combined measure of longevity and morbidity — a number of **quality-adjusted life years (QALYs)**.

Definition. The number of **quality-adjusted life years (QALYs)** is the number of years at full health that would be valued equivalently to the number of years of life as experienced.

Since some years as experienced are typically at less than full health, the number of QALYs is typically smaller than the number of years experienced. A year at full health would count as 1.0 QALY, but two years, each valued at 0.4, would count together as 0.8 QALY.

The method by which the value of a year at any given health status may be measured against a year at full health is analogous to the method of utility assessment presented in Chapter Seven. Two possible approaches are the **time-trade-off method** and the **lottery method.*

In the time-trade-off method, the following question is asked:

If disability, lost earnings, limitation of activity, pain, and suffering are taken into account, what is the smallest fraction, P, of a year of life at full health that you would accept in exchange for a year of life at health status S?

The closer to 1 the answer is to this question, the nearer to perfect health is the health status that is experienced. An answer near 0 implies the status is nearly as bad as death.

The lottery method presents the following question:

Suppose that you face a lifetime of impaired health status S but that you have the opportunity to take a gamble that might relieve you of the morbidity, at some risk of immediate death. In particular, suppose that this gamble involves a probability of P of having a healthy life (of the same length) and a probability of one minus P of death. What is the smallest value of P that would persuade you to choose the lottery?

The answer P to either the time-trade-off question or the lottery question then corresponds to the value attached to that year as experienced.

This method for determining QALYs may also be used to compare the quality of life at different ages. For example, it may be that one year of life in one's 90s is valued the same as 0.8 years of life in one's 30s. In that case the 92nd year of life might be valued as, at most, 0.8 QALYs. This is one way of taking into account the morbidity of old age without explicitly itemizing the effects

---

*This discussion is adapted from Raiffa et al.[205]

on health status. On the other hand, if morbidity is held constant, the value placed on an additional year of life may increase rather than decrease with age.

The QALY scale is subjective and liable to all of the shortcomings of utility assessment. For example, persons may not have experienced or be able to imagine the meaning of various states of morbidity. While human capital measures may be more objective, the QALY scale embraces more aspects of health status and avoids the distasteful monetary valuation of life.

DISCOUNTING HEALTH BENEFITS

Discounting health benefits to their present value is more controversial than discounting costs. We believe that it is proper to discount benefits as well as costs as long as we assume that the increase in the number of years of life owing to a given expenditure will be the same in the future as it is today.

The reason for discounting future years of life saved is not because life years can, in any sense, be invested to yield more life years, as dollars can be invested to yield more dollars. Nor is it necessary to assume that life years in the future are less valuable than life years today in any absolute utilitarian sense. Rather, the main reason for discounting future years of life in cost-effectiveness and benefit-cost analysis is because they are being valued relative to dollars, and, since a dollar in the future is discounted relative to the present value of dollar, so must a future life year be discounted relative to a present life year.

This line of reasoning assumes that opportunities for purchasing health benefits for dollars do not change over time. If it is expected that technology will improve such that it becomes less expensive to save lives, this would suggest an even higher effective discount rate for life years than for resource costs. If it is expected that environmental or other factors will conspire to make life-saving more expensive — that is, more valuable — in the future, a lower discount rate might be in order.*

For programs involving screening for disease in which the life years saved are far in the future, it matters a great deal whether expected benefits are discounted. Without discounting, a program that saves one life year 40 years hence at a present-value cost of $10,000 would have a cost-effectiveness ratio of $10,000 per life year. With discounting at 5 per cent per year, the present value of that future life year is reduced to $1/(1.05)^{40}$, or about 0.14, and the ratio becomes $70,000 per life year, which is a remarkable difference. Since discounting benefits is controversial, the best practical approach is to include a sensitivity analysis in which the rate of discount is varied from 0 to perhaps 10 per cent.

8.6 COSTS AND BENEFITS TO WHOM? THE QUESTION OF EQUITY

When resource costs are computed as part of a cost-effectiveness or benefit-cost analysis, the *distribution* of those costs and benefits may be as important as, or more important than, the aggregate *amount* of those costs and benefits.

---

*A more extensive treatment of the issue of discounting health benefits may be found in Raiffa et al.[205]

We discussed earlier in this chapter (Section 8.2) the perspectives of different participants on the costs and benefits of health care. From a societal perspective, there are basic questions of equity in the distribution of services and their costs and benefits.

Of course, all people may value the concept of "equity" in the abstract but disagree over what is and is not equitable in the distribution of costs and benefits. Is it more equitable for services to be equally available to everyone or more equitable for those who contribute more of the resource costs to obtain more of the benefits? What parts, if any, of health care should be available to everyone, and what parts, if any, should be considered luxuries for those who can afford them?

These are questions that reach beyond the realm of health care and touch fundamental value choices in society. They are answered implicitly in our choices and manner of choosing among alternative health resource investments. We return briefly to the issues of rights and interests in health in Chapter Ten.

8.7 COST-EFFECTIVENESS: STEPS IN ANALYSIS AND ILLUSTRATIVE EXAMPLES

In this section we will summarize the basic approach in cost-effectiveness analysis and offer two examples of analysis that illustrate particular aspects. The first highlights the incremental nature of costs and benefits, and the second demonstrates the importance of considerations of the quality of life.

SUMMARY OF STEPS IN COST-EFFECTIVENESS ANALYSIS

A valid and complete cost-effectiveness analysis would meet the following criteria:

1. The analysis should specify the decision maker and perspective from which the assessment of costs and benefits will be conducted. Usually, a societal perspective is adopted.

2. An explicit description of the procedures or programs to be evaluated should be provided. Alternatives should be clearly specified, and viable options should not be ruled out prematurely.

3. A complete and clear specification of the items included in the calculation of both costs and benefits should be given.

Procedures for calculating costs should be described. The distinction between incremental and average costs should be maintained, especially in cases in which equipment or facilities are involved, as should the distinction between charges and costs. Care should be taken to avoid counting the same cost twice. Decisions, in general, should be based on incremental benefits and incremental resource costs. The use of charges in lieu of costs is permissible if it can be argued that the discrepancy is not quantitatively great in a given instance.

The measure or measures of benefits should reflect the attributes that are relevant to the decision maker. Final outcomes, such as lives saved, life years gained, or days of disability averted, are usually preferable to intermediate outcomes, such as cases of disease identified. The incorporation of preferences to facilitate aggregation into a composite measure of utility (e.g., quality-adjusted life years) may be valuable, but care should be taken to provide a sensitivity analysis over a range of possible utility values.

4. Assumptions underlying the estimated relation between inputs and outputs should be made explicit and should be consistent with the available empirical evidence. Subjective estimates based on common sense or theoretical considerations should not necessarily be avoided, but the uncertainty in those estimates should be noted and appropriate sensitivity analyses should be reported.

5. The analysis should make clear the timing of the receipt of benefits in relation to that of the costs. Appropriate discounting procedures should be employed, and a sensitivity analysis with respect to the discount rate should be reported.

6. Before making policy recommendations based on such analyses, the distribution of costs and benefits among the major segments of the population should be examined. Major imbalances between those who benefit and those who pay should be identified.

INCREMENTAL BENEFITS AND COSTS: ALTERNATIVE SCREENING STRATEGIES FOR COLON CANCER

The purpose of this example is to probe further into the distinction between the average and the incremental cost in decisions involving the allocation of health resources. In particular, the example demonstrates that it is the incremental cost per unit of benefit derived, and not the average cost, that should be the basis for deciding whether a particular procedure or set of procedures is worth its opportunity cost.

Digital examination of the rectum, a test for occult blood in the stool, and sigmoidoscopy are three screening procedures for the detection of asymptomatic colon cancer. Their costs, estimated by the procedures described in the section on production costs (p. 242), are as follows: test for occult blood, $0.50; digital examination, $2.00; and sigmoidoscopy, $25.00. Suppose that in a population between 60 and 80 years of age, the number of true cancers is one per 1,000 patients examined. The problem is to decide which test or combination of tests to use to detect cases of cancer as efficiently as possible.

None of these tests is perfectly sensitive, however. Digital examination and sigmoidoscopy have limited range, and the test for occult blood detects only cancers that bleed. Specifically, digital examination (DE) finds the 10 per cent of cancers that are at the very lower end of the colon and rectum; sigmoidoscopy (SIG) finds the 85 per cent of cancers that are within 25 to 30 cm of the rectum; and the test for occult blood (OB) finds 80 per cent of cancers throughout the colon and rectum.

If we assume that all colon cancers are equally likely to bleed, the detection of 100 cases of cancer might break down as shown in Figure 8–4. Thus, any cancer found by digital examination would be found by sigmoidoscopy, because these examinations are performed at the lower end of the colon or rectum; only 3 per cent of cancers would be undetected by all three examinations.

For purposes of simplifying the example, we will assume that digital examination and sigmoidoscopy are perfectly specific but that the test for occult blood has a false-positive rate of 10 per cent. We shall also assume that all patients who have a positive test result for occult blood only will receive a barium enema (BaE), which is a confirmatory test for colon cancer that is assumed to be perfectly sensitive and specific. Based on our earlier calculation, we take the cost of a BaE to be approximately $80.

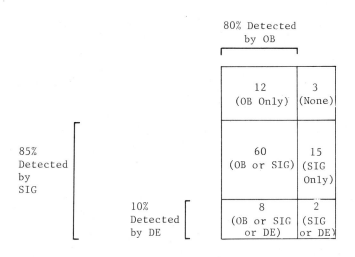

Figure 8-4 *The detection of 100 cases of cancer by digital examination (DE), sigmoidos-copy (SIG), and a test for occult blood (OB).*

With this information let us consider the following possible strategies:

1. DE only;

2. OB only, followed by BaE for all patients with positive test results;

3. OB and DE, followed by BaE for all patients with positive results on the test for OB only;

4. DE, followed by SIG for patients with negative results on DE;

5. OB and DE, followed by SIG for patients with negative results on both tests or by BaE for patients with positive results on the test for OB only.

These strategies assume that sigmoidoscopy would be done only if the results of less expensive tests were negative and that sigmoidoscopy is always preceded by a digital examination. We also assume that if a test for occult blood and a digital examination are performed, they are done at one time and not sequentially.

If we assume a prevalence of one true cancer per 1,000 patients, 100,000 patients will have 100 true cancers. Consider the possible approaches to finding cancer in a population of 100,000 men between the ages of 60 and 80, as shown in Table 8-7.

The expected cost for the DE only strategy is simply the unit cost of $2 multiplied by the population of 100,000, or $200,000. The expected number of cases of cancer found is ten (Figure 8-4).

The expected cost for the OB only strategy includes the cost of the screening test in the full population of 100,000 and the cost of a BaE in all those with positive test results. The expected number with positive test results is equal to

$$(0.8)(100) + (0.1)(99,900) = 10,070.$$

Therefore, the expected cost of this strategy is

$$(\$0.50)(100,000) + (\$80)(10,070) = \$855,600.$$

TABLE 8-7   COSTS AND FINDINGS IN FIVE STRATEGIES
OF TESTING 100,000 PERSONS FOR COLON CANCER

STRATEGY*	TOTAL COSTS	TOTAL CANCERS FOUND	AVERAGE COST PER CANCER FOUND
DE only	$ 200,000	10	$20,000
OB only†	855,600	80	10,695
OB + DE†	1,054,960	80 + 2 = 82	12,865
DE → SIG‡	2,699,750	10 + 75 = 85	31,762
OB + DE → SIG†‡	3,303,160	80 + 2 + 15 = 97	34,053

*OB = occult blood test; DE = digital examination; SIG = sigmoidoscopy.

†Under these strategies a barium enema is done on patients in whom only the test result for OB is positive.

‡Under these strategies sigmoidoscopy is done on patients in whom the earlier test results were negative.

The expected number of cases of cancer detected is 80 (Figure 8–4).

The expected cost for the OB plus DE strategy includes the cost of both screening tests in the full population and the cost of a BaE in those patients with positive results on the test for OB but not on the DE. The expected number with positive results on the test for OB is 10,070, as determined previously, but of these eight would also have positive results on the DE and hence would not need a BaE for confirmation. Therefore, 10,062 barium enemas would have to be performed, and the total expected cost of the strategy would be

$$(\$2.50)(100,000) + (\$80)(10,062) = \$1,054,960.$$

The expected number of cases of cancer detected would be 80 plus 2, or 82 (Figure 8-4).

The expected costs for the DE followed by SIG strategy are computed as the sum of $2 per digital examination in all patients and the cost of sigmoidoscopy in all but the ten patients in whom cancer is detected by DE:

$$(\$2.00)(100,000) + (\$25.00)(99,990) = \$2,699,750.$$

The expected number of cases of cancer found is 10 plus 75, or 85 (Figure 8–4).

Finally, the expected costs for the OB plus DE followed by SIG strategy include the costs of both screening tests in the full population, the cost of sigmoidoscopy in the 89,928 (100,000 − 10,062 − 10) patients with negative results on both tests, and the cost of a BaE in patients with positive results on the test for OB but negative results on the DE:

$$(\$2.50)(100,000) + (\$25)(89,928) + (\$80)(10,062) = \$3,303,160.$$

The expected number of cases of cancer found is 80 plus 2 plus 15, or 97 (Figure 8–4).

The next step in assessing a table of costs and benefits is to determine whether any of the strategies is dominated by another, that is, whether any strategy costs more and yields fewer benefits than another. In this example (Table 8–7), each successively more expensive strategy also detects more cases of cancer, so that none can be eliminated on the basis of dominance. This leaves us with the five strategies listed in ascending order of both total cost and total number of cancers found.

To obtain the incremental costs of finding more cancers as we move from a less costly and less sensitive approach to a more costly and more sensitive approach, we need to perform the analysis shown in Table 8–8. The number of additional cases of cancer found with each strategy is the difference between the total number detected by that strategy and the number detected by the strategy with the next lower total cost. The incremental cost of a strategy is the difference between its cost and that of the strategy with the next lower total cost. The incremental cost per additional case of cancer is simply the ratio of incremental cost to the number of additional cases of cancer. This ratio may be considered a measure of the cost-effectiveness of using the resources required to obtain the additional benefits gained by moving to the next more costly strategy.

TABLE 8–8 ADDITIONAL CASES OF CANCER AND INCREMENTAL
COSTS FOR FIVE TEST STRATEGIES FOR COLON CANCER

STRATEGY*	ADDITIONAL CANCERS FOUND	INCREMENTAL COST	INCREMENTAL COST PER ADDITIONAL CANCER FOUND
Do nothing	0	$ 0	$ 0
DE only	10	200,000	20,000
OB only†	70	655,600	9,366
OB + DE†	2	199,360	99,680
DE → SIG‡	3	1,644,790	548,263
OB + DE → SIG†‡	12	603,410	50,284

*OB = occult blood test; DE = digital examination; SIG = sigmoidoscopy.

†Under these strategies a barium enema is done on patients in whom only the test result for OB is positive.

‡Under these strategies sigmoidoscopy is done on patients in whom the earlier test results were negative.

While the strategies were originally arrayed in increasing order of the total number of cases of cancer found (Table 8–7), the incremental costs per additional case of cancer do not necessarily increase from one strategy to the next. In fact, in this example the incremental cost per case of cancer detected by a test for OB only is less than the incremental cost per case of cancer detected by DE only; similarly, the incremental cost per case of cancer found by the OB plus DE followed by SIG strategy is less than that for the DE followed by SIG strategy. These observations imply that DE only and DE followed by SIG may be eliminated from further consideration. If our objective were to detect the first ten cases of cancer as inexpensively as possible, rather than using DE only we would be better off applying the OB only strategy to one eighth of the 100,000 people; the total cost of this approach would be

$$\$855,600/8 = \$106,950,$$

or $10,695 per case of cancer found, which is just over half the cost of performing a DE only. By this reasoning we can eliminate the DE only and similarly the DE followed by SIG strategies.

Finally, we reanalyze the remaining strategies in terms of incremental cost per case of cancer found (Table 8–9). The decision as to the appropriate strategy now depends on how much you, the patient, or society is willing to spend per case of cancer found — $10,695, $99,680, or $149,880 — and on the value of these resources in other areas of health care. It may also be determined by the total resources available for screening this population for colon cancer. For example, with up to $855,600 (Table 8–9), the most cost-effective strategy would be to test for OB only on all 100,000 patients, which would detect an expected total of 80 cases of cancer. With a budget of $1,054,960, it becomes possible to use the OB plus DE strategy on all 100,000 patients, which will identify an expected total of 82 cases of cancer. With a budget of $955,280, we can compute the most cost-effective strategy in the following way. If we tested for OB only on all patients, we would have $99,680 remaining. With this money we could use on some patients the OB plus DE strategy instead of the OB only strategy. From Table 8–9 we find that the expected incremental cost per patient of the OB plus DE strategy relative to the OB strategy only, is

$$\$199,360/100,000 = \$1.9936.$$

Therefore, the number of patients who can be given the more sensitive screen is

$$\$99,680/\$1.9936 = 50,000.$$

Hence, with a budget of $955,280, we would find the most cases of cancer by screening half of the patients with the OB plus DE strategy and the other half with the OB only strategy. (Of course, the opportunity to screen some patients more intensively than others raises ethical questions about the equity of resource allocation.)

TABLE 8–9   ADDITIONAL CASES OF CANCER AND INCREMENTAL
COSTS FOR THREE TEST STRATEGIES FOR COLON CANCER

STRATEGY*	CANCERS FOUND	TOTAL COST	ADDITIONAL CANCERS FOUND	INCREMENTAL COST	INCREMENTAL COST PER CANCER FOUND
Do nothing	0	$ 0	0	$ 0	$ 0
OB only[†]	80	855,600	80	855,600	10,695
OB + DE	82	1,054,960	2	199,360	99,680
OB + DE → SIG[†‡]	97	3,303,160	15	2,248,200	149,880

*OB = occult blood test; DE = digital examination; SIG = sigmoidoscopy.
[†]Under these strategies a barium enema is done on patients in whom only the test result for OB is positive.
[‡]Under these strategies sigmoidoscopy is done on patients in whom the earlier test results were negative.

The total budget allocated to screening for colon cancer might itself be determined by comparing the cost-effectiveness of using incremental resources to intensify this screening program with that of using those resources in other areas. Of course, in reality many considerations other than demonstrated cost-effectiveness determine the use of health resources.

In summary, when comparing alternative strategies for obtaining a certain type of benefit, it is most appropriate to analyze the choices in terms of their incremental costs per additional unit of benefit. Some choices may be dominated or eliminated by others because they attain fewer benefits for more cost in the total population or in some fraction of the total. For the remaining alternatives, the preferred choice depends on the total budget available and on the cutoff level of incremental cost per additional unit of benefit.

LONGEVITY AND THE QUALITY OF LIFE: THE TREATMENT OF HYPERTENSION VERSUS CORONARY ARTERY BYPASS SURGERY

Consider the question of whether a health maintenance organization should offer coronary artery bypass graft (CABG) surgery to men between the ages of 40 and 50 years with mild symptoms of angina and signs of reduced cardiac output. The alternative would be to use the resources to treat men in the same age group with mild or moderate hypertension.

Table 8–10 shows estimates of life expectancy and costs for the alternative resource expenditures. The treatment cost for CABG is primarily for surgery, including hospital costs, the surgeon's fee, and subsequent medical care. The treatment cost for hypertension is for medications, physicians' fees, and laboratory expenses for the remainder of the patient's life. Costs and benefits are expressed in terms of present value; at a discount rate of 5 per cent, one year of life saved 15 years from now is approximately equivalent to one-half year saved now. According to these estimates, it appears to be more cost-effective to treat hypertension, either mild (diastolic pressure, 90 mm Hg) or moderate (diastolic pressure, 110 mm Hg) than to offer CABG surgery to the type of patient described. For other candidates for CABG surgery (e.g., those with more severe angina and good cardiac output), the cost-effectiveness of surgery might exceed that of treatment for asymptomatic mild hypertension.

TABLE 8-10 LIFE EXPECTANCY AND COSTS FOR CABG SURGERY AND MEDICAL MANAGEMENT OF HYPERTENSION*

TREATMENT	INCREASED YEARS OF LIFE EXPECTANCY	TREATMENT COST	COST PER YEAR OF LIFE SAVED
CABG surgery	0.10[†]	$15,000[†]	$150,000
Medical management of hypertension			
DBP = 90 mm Hg	0.20[‡]	2,700[‡]	13,500
DBP = 110 mm Hg	0.40[‡]	2,500[‡]	6,250

*The present value for columns 2, 3, and 4 is calculated at a 5 percent discount rate. CABG indicates coronary artery bypass graft, and DBP, diastolic blood pressure.

[†]Based on Weinstein et al.[271]

[‡]Based on Weinstein and Stason.[272] The expected lifetime treatment costs for a patient with a diastolic blood pressure of 110 mm Hg are lower than those for a patient with a diastolic blood pressure of 90 mm Hg, because life expectancy is shorter at the higher pressure.

When quality-adjusted life expectancy is used as the effectiveness measure, the situation changes. Improvement in the quality of life (relief from disabling angina pectoris) may be the major reason for CABG surgery. Assuming a life expectancy of 20 years, an average improvement in quality of life of 5 per cent would add approximately one quality-adjusted year of life for each patient operated on. The net effects on the quality of life owing to the treatment of hypertension may even be negative, because the positive effects that are due to the prevention of cardiovascular morbid events may be outweighed by the side effects of antihypertensive drugs. It appears that the first priority should be to treat moderate hypertension but that CABG surgery may be a more cost-effective way to use resources than the treatment of mild hypertension. The potential importance of quality-of-life outcomes is largely responsible for this change in results.

TABLE 8–11 QUALITY-ADJUSTED LIFE EXPECTANCY AND COSTS FOR CABG SURGERY AND MEDICAL MANAGEMENT OF HYPERTENSION*

TREATMENT	INCREASED YEARS OF QUALITY-ADJUSTED LIFE EXPECTANCY	TREATMENT COST	COST PER YEAR OF QUALITY-ADJUSTED LIFE EXPECTANCY
CABG surgery	0.75[†]	$15,000[†]	$20,000
Medical management of hypertension			
DBP = 90 mm Hg	0.08[‡]	2,700[‡]	33,750
DBP = 110 mm Hg	0.34[‡]	2,500[‡]	7,350

*The present value for columns 2, 3, and 4 is calculated at a 5 percent discount rate. CABG indicates coronary artery bypass graft, and DBP, diastolic blood pressure.

[†]Based on Weinstein et al.[271]

[‡]Based on Weinstein and Stason.[272]

8.8 SUMMARY OF CHAPTER EIGHT

Given limited health resources, one should try to use those resources to gain the greatest total health benefits for all patients. There is usually little concern for limited resources in medical decisons for an individual patient in situations in which that person does not bear the true resource cost of care. From a societal point of view, however, limits on total resources are very important considerations. This difference in valued objectives between the perspective of "individual" patients and the perspective of "all" patients constitutes a genuine dilemma for physicians and health-care planners.

All analysis of the efficient use of resources requires the measurement of costs and benefits. Two related but distinct analytic approaches are **cost-effectiveness** and **benefit-cost** analysis.

Resource costs that are attributable to a particular health service include production costs and induced costs. Production costs typically include components for equipment, labor, and materials as well as overhead. These production costs may be classified as fixed, semivariable, or variable, depending on the relation between costs and increases in the volume of services. Induced costs are the resources consumed in tests and treatments undertaken as a consequence of the initial service. Each induced procedure has its own production costs, and there may be induced savings as well as costs.

The measurement of **health benefits** is more controversial than the measurement of health costs. A variety of monetary approaches have been proposed, including measures of lost earnings and willingness to pay. These are subject to philosophic and practical objections. A nonmonetary measure favored by the authors is **quality-adjusted life years,** a utility scale that combines longevity and morbidity considerations. Nonmonetary measures suffice for **cost-effectiveness** analysis, but **benefit-cost** analysis requires that monetary valuations be placed on health benefits.

Cost-effectiveness analysis is a means of determining the most efficient allocation of limited resources. It entails assessing the ratio of benefits to resources consumed for each alternative choice and then selecting alternatives in ascending order of the ratio of costs to benefits until resources are exhausted. The decision maker's perspective is very important; usually a societal perspective is adopted. In conducting cost-effectiveness analysis, one should distinguish **resource costs** from charges for services, stress **incremental** (as distinct from **average**) costs and benefits, and use **discounting** to measure future streams of costs and benefits in terms of present value. Appropriate **sensitivity analyses** should be included and attention should be paid to equity considerations in the distribution of costs and benefits. Several examples illustrated these points and demonstrated the techniques of cost-effectiveness analysis.

Benefit-cost analysis provides an explicit comparison of resource costs and health benefits in terms of a common unit of measurement, usually monetary. It offers the decision maker a means of comparing the benefits and costs of health services with the benefits and costs of nonhealth programs.

EXERCISES FOR CHAPTER EIGHT

EXERCISES FOR SECTION 8.3

1. *Surgery for Pancreatic Cancer*
   Recall the question of palliative surgery for patients with pancreatic cancer. The simplified decision tree given in Figure 8–1 does not consider quality-adjusted years of survival. If each day of survival without surgery has a quality-adjusted value of 0.5 days following surgery, how long would survival without surgery have to be to make you indifferent about surgery?

2. *Screening for a Rare Disease*
   Pilfadactyly is a rare, asymptomatic, hypothetical disease that can lead to sudden death if it is not diagnosed early. The result of the screening test for the disease is positive in 95 per cent of patients who have the condition, but it is also positive in 1 per cent of patients without the disease. The prevalence of pilfadactyly in the general population is $1/100,000$ (10^{-5}). The treatment of pilfadactyly is surgery; the operative mortality is 0.1 per cent, and the cure rate is 100 per cent among survivors of the operation. Untreated pilfadactyly will result in death within the year for 50 per cent of the patients; the rest of the cases will be cured spontaneously.

a. If the cost is disregarded and the objective is to minimize the probability of death, is surgery indicated for those patients with positive test results? Why?

b. Suppose the prevalence of pilfadactyly were $1/10,000$ (10^{-4}). Is surgery indicated for those with positive test results? Why? What is the net benefit of surgery for those with positive test results?

c. Continue to assume a prevalence of $1/10,000$. Surgery costs $15,000 and the test for pilfadactyly costs $100. Assess the cost per life saved by screening for pilfadactyly in this population. (Hint: Use a decision tree to compute expected mortality, both with and without the test.)

d. Interpret your findings, and discuss the sensitivity of your result to changes in the prevalence of disease and the cost of surgery.

EXERCISE FOR SECTION 8.4

3. *Discounting Program Costs*
Consider the three hypothetical programs in Table 8—6.

a. What is the present-value cost of each program at an annual discount rate of 0 per cent, 5 per cent, and 10 per cent?

b. What is the annual cost of each program amortized over five years at an annual discount rate of 0 per cent, 5 per cent, and 10 per cent?

EXERCISE FOR SECTION 8.5

4. *Choice of Treatment for Blastobliticosis*
Blastobliticosis is a severe, disabling, hypothetical disease of the circulatory system. Without treatment a 40-year-old patient has a life expectancy of only five years, is in severe and continuous pain, and is confined to bed. Fortunately, however, there are two treatment options: surgery and medical management. Your task is to assess the cost-effectiveness of surgical and medical management as alternative treatment policies for 40-year-olds with incipient blastobliticosis.

Medical management arrests progress of the disease; under such care the patient's life expectancy is increased to 15 years, and the pain and disability are reduced to a mild level. The cost of medical management is $200 per year for each remaining year of life.

Surgery can result in a total cure of the disease, but it presents risks. Operative mortality is 5 per cent. Of those who survive, it is estimated that 50 per cent are cured, but this varies from surgeon to surgeon. Whether the patient is cured becomes known at surgery. Those who survive surgery but are not cured are immediately treated by medical management and have the same prognosis that they would have if they had never been operated on (15 years of life with some disability). Those who are cured of blastobliticosis, however, face a 10 per cent risk of stroke, which occurs, on the average, ten years after the operation. Mortality from these strokes is 50 per cent, and those who survive the stroke can expect to live ten more years following the stroke (i.e., 20 years from the time of the operation), but at a moderate level of disability. The patients who are cured and who avoid the stroke, however, have a normal life expectancy of 30 years without disability.

The cost of surgery is $12,000. The expected lifetime cost of treating a nonfatal stroke, should it occur, is estimated to be $10,000; this sum is calculated as a discounted present value from the time the stroke occurs (e.g., an annual expenditure of $1,233 for each of the ten years of life expectancy has a present value, at a 5 per cent discount rate, of $10,000). The cost of treating a fatal stroke is estimated to be $3,000.

A survey of 14 patients indicates that they consider a year of life with the severe symptoms of untreated blastobliticosis to be the equivalent of only 0.2 years of life in normal health. They consider a year with the symptoms and disability of stroke to be the equivalent of 0.7 years of life in normal health. A year with the mild disability of medically managed blastobliticosis is considered to be the equivalent of 0.9 years of life in good health. Surgery results in the same degree of disability as medically managed blastobliticosis does, but for only one year.

Assume a discount rate of 5 per cent per annum.

a. Analyze the cost-effectiveness of the surgical and the medical management of blastobliticosis, ignoring considerations of the quality of life. Make any assumptions you feel you need in order to complete the analysis, but make them explicit. Interpret your results.

b. Introduce considerations of the quality of life and reanalyze the cost-effectiveness of the alternative interventions.

In your analysis you will need to use present values for constant cost streams (i.e., $200 per year for 15 years) and for life spans. For example, the present value of five years at a discount rate of 5 per cent is

$$1 + \frac{1}{1.05} + \frac{1}{(1.05)^2} + \frac{1}{(1.05)^3} + \frac{1}{(1.05)^4} = 4.55.$$

An expenditure of $200 for each of five years would have a present value, therefore, of ($200) (4.55) or $910. The present value of five years of life expectancy would be 4.55 years. The following table gives the present value of an annual expenditure of one dollar for each of N years, or, equivalently, the present value of N years of life.

	Discount Rate	
N (Years)	0 Per Cent	5 Per Cent
1	1	1
5	5	4.55
10	10	8.11
15	15	10.90
20	20	13.09
30	30	16.14

Chapter Nine

Applications of Clinical Decision Analysis

9.1 THE RANGE OF FORMAL APPLICATIONS

The principles of clinical decision analysis can serve many purposes. They can help physicians to think more cogently about a clinical situation, help to clarify reasons for disagreement among physicians about the best course of management for a patient's condition, help to determine the optimal strategy for the care of an individual patient, and help to choose the most socially cost-effective medical strategy for a population of patients. In this chapter we offer several examples of how the principles of decision analysis have been applied in medical care.

The examples we have chosen illustrate several decision-analytic approaches to problems of diagnosis and treatment. Being published reports, they are more representative of formal decision-analytic studies than of informal uses of decision analysis in clinical settings. Our bibliography includes a larger selection of articles and monographs that encompass a variety of formal and less formal applications of clinical decision analysis.

Our first example is an analysis of the value of a diagnostic test — exercise stress testing — in the detection of coronary artery disease. It is a partial analysis that focuses on issues of probability revision and test discrimination and not on the overall decision problem that would require consideration of the timing and efficacy of subsequent treatment decisions and of the values and costs associated with outcomes.

The second example is based upon two analyses of a treatment decision — whether to perform coronary artery bypass graft surgery for patients with coronary artery disease. The two articles discussed in that section[190,271] can be read profitably either before or after reading this chapter. A comparison of the studies gives us an opportunity to explore in some detail the methodologic choices that go into any relatively comprehensive decision analysis.

The final section of the chapter gives a brief overview of the application of computers in clinical decision making.

9.2 EXERCISE STRESS TESTING: AN ANALYSIS OF DIAGNOSTIC TEST INFORMATION

As we saw in Chapter Four, the clinical meaning of a diagnostic test can be expressed in terms of the probability of disease given a particular test result. Bayes' theorem shows that this *posterior* probability of disease depends upon the likelihood of the observed test result in patients with and without the disease as well as on the *prior* probability of disease (the assessed probability that the patient has the disease before the test is conducted). We also saw in Chapter Four how it is theoretically possible to adjust the *positivity criterion* for a test so as to make it more *sensitive* or more *specific*. One test for which various positivity criteria may be chosen is the exercise stress test which is used for the diagnosis of obstructive coronary artery disease.

Rifkin and Hood[211] applied Bayes' formula and the notion of an adjustable positivity criterion to a review of previously published trials of exercise stress testing. Their report criticizes a simple dichotomous "positive-negative" classification of test results and points out apparent inconsistencies in the results of earlier studies. Their paper is instructive not only because it clarifies the value (and limitations) of exercise stress testing but also because it demonstrates the usefulness of a systematic, quantitative interpretation of diagnostic tests. The same type of analysis can be applied to any diagnostic test whose results are arrayed along a continuous scale.

THE CLINICAL RATIONALE AND THE METHOD FOR EXERCISE STRESS TESTING

Exercise stress testing is a relatively safe and simple means of testing the adequacy of blood flow through the coronary arteries. The test instrument is the patient's electrocardiogram (EKG), which is recorded while the patient performs exercises such as walking on a treadmill. During the test the patient normally exercises until a certain heart rate is achieved or until changes occur in the EKG. The part of the EKG that is of special interest is the ST segment, the portion of the tracing that signifies the first phase of electrical repolarization of the heart following each beat. Normally, the ST segment is isoelectric, which is indicated by a flat line at the level of the EKG base line. When blood flow to the heart is inadequate, the ST segment may be depressed. In exercise stress testing the degree of *ST-segment depression* below the horizontal level is the commonly measured test result. Traditionally, ST-segment depression greater than 1 mm (which is equivalent to 1 mV of electrical force) is considered positive, that is, indicative of obstructive coronary artery disease.

The degree of obstruction in the coronary arteries can be visualized in a separate imaging examination, coronary angiography. In this examination a catheter is inserted into an artery and threaded to the entrance of the coronary vessels, a radiopaque dye is injected, and a rapid series of x-ray pictures is taken to depict blood flow through the heart's own vessels. If the coronary vessels show greater than 50 per cent (or, in some studies, 70 per cent) narrowing, this is usually taken as diagnostic of obstructive coronary artery disease. In the studies analyzed by Rifkin and Hood, angiography was the "truth" measure that confirmed or denied the presence of disease. Although angiography is the more definitive test for disease, it is also more risky and costly than exercise stress testing.

The typical patient who is considered a candidate for exercise stress testing is someone who has chest pain of uncertain origin and a normal EKG when at rest. In nearly all cases, patients with evidence of other kinds of heart disease, high blood pressure, or resting EKG abnormalities were excluded from the trials reviewed by Rifkin and Hood.

BAYESIAN ANALYSIS OF EXERCISE STRESS TESTING

Rifkin and Hood introduce their analysis by acknowledging controversy over the diagnostic value of ST-segment depression during exercise stress testing as a predictor of obstructive coronary artery disease. They cite some studies showing a close relation between ST-segment depression and angiography results, but they cite others questioning the predictive value of exercise stress testing. They raise the following question: Are these different results explicable in terms of different patient populations, or is the test measure itself unreliable as applied to different patients by different investigators?

To answer this question, the authors first reanalyze data from three major trials of exercise stress testing conducted since 1970. Each study involved more than 100 patients, and each presented data on the results of angiography in patients with varying degrees of ST-segment depression. In each study the scale of ST-segment depression was divided into discrete intervals of 0.50 mm in width. In fact, this reporting of the ST-segment depression was a distinctive feature of these three studies; many others simply classified patients as having a depression of less than 1.00 mm ("negative") or a depression of greater than or equal to 1.00 mm ("positive").

Based on combined data from the three studies, the authors compute the overall likelihood ratio for each degree of ST-segment depression. Recall from Chapter Four that the numerator of the test likelihood ratio is the probability of a test result (R) in patients with disease (D) and that the denominator is the probability of the same test result in patients without disease. Recall that the likelihood ratio, L, is defined as follows:

$$L = \frac{P[R \mid D]}{P[R \mid \overline{D}]}.$$ (9–1)

Bayes' formula can be used to define the posterior probability of disease, $P[D \mid R]$, as a function of the prior probability of disease, $P[D]$, and the likelihood ratio, L, for the observed test result. For this purpose, Rifkin and Hood use a slightly modified form of Bayes' formula:

$$P[D \mid R] = \frac{P[D]}{P[D] + (1 - P[D])/L}.$$ (9–2)

You might wish to verify that Equation 9–2 is mathematically equivalent to Equation 4–9 in Chapter Four.

From Equation 9–2 the authors generated a family of curves showing the post-test (i.e., posterior) probability of disease as a function of the pre-test (i.e., prior) probability, with each curve representing a different test result and its corresponding likelihood ratio (Figure 9–1). These curves graphically illustrate the extent to which the predictive value of the test depends upon both the prior probability of disease and the likelihood ratio. If a patient's prior probability of disease is 0.6 and the ST-segment depression is between 1.00 and 1.49 mm, then the posterior probability of disease is approximately 0.77. If a second patient has only half as great a prior probability of disease (0.3) but has an ST-segment depression between 1.50 and 1.99 mm, the posterior probability of disease is just slightly higher, about 0.81. Notice that the curves also can be taken to indicate the predictive value negative of a test result, or the posterior probability that the patient does not have the disease. In particular, an ST-segment depression of less than 1.00 mm is associated with a reduced probability of disease, but the reduction is relatively modest.

These curves are illuminating, but they do not bear directly on the question of discrepant results from different investigators. Rifkin and Hood also compute a combined likelihood ratio curve, for which they pool the test results with an ST-segment depression of greater than 1.00 mm for all patients in their three major studies. This curve (Figure 9–2) depicts the expected results if all patients with a depression of greater than or equal to 1.00 mm are considered to be "positive" and all others are considered to be "negative." On this curve the authors superimposed additional data points from other studies in the literature in which patients were classified as showing an ST-segment depression of greater or less than 1.00 mm.

The correspondence of data from additional studies with the derived curve is striking. It suggests that variation in the patient population (reflected in the prior probability of disease) is a sufficient explanation for most of the observed discrepancies in the predictive value of exercise stress testing.

A COMMENT ON BAYESIAN ANALYSIS
OF DIAGNOSTIC TEST INFORMATION

The data requirements for a Bayesian analysis of diagnostic tests are straightforward, but they are often not available in reports of clinical trials. In discussing

Figure 9–1 Curves showing the post-test (posterior) probability of disease as a function of the pre-test (prior) probability of disease for various test results. L indicates the likelihood ratio. (Modified from Rifkin and Hood, p. 684.[211])

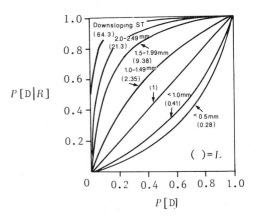

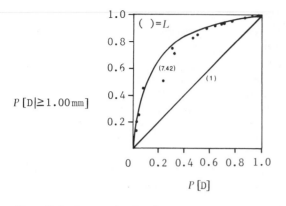

Figure 9-2 *A curve showing the post-test (posterior) probability of disease as a function of the pre-test (prior) probability of disease for a test result greater than or equal to 1.00 mm of ST-segment depression. L indicates likelihood ratio. (Modified from Rifkin and Hood, p. 683.[211])*

their study, Rifkin and Hood note the "paucity of data in the literature that are amenable to analysis in the format of half-millimeter ranges of ST-segment depression." It is indeed frustrating to search the literature for information on a particular test, uncover carefully conducted clinical trials, and then find that results have been inappropriately aggregated so as to obscure important relations of degree. At other times a critical numerator or denominator may be missing from one of the probabilities needed to compute sensitivity, specificity, or predictive value. Occasionally it seems clear that such information was available to the investigators, but they simply did not think to include it. These lapses could be substantially reduced if investigators kept in mind the requirements of Bayes' formula, which are really no more than the requirements for logical inference from test results.

Bayesian analysis in general and the exercise stress testing example in particular emphasize the salience of the prior probability of disease. One implication is that different medical centers should adjust their diagnostic judgments according to the underlying prevalence of different diseases in the populations they serve. Another implication is the importance of gaining for individual patients some quantitative understanding of this predictive value of pre-test information from the patient's history and physical examination. In some clinical areas there have been notable efforts to identify and quantify "risk factors."[5] Indeed, Rifkin and Hood argue that results of exercise stress testing should be treated as just another risk factor for coronary artery disease. Semantics aside, risk factors from epidemiologic surveys, information from a patient's history, physical findings, and diagnostic test results all work toward the same goal, which is to help the clinician better predict the presence or absence of disease in the patient. Bayes' formula describes how they all come together.

9.3 CORONARY ARTERY BYPASS GRAFT SURGERY

Decision analysis can be helpful in clinical situations for which a rather complete data base exists and in which the need is to structure the information into a format that is useful for decision making. Were those the only situations in which clinical decision analysis is helpful, however, the value of the approach would be very limited. Most clinical decisions must be based on incomplete data and must incorporate what inevitably are subjective value judgments. It is in these latter circumstances that decision analysis — the process of structuring the decision problem in the form of a simple tree and forcing oneself to marshal all the evidence and values in a coherent way — may exhibit its greatest advantage. When the uncertainty is great, the process of analysis can highlight the data to which the decision is most sensitive and suggest specific pieces of information that the physician should seek from the literature and from the opinions of peers. Debates can be focused upon particular probability or utility assessments rather than diffused into generalities. These, of course, are the values of breaking the problem down into component parts — structure, probabilities, and utilities — and then reassembling them after each has been analyzed.

With this motivation in mind, we turn to our second major application, that is, the decision whether to perform coronary artery bypass graft (CABG) surgery for a patient with documented coronary artery disease. As this book goes to press, the efficacy of CABG is very much debated, both in terms of its effect on survival and in terms of its long-term ability to relieve the symptoms of angina pectoris. And yet, thousands of decisions to operate continue to be made, despite the uncertainty.

A DESCRIPTION OF CABG SURGERY AND THE DECISION PROBLEM

The CABG procedure itself involves grafting a piece of vein, usually taken from the patient's leg, onto one of the major coronary arteries in order to bypass an atherosclerotic obstruction. Sometimes two or three bypasses are created during a given procedure. If a patient with angina is considered to be a candidate for a CABG, the physician would first submit the patient to coronary angiography. If an obstruction is found in one or more of the three major coronary arteries (left anterior descending, left circumflex, or right) and if the indications are that the lesions are operable and that the patient's heart is strong enough to withstand surgery, then a CABG may be prescribed. The purpose of CABG surgery is to relieve the disabling symptoms of angina and possibly to enhance long-term survival. Against these hoped-for benefits must be weighed the risk of operative mortality and the possibility that the patient's condition may worsen, not improve. The major reason for the latter possibility would be lack of patency (graft failure).

The alternative to surgery is medical management with drugs, including standard treatments for angina such as nitroglycerin. Usually, a patient who undergoes surgery will receive some continued drug therapy as well.

Three sets of issues surround this decision problem, and as usual they can be structured into questions of (1) probabilities, (2) personal utilities, and (3) cost and cost-effectiveness.

The probability issues concern the efficacy of the procedure: What does a CABG do for the patient? Included are questions as to the operative mortality, the probabilities of short-term and long-term pain relief, and the probabilities of long-term survival. These probabilities vary considerably from individual to individual, depending on such factors as the number of coronary arteries involved, the ability of the patient's heart muscle to pump blood, prior heart attacks, and perhaps the patient's age, sex, and other cardiovascular risk factors. Parallel to these probability assessments (except for operative mortality) are those for medical management, the alternative course of treatment.

Controlled clinical trials, such as the study completed by the Veterans Administration in 1977,[178] can be an important source of probability estimates, but trials are never definitive for all patients in all settings. Each clinical setting has certain unique characteristics, so that probabilities derived from a trial may not apply. For example, hospitals differ in their operative mortalities. Moreover, a clinical trial rarely can shed light on all of the important probabilities. For example, long-term survival cannot be assessed objectively for many years after the initiation of a trial. Beyond probabilities, clinical decisions must take into account personal values and preferences, as reflected perhaps by utility assessments.

Clinical trials do provide valuable information for clinical decision analysis, but neither is a substitute for the other. The trial provides some objective data; the analysis provides a structure for interpreting the data that exist and for evaluating the implications of probabilities and value judgments that cannot be assessed objectively.

The utility issues in the CABG decision are of two kinds. One has to do with the relative values assigned to early and later mortality. Two procedures that have a 90 per cent survival rate after five years may not be viewed equivalently if one involves 10 per cent immediate mortality and the other involves 2 per cent mortality in each of the first five years. The latter would yield a greater life expectancy. Moreover, the patient may wish to assign greater value to the more proximate years than to the later years, which would further favor the latter procedure. The second utility issue in the CABG context has to do with the trade-off between relief from pain and disability, and survival. Any given outcome can be described as some number of years of survival, each at some level of pain and disability (e.g., 15 years of survival, during 10 of which the patient is free of pain and 5 of which the patient is in pain). In assigning utilities to these outcomes, trade-offs between early operative mortality and the promise of pain relief should the patient survive are taken into account. Quality-adjusted life years (introduced in Chapter Seven) is one utility measure that captures this trade-off but is not the only possibility, as we shall see later in this chapter. Differences in attitudes concerning this trade-off can lead to very different decisions, even assuming the same data base for the probabilities.

Finally, the cost-effectiveness issue is raised strikingly by CABG. The cost of the procedure in 1978 was about $15,000. CABG alone accounts for nearly 1 per cent of all medical expenditures in the United States. Is this cost justified? If the equivalent resources could yield greater improvements in longevity and quality of life by other means, would it not be appropriate to reserve those resources for the other uses? An explicit assessment of cost-effectiveness permits these questions to be addressed.

Before turning to the analysis itself, we should stress that no decision analysis should be accepted unthinkingly. Data change, values differ, and conditions vary. In evaluating the analysis of another physician or analyst, a physician may or may not agree with the assumptions, probabilities, and utilities. A good analysis will be accompanied by sensitivity analyses, and this should help. But even the most thorough analysis is no more than a prescriptive guide to decision making and should be continually revised in light of new evidence or changing values.

The rest of this section will be devoted largely to a comparison of two independently developed but conceptually and philosophically very similar analyses of the CABG decision.[190,271] They differ in some interesting ways with respect to structure, probability assessment, and utility assessment. We explore these differences to illustrate how two analysts coped with the need to simplify the problem so as to highlight the central issues. In addition, we shall illustrate the interpretation of clinical data in the context of decision analysis. We do this by relating the findings of various uncontrolled clinical series[25,103,159,229] to the analyses and discuss their limitations in the process. Then we turn to the findings of a randomized clinical trial[178] and illustrate how these data complement but do not substitute for the clinical decision analysis. In this context we illustrate how sensitivity analyses, by suggesting those probability estimates to which the decision is most sensitive, can feed back to the process of data collection and contribute to the design of clinical trials.

STRUCTURING AND ANALYZING THE CABG DECISION

To facilitate our exposition, we shall refer to the two published analyses as study A (Pauker[190]) and study B (Weinstein et al.[271]).

Before describing the details of — and differences between — the two studies, we would like to highlight the similarities. The two independent analyses share what is really a very similar approach, even to the extent that the decision trees analyzed are not that much different from each other. Seven common elements can be identified, as follows:

The Clustering of Cases by Patient Characteristics. Both studies, recognizing the importance of patient characteristics in assessing both probabilities and utilities, develop a patient typology from which are selected some cases for analysis. The typologies are described by such characteristics as the preoperative severity of angina, the operability and nature of the disease, the function of the left ventricle (i.e., the strength of the heart), and, importantly, the preferences of the patient.

The Basic Structure of the Decision Tree. The decision trees actually analyzed are so similar that it is possible to draw a generic tree that incorporates the common elements (Figure 9–3). These elements are the decision whether

Figure 9–3 A simplified general structure of the CABG decision problem.

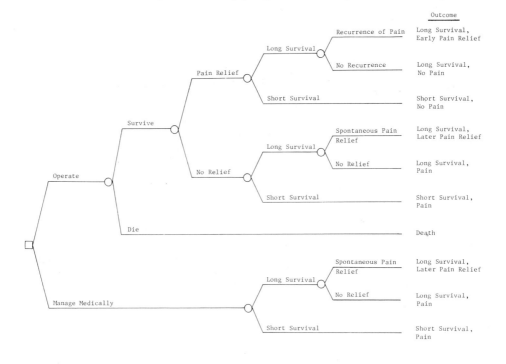

to operate, the possibility of operative mortality, short-term and long-term pain relief, and short-term and long-term survival. The differences, which are subsequently discussed, include the handling of graft patency and of nonfatal surgical complications as well as the classifying of different levels of pain relief and the timing of mortality and pain relief outcomes.

Outcomes and Utilities.   As seen in Figure 9–3, all outcomes are described along two dimensions: survival and degree of pain. Both analyses assign to each possible outcome a utility that reflects the possible trade-offs between these two attributes. Indeed, both analyses allow for variations in patient preferences, such that some patients might assign virtually full weight to survival while others might assign substantial weight to pain relief (i.e., would accept a major reduction in longevity in exchange for pain relief while alive).

Probability Assessments.   Both studies rely on published clinical series for data on short-term survival and pain relief and are supplemented by expert subjective assessments to fill in the gaps in such areas as long-term survival. Ultimately, both sets of assessments are highly subjective, given the paucity of data and the discrepancies and distortions in the existing data. Both were completed prior to the publication of the Veterans Administration randomized trial and therefore do not incorporate those results.

The Calculation of Optimal Action Conditional Upon Patient Characteristics. Given assessments of utilities and probabilities, both analyses employ the usual averaging-out procedure to derive expected utilities. On that basis, the preferred course of action is determined for each set of patients. In both analyses the preferred course depends upon patient preferences and other characteristics. The measure of expected utility under the surgical or medical strategy can be given an interpretation analogous to quality-adjusted life expectancy.

Sensitivity Analysis.   Both studies include sensitivity analysis, which permits the user to see the effect of changes in such probabilities as those for operative mortality or long-term survival as well as in preference characteristics.

The Underlying Philosophy.   Both analyses reflect a similar philosophy with regard to the role of analysis in clinical decision making. Both seek to be explicit about the underlying rationale for decisions. They share a flexible attitude toward the incorporation of new evidence and personal preferences and point out the caveats of accepting the results of the analysis too rigidly.

In the next several sections, the two studies are compared and contrasted along each of these dimensions to illustrate the variety of choices that a decision analyst has in structuring a medical decision problem.

Patient Characteristics

Table 9–1 lists the patient characteristics considered in each of the two studies. The characteristics fall into four broad categories: demographic characteristics, symptoms and history, severity of disease, and preferences. In each study a set of hypothetical patient categories varying along these dimensions is constructed and analyzed. In general, study A defines patient categories more broadly than study B. There is a trade-off here, and a judgment is made by each analyst. The more narrowly one specifies patient categories, the more specific are the implications of the analysis but the greater are the demands for specific information.

TABLE 9-1 PATIENT CHARACTERISTICS CONSIDERED IN DEFINING
HYPOTHETICAL CATEGORIES*

PATIENT CHARACTERISTICS	STUDY A[190]	STUDY B[271]	DEFINITION OF CHARACTERISTICS
Demographic Characteristics			
Age	0	+	Study B: age 40, 50, or 60
Symptoms and History			
Severity of angina	+	+	Study A: "disabling" or "asymptomatic"
			Study B: "severe," "moderate," or "asymptomatic"†
Congestive heart failure	0	+	Study B: present or absent
History of MI	0	+	Study B: present or absent
Severity of Disease			
Number of vessels	0	+	Study B: 0, 1, 2, or 3 vessels obstructed at least 70 per cent
Anatomy/operability	+	+	Study A: "good" (localized occlusion) or "fair" (diffuse occlusion)
			Study B: 0, 1, 2, or 3 vessels "operable"
Specific vessels involved	+	0	Study A: asymptomatic patients with obstruction of the left anterior descending (LAD) artery considered as a distinct category
Cardiac output	+	+	Study A: "good" (cardiac ejection fraction greater than 40 percent), "fair" (ejection fraction between 25 and 40 percent), or "poor" (ejection fraction less than 25 percent)
			Study B: same as Study A, except the ranges are greater than 45 percent, between 35 and 45 percent, and less than 35 percent, respectively
Preferences			
Trade-offs between pain and survival	+	+	See text, page 279.

*A plus sign denotes that the characteristic was considered in the study, and a zero denotes that it was not. MI indicates myocardial infarction.

†"Severe" denotes New York Heart Association (NYHA) classes III and IV; "moderate" denotes NYHA classes I and II.

The Structure of the Decision Tree and Simplifying Assumptions

To be useful, a decision analysis must simplify the clinical situation. However, the simplifications must not be so severe as to rob the representation of the problem of its most salient features. Both studies invoke simplifying assumptions, but each does so in a rather different way.

The common features, in their most general form, are displayed in Figure 9–3. The basic decision is the same: to operate or to manage medically. Both studies suppose that coronary angiography has already been done, that the patient has survived that procedure, and that the findings from the procedure (e.g., number of arteries occluded, severity and operability, ventricular function) are known and become part of the patient characteristics entering the decision. Both make the simplifying assumptions that a second operation after graft closure is not considered and that a delay in the operation to await developments is not possible. The former assumption tends to favor medical management, while the latter tends to favor surgery. Each assumption could be relaxed, but at a substantial cost in terms of complicating the decision tree; hence, both analysts choose to invoke the simplifications.

The basic decision trees for the two studies are shown in Figure 9–4A (study A) and Figure 9–4B (study B). Let us interpret them and examine them in detail.

Consider first the initial decision point ($\boxed{A}$) in both decision trees. In each case the choice is whether to operate or to manage medically.

Consider next the "operate" branch. Both formulations (at point Ⓑ) provide for the possibility of operative death, defined by each as death within 30 days of surgery. Study B also allows for the possibility of nonfatal complications of surgery. Specifically, the possibility of perioperative myocardial infarction and of "other complications" (such as stroke, pulmonary embolism, and infection) is considered. If the "other complication" is a stroke, the possibility of permanent chronic limitation is included. Considering complications of surgery requires the analyst in study B to assess additional probabilities and utilities: First, the subsequent probabilities of survival and pain relief depend on whether the patient has suffered a heart attack during surgery, and second, a negative adjustment is made to the utility of each outcome following complications to allow for a reduction in the quality of life. Whether these additional assessments will alter the preferred strategy cannot be foretold prior to analysis and sensitivity testing, but they certainly complicate the analysis.

Following the "survive" branch from Ⓑ in each figure (and skipping past the surgical complications in study B), we come to point Ⓒ. This is the point

Figure 9–4A A decision tree for the CABG decision problem (study A). Outcomes describe the first two years only. Subsequent years are determined by recycling through the tree from the dashed line to the right. Outcome descriptions followed by an ellipsis (...) indicate that the outcome is not completely described as of year 2. Branches to the right of the dashed line recycle every year for years 1 through 5, with the probabilities dependent on the current state: patent or not patent and pain or no pain. (Modified from Pauker.[190])

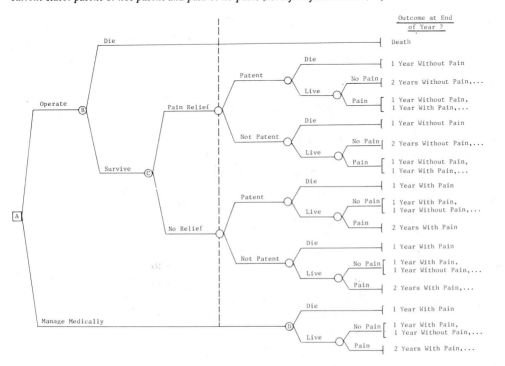

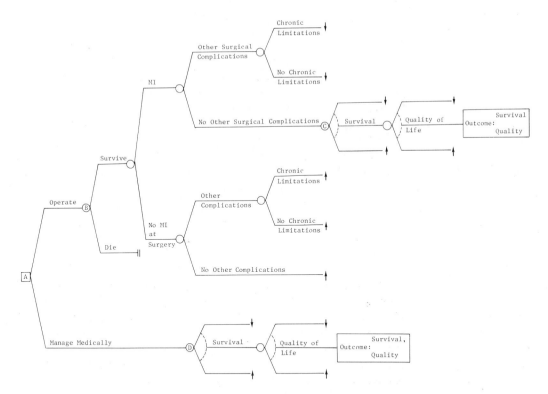

Figure 9–4B *A decision tree for the CABG decision problem (study B). An arrow (↑ or ↓) indicates that the branching structure beyond that point is similar to that found at the prototypical node in the direction of the arrow. A double bar (‖) indicates a terminal branch. Dotted curved lines at a chance point (⤎) indicate a range of possible outcomes, the one shown being representative only of that range. (Modified from Weinstein, Pliskin, and Stason.[271])*

at which the outcomes begin to unfold: survival and quality of life. Here the two studies take rather different technical approaches, although the overall concept is the same.

Consider the unfolding of outcomes in Figure 9–4A first. The first chance node (at Ⓒ) describes whether the operation has succeeded in relieving the anginal pain. Two levels of pain are considered: no pain and the level of pain that the patient had experienced at the outset. Following this resolution of uncertainty, there begins a sequence of events that are assumed to occur at the end of each year following surgery.

Specifically, it is first revealed whether the graft remains patent. Next, depending on patency, there is a probability of death (from myocardial infarction). Finally, if the patient survives the end of the year, then, depending on the patency of the graft, the pain that had been relieved may recur, or the pain that had not been relieved may disappear. Recurrence is assumed to be associated with lost patency, whereas spontaneous relief is assumed to occur with some probability independent of the patient's prior history. One iteration through the tree thus establishes the prognosis up to the end of year 2. For example, if the patient survives through the end of year 1 with no recurrence of pain, then the outcome is at least two years of life, both of which are pain free. The outcome for year 3 is revealed by the next iteration of events, which are assumed to occur just at the end of year 2. Each iteration consists of the evolution of the underlying patency of the graft (which is not observed, but which determines the subsequent probabilities), the possibility of death at the end of the corresponding year, and the possibility of the presence or the absence of pain, as indicated by the branching to the right of the dashed line. The time horizon is five years; thus, four iterations through this part of the tree are required. Outcomes (survival, pain level) after five years are not considered and are therefore implicitly assumed to be comparable between surgery and medical management.

Before we contrast this approach with that taken in study B, consider the medical management branch in Figure 9–4A. Here the same kind of recursive cycling through the tree occurs, except that patency is not an issue. It is assumed that spontaneous pain relief occurs at the same annual rate following medical management as following surgical failure; that pain recurrence occurs with graft closure and may occur in subsequent years following spontaneous pain relief; that surgery decreases the annual mortality as long as the graft remains patent, but that mortality becomes greater if the graft closes; and all probabilities in the recursive part of the tree (i.e., to the right of the dashed line) are considered constant from year to year.

Note that the *recursive* approach taken in study A (i.e., recycling through part of the tree at yearly intervals) could have been represented by tacking end-to-end, four times, the portion of the tree to the right of the dashed line. Conceptually and technically that is how the analysis was actually done. However, for purposes of presentation it is neater to indicate such repeated tree structures as the author of study A has done. The disadvantage of the recursive structure, however, is that it assumes the probabilities to the right of the dashed line remain constant from year to year. That simplifying assumption is the price for conceptual clarity and computational ease.

Now consider the decision tree in study B (Figure 9–4B). There are several differences in approach from points Ⓒ and Ⓓ on (in the surgical and medical management branches, respectively). Instead of looking at outcomes on a yearly basis and truncating the decision tree at five years, study B divides time into the following intervals: the first year, the second through fifth years, and the rest of the patient's life. Survival in year 1 and the degree of pain relief in year 1 are assessed conditionally upon the presence or absence of perioperative heart attack. Three levels of angina are designated: severe, mild to moderate, and none. Transitions from any initial level to any other level are possible. Next, the annual probabilities of survival in years 2 through 5 are estimated. Unlike study A, study B fails to consider the explicit relation between mortality and patency. However, the annual mortality, which was assumed constant in study A, can vary in study B. Next, the probabilities of various degrees of angina in years 2 through 5 and beyond year 5 are considered in study B. However, while study B assumes a constant degree of angina for any one patient within years 2 through 5, study A permits transitions from one year to the next. The survival rate in each year beyond year 5 is obtained in study B by extrapolating the two-year and five-year survival rates according to a standard statistical model that provides for the annual mortality probability to grow at a constant rate from year to year. Each possible outcome at the tip of each extensive branch of the tree (summarized conceptually by the "fans" following Ⓒ and Ⓓ in Figure 9–4B) is described by the length of life (survival) and the degree of angina (quality of life) in each year of the patient's lifetime.

Thus, the key differences of study B from study A are (1) the inclusion of surgical complications; (2) the use of three, rather than two, degrees of angina; (3) the use of an extensive, rather than recursive, approach; (4) the omission of patency as a separate variable; (5) the assumption of an unchanging degree of angina during years 2 through 5; and (6) a time horizon spanning the patient's entire lifetime rather than five years.

Truncation of the time horizon at five years presumes that the outcomes of the two alternatives become the same at five years and remain the same thereafter. If the estimated five-year survival rate is comparable in the two groups, the only assumption needed would be that annual mortalities beyond five years are equal. The evidence to that effect is equivocal for CABG surgery versus medical management, and we shall return to this question in light of the randomized trial of the Veterans Administration. If the survival rate at five years is different, for example, a 60 per cent survival rate with surgery versus a 50 per cent survival rate with medical management, truncation would presume not only that the annual mortalities with surgery and medical management were equal beyond five years but also that 16.7 per cent of the remaining surgical patients (i.e., 10 per cent out of 60 per cent) would die immediately after the end of year 5 to equalize the cumulative survival rate in the two groups. The difference in the expected number of years of survival attained by each group depends not only on the difference in the survival rate at five years but also on the length of life expectancy thereafter. Even if annual survival rates (and, hence, life expectancy) beyond five years were the same for both groups, the longer the common life expectancy ahead, the greater the difference would be in the expected number of years of life between the two groups. The difficulty with extending the probabilities of life expectancy beyond five years is that the probabilities to be assessed are inevitably less objective because of the lack of clinical data.

Outcomes and Utility Assessments

In both analyses, outcomes are described by the number of years of survival and the degree of angina in each of those years. The assignment of utilities to these outcomes is carried out in rather different ways, but both are entirely consistent with the methodology we have described in Chapter Seven, and both can be interpreted in terms of the concept of quality-adjusted life years.

In study A, four different types of individual preference patterns — and hence utilities — are considered. The first describes the patient who is concerned only with longevity; quality of life (pain relief) is not a factor. However, this type of patient is risk averse with respect to longevity; a certainty of 2.5 years is preferred to an even gamble at five years versus immediate death. In the example used in the study, if 0 years has a utility of 0 and 5 years (out of a possible 5) has a utility of 100, then 3 years is given a utility of 88 for this patient.*

The second type of patient in study A is one who cares only about pain-free years of life; years with pain, in this extreme case, are no better than death. This patient type is also risk averse, but with respect to pain-free years. Thus, the outcome of five years of life, the first two of which are pain free, would have the same utility as the outcome of two years of pain-free life, which in this case is 52 on the same scale of 0 to 100 between five pain-free years and no pain-free years.

---

*Actually, the utilities were derived from a hypothetical utility function, $u(Y) = K_0(1 - e^{-K_1 Y})$, where Y is survival. The number K_1 reflects the degree of risk aversion, and K_0 is a scale factor to ensure that $u(5) = 100$.

The third and fourth types of patient preference in study A are intermediate between the first two in the sense that both life years and pain relief are valued positively. In one case the utility for the patient is the arithmetic average of the utilities for the first two patient types. In the other, which weighs pain relief somewhat more heavily, the utility is the geometric average of the first two types. Thus, the outcome of three-year survival, two years of which are pain free, would have a utility of

$$\frac{88 + 52}{2} = 70$$

in the former case and a utility of

$$\sqrt{(88) \cdot (52)} = 67.6$$

in the latter. The utilities for all four patient types are shown in Figure 9–5.

In study B all of the patients are assumed to be concerned with quality-adjusted life years. That is, each year of survival is weighted by a number (from 0 to 1) corresponding to the quality of life in that year. For death the weight is 0. For severe angina the weight depends on patient preferences: For active patients this weight is relatively low (0.7), because angina implies a high cost in terms of the ability to perform normal activities; for sedentary patients this weight is higher (0.8), because the angina is less disabling for less active persons. Mild angina is assigned a weight intermediate between those for severe angina

Figure 9–5   Utility curves for the four patient types in study A. Types "pain" and "life" consider only a single factor. The type "life" curve is steeper (more risk averse) than the type "pain" curve. Types "either" and "both" consider both survival and freedom from pain. For each of these latter types, the curve is determined by the number of years of survival, and the position on the curve is determined by the number of years free of pain. (Modified from Pauker, p. 11.[190])

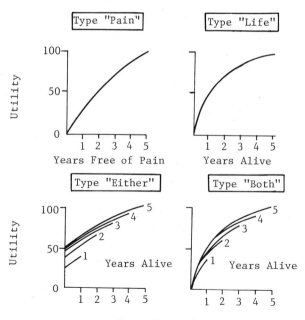

and total pain relief (the latter being 1.0). Thus, an outcome of ten years survival, three of which involve severe angina, would have a utility of

$$(3) (0.8) + (7) (1) = 9.4$$

for a sedentary patient and a utility of

$$(3) (0.7) + (7) (1) = 9.1$$

for an active patient. Patients are assumed to be risk neutral with respect to these quality-adjusted life years (QALYs); expected utility corresponds to quality-adjusted life expectancy.

The interpretation of the weights assigned to the quality of life is consistent with the constant proportional trade-off assumption described in Chapter Seven. Thus, the weight of 0.7 for severe angina implies that 10 years with severe angina are valued the same as 7 years with no angina, and 20 years with severe angina are valued the same as 14 years with no angina.

The utility scales used in the two studies are not as different as they may seem. The first patient type in study A (i.e., the one who cares only about life years, not pain) is analogous to a patient in study B who assigns a weight of 1.0 to severe angina. The only difference is that the patient in study A is assumed to be risk averse with respect to longevity, while the patient in study B is risk neutral (i.e., a life-expectancy maximizer). By the same line of reasoning, the second patient type in study A (i.e., the one who cares only about pain-free years) is analogous to a patient in study B who assigns a weight of 0 to any year with angina. (The lowest weight actually considered in study B is 0.7 for chronic severe angina in the active patient.) Again, the difference lies in the assumption about risk aversion in study A. Finally, the utilities for the intermediate patient types in study A correspond roughly to the intermediate weights in study B. For example, the patient in study A whose utility is a simple average of those for the first two types is similar to the patient in study B whose weight for severe angina is 0.5, the only difference being the assumption of risk aversion in study A. The final patient type in study A has no exact analogue in study B, nor do the patients with weights between 0.5 and 1.0 in study B have analogues in study A.

There is one more factor contributing to the utility assigned to each outcome, namely, the effect of surgery itself and its complications, if any. Study A accounts for the disability owing to surgery by reducing the quality of one year without pain to one year with pain. Thus, an outcome of four years, two of which are without pain, would be valued as if it were four years, one of which is without pain, if the outcome followed surgery; no such adjustment would be made, obviously, if the outcome followed medical management. In study B, however, this adjustment is less radical. Specifically, the quality level in the first year (on the same scale of 0 to 1) is assumed to be reduced by 10 per cent by uncomplicated surgery and by 20 per cent by postoperative complications. If chronic disability occurs owing to perioperative stroke, the quality level of all remaining years is reduced by half, so that a year with severe angina in a sedentary patient (a quality-adjusted value of 0.8) would be reduced to an equivalent of 0.4 years of health if the patient suffers a stroke owing to surgery.

In both studies the utilities assessed may be interpreted in terms of quality-adjusted life years, but the interpretation is more direct in study B. The utility value in study B is itself the equivalent number of years of health (free of pain or disability). In study A the utilities are on an arbitrary scale of 0 to 100 (rather than on a scale of 0 to 5 corresponding to zero to five equivalent years free of pain); therefore, the conversion to quality-adjusted life years takes an extra step. Consider the outcome of five years, two of which are pain free, for a patient of the third type in study A (i.e., whose utility is an average of those for the first two patient types). Suppose this outcome has a utility of 75 for this patient type. We find in Figure 9–5 the outcome of the form "X life years, all pain free," that has a utility of 75. We find that a value of X of three years has this property. Hence, for this patient type the outcome (five years, two of which are pain free) is the equivalent of three quality-adjusted life years. For the active patient who weights a year of severe angina at 0.7 in study B, the same outcome would be equivalent to

$$(3) (0.7) + 2$$

or 4.1 quality-adjusted life years.

Our reasons for mentioning this interpretation of the utilities are twofold. First, when utilities are assigned it is good to use as many checks on consistency as possible. (Did you really mean your utility scale to have these implications?) Second, it is helpful to be able to interpret results (expected utilities) in meaningful terms rather than just as utilities. After all, a difference of 5.7 on a utility scale of 0 to 100 is difficult to interpret, but the statement that surgery yields 1.3 more quality-adjusted life years than medical management yields is interpretable and quite suggestive.

The Assessment of Probabilities

In both studies the probabilities were assessed ultimately by subjective means, by experts in cardiac disease who had knowledge of the literature. The reasons for not relying on the literature exclusively are, first, that most studies are too small to provide reliable probability assessments suitable for patients with specific characteristics and, second, that some outcomes (such as the later recurrence of angina) are not reported in most studies. In areas in which the literature does provide reliable data (e.g., the operative mortality, the graft patency rate, the two-year survival rate), these are used as the basis for the assessments in the studies.

As suggested previously, study A required the assessment of two initial probabilities and six annual probabilities. The initial probabilities are operative mortality and postoperative pain relief. The annual probabilities are the annual graft closure rate, the annual mortality with a patent graft, the annual mortality with a closed graft, the rate of spontaneous pain relief per year, the rate of spontaneous pain recurrence per year, and the annual mortality under medical management. Spontaneous pain relief and recurrence are assumed to occur at the same rate under medical management as they do following surgery with graft closure.

In study A these eight probabilities are assessed for each set of patient characteristics considered: the presence or absence of symptoms, good or fair coronary anatomy, and good or fair ventricular function. For asymptomatic patients the only coronary anatomy considered is occlusion of the left anterior descending artery, and the anatomy in those cases is assumed to be good.

As a kind of sensitivity analysis in study A, probability assessments are made separately for three classes of surgical teams to account for differences in skills and past results. Since the literature suggests wide variation in the frequency of such events as operative mortality, it is useful to analyze the effects of better or worse than typical performance so that the results are meaningful in different hospital settings.

The full set of probabilities used in study A is shown in Table 9–2.

TABLE 9-2 PROBABILITIES ASSESSED IN STUDY A*

	DISABLING ANGINA									ASYMPTOMATIC		
Patient Characteristics												
Coronary anatomy	Good	Good	Good	Fair	Fair	Fair	Good	Good	Good	LAD	LAD	LAD
Ventricular function	Good	Good	Good	Good	Good	Good	Fair	Fair	Fair	Good	Good	Good
Past surgical results	Exc	Good	Avg	Exc	Good	Avg	Exc	Good	Avg	Exc	Good	Avg
Probabilities												
Surgical Outcome												
Operative mortality	0.01	0.03	0.06	0.02	0.06	0.12	0.04	0.12	0.24	0.02	0.04	0.08
Operative success with pain cure	0.90	0.85	0.80	0.80	0.70	0.60	0.88	0.80	0.70	0.95	0.90	0.85
Graft closure/year	0.05	0.10	0.15	0.10	0.20	0.30	0.07	0.15	0.25	0.05	0.10	0.15
Annual mortality with patent graft	0.04	0.04	0.04	0.07	0.07	0.07	0.12	0.12	0.12	0.05	0.05	0.05
Annual mortality with closed graft	0.07	0.07	0.07	0.12	0.12	0.12	0.18	0.18	0.18	0.12	0.12	0.12
Spontaneous pain cure/year	0.03	0.03	0.03	0.02	0.02	0.02	0.03	0.03	0.03	0.03	0.03	0.03
Spontaneous pain recurrence/year	0.04	0.04	0.04	0.04	0.04	0.04	0.04	0.04	0.04	0.04	0.04	0.04
Natural History												
Annual mortality	0.05	0.05	0.05	0.10	0.10	0.10	0.15	0.15	0.15	0.10	0.10	0.10
Spontaneous pain cure/year	0.03	0.03	0.03	0.02	0.02	0.02	0.03	0.03	0.03	0.03	0.03	0.03
Spontaneous pain recurrence/year	0.04	0.04	0.04	0.04	0.04	0.04	0.04	0.04	0.04	0.04	0.04	0.04

*LAD indicates proximal obstruction to the left anterior descending coronary artery; Exc, excellent; and Avg, average. (Modified from Pauker.[190])

In study B it is necessary to assess more probabilities than in study A, because such rates as annual mortality are not necessarily assumed to be constant from year to year. The survival rates to year 1, year 2, and year 5 are assessed independently, as is operative mortality. Similarly, the probability of each degree of angina in each time interval (year 1, years 2 through 5, years 6 and beyond) is assessed conditionally upon the severity of angina in the previous interval. For example, for one patient type, operative mortality is assigned a probability of 0.03, relief from angina postoperatively is assigned a probability of 0.70, survival through year 1 is assigned a probability ranging from 0.93 to 0.97, depending on the degree of angina postoperatively and on whether there was a perioperative myocardial infarction, and so forth. The full set of survival probabilities through each year of life is generated by a statistical "curve-fitting" procedure, whereby the estimates of the two-year and five-year survival rates are extrapolated to a full survival curve based on a standard probability distribution.* The probability distribution used has, as a special case, the constant-mortality-rate, or exponential, distribution implicitly assumed in study A.

---

*The actual probability distribution used was the Weibull distribution, which is defined by $P[Y \leq y] = 1 - e^{-ay^b}$

Thus, the survival probabilities in study B are based on slightly more flexible assumptions under which the mortality may increase from year to year. The price of such flexibility is an increase in the number of assessments required.

Results

Both studies present results that are rather favorable to surgery, especially for patients who value pain relief highly. Results in terms of expected utilities are shown in Tables 9–3 and 9–4.

TABLE 9–3   RESULTS OF ANALYSIS OF THE CABG DECISION IN STUDY A: EXPECTED UTILITIES AND UTILITY DIFFERENCES*

	DISABLING ANGINA									ASYMPTOMATIC		
Patient Characteristics												
Coronary anatomy	Good	Good	Good	Fair	Fair	Fair	Good	Good	Good	LAD	LAD	LAD
Ventricular function	Good	Good	Good	Good	Good	Good	Fair	Fair	Fair	Good	Good	Good
Past surgical results	Exc	Good	Avg	Exc	Good	Avg	Exc	Good	Avg	Exc	Good	Avg
Patient Type†												
Pain												
	58.2‡	47.4	37.9	43.8	28.5	17.1	44.2	30.0	16.7	−15.7	−26.5	−36.6
	64.0§	53.3	43.7	47.2	31.9	20.5	48.5	34.3	21.0	80.0	80.8	80.8
Life												
	−0.4‡	−2.5	−5.6	−0.3	−4.6	−10.5	−1.9	−9.4	−20.5	1.9	−0.4	−4.6
	95.4§	95.4	95.4	91.1	91.1	91.1	87.0	87.0	87.0	93.0	91.1	91.1
Either												
	28.9‡	22.5	16.1	21.8	12.0	3.3	21.1	10.3	−1.9	−6.9	−13.4	−20.6
	79.5§	73.1	66.7	69.0	59.2	50.5	66.8	55.9	45.7	85.9	85.9	85.9
Both												
	63.9‡	53.5	43.9	50.2	34.5	22.0	50.6	35.7	21.0	−12.3	−22.8	−33.2
	71.4§	61.0	51.4	54.6	38.9	26.4	56.2	41.3	26.6	85.2	85.2	85.2

*LAD indicates proximal obstruction of the left anterior descending coronary artery; Exc, excellent; and Avg, average. (Modified from Pauker.[190])

†Patient type indicates the type of patient preferences (utilities). Type "pain" is concerned with freedom from pain; type "life" is concerned with life expectancy; and types "either" and "both" are concerned with both. For details see the text and Figure 9–5.

‡The first number is the benefit of surgery ($EV_{Surg} - EV_{No\ Surg}$), where EV_{Surg} is the expected value of surgery and $EV_{No\ Surg}$ is the expected value of medical therapy; a positive benefit implies that surgery is preferable, whereas a negative benefit implies that medical therapy is preferable.

§The second number is the expected value of the better choice.

Recall that the utilities in study A are calibrated on a scale of 0 to 100, with 100 representing five-year survival without pain. Hence, the expected values in Table 9–3 should be interpreted in terms of that scale. The certainty-equivalent numbers of quality-adjusted life years corresponding to these utility values may be obtained from Figure 9–5 by the procedure indicated in the section on outcomes and utility assessments (p. 279). Note that surgery is generally preferred, unless the patient is not concerned at all about pain relief (i.e., the second patient type).

The results from study B are shown in Table 9–4 for five specific patient types corresponding to different coronary anatomy, symptoms, age, and ventricular function. Both the active and sedentary counterparts of these five types are analyzed.

TABLE 9-4   RESULTS OF ANALYSIS OF THE CABG DECISION IN STUDY B:
EXPECTED UTILITIES AND UTILITY DIFFERENCES[271]

PATIENT TYPE*	TREATMENT	EXPECTED UTILITY† FOR ACTIVE PATIENT	DIFFERENCE	EXPECTED UTILITY† FOR SEDENTARY PATIENT	DIFFERENCE
1	Surgical	12.3	−0.2	12.7	−0.8
	Medical	12.5		13.5	
2	Surgical	12.6	0.4	12.9	−0.1
	Medical	12.2		13.0	
3	Surgical	1.2	0.4	1.2	0.3
	Medical	0.8		0.9	
4	Surgical	13.4	0.3	13.7	0.3
	Medical	13.1		13.4	
5	Surgical	15.2	8.5	15.6	8.1
	Medical	6.7		7.5	

*Type 1 is a 50-year-old man with moderate angina, fair heart function, an old myocardial infarction, and one operable vessel; type 2 is a 60-year-old man with moderate angina, good heart function, and two operable vessels; type 3 is a 50-year-old man with severe angina, poor heart function, an old myocardial infarction, and three operable vessels; type 4 is an asymptomatic 50-year-old man with good heart function and two operable vessels; and type 5 is a 40-year-old man with severe angina, good heart function, and one operable vessel.

†In quality-adjusted life years.

The expected utilities in Table 9–4 represent quality-adjusted life expectancy. Hence, for patient type 5 with the active preference structure, surgery offers an increase of 8.53 quality-adjusted life years compared with 8.14 for the sedentary preference structure. Note that for patient type 2 the choice is surgery for an active patient and no surgery for a sedentary patient, thus corroborating study A as to the importance of differences in preferences.

It is noteworthy that study A seems to find surgery contraindicated if life expectancy alone is of concern, while study B finds surgery strongly preferred for some patients (e.g., type 5), even if pain relief is not a consideration. The reason for this divergence of results may be attributed, in part, to the longer time horizon in study B. If surgery results in a high survival rate at five years, this benefit may not have a chance to cancel out the effects of operative mortality if the years only through year 5 are monitored. If, as the probability assessments and most current clinical studies suggest, surgery catches up to or surpasses medical management after three to five years, the longer time horizon will allow for the fact that a death averted at year 4 saves more than just one year of life expectancy and will thus tend to favor surgery.

Sensitivity Analyses

Sensitivity to Probabilities.   Both studies reported sensitivity analyses of their results with respect to changes in probability assessments. In study A these sensitivity analyses were reported in a particularly useful way: by means of a *threshold analysis*. Recall that in threshold analysis, the probability in question (e.g., the operative mortality) is varied in the direction unfavorable to the currently optimal decision (e.g., the assessment of operative mortality is increased if surgery is currently favored by the analysis) until the point is reached at which the two alternatives are equally desirable (i.e., have the same expected value).

For example, consider the patient who values only life years and not pain relief, who has good coronary anatomy and heart function, and who is operated on by an excellent surgical team. The base probability of annual mortality with a patent graft was 0.04 (Table 9–2), and medical management was preferred (Table 9–3). However, the threshold for switching the result is 0.03; that is, if the annual mortality with a patent graft in such patients were 0.03 rather than 0.04, surgery would become the therapy of choice. Study A reports thresholds for all of the major probabilities; for some, of course, there is no threshold because the extreme values of 0.00 and 1.00 fail to change the decision. A threshold value very close to the base probability indicates that the decision is very sensitive to that probability assessment; where there is no threshold, the decision is not at all sensitive to that particular probability.

Of course, the assessment of separate sets of probabilities for different hypothetical surgical skill levels is also a form of sensitivity analysis. In particular, that sort of analysis permits variation in more than one probability at a time and is therefore particularly useful if one suspects that the probabilities are too optimistic or too pessimistic across the board. Hence, a comparison of the first three columns of Table 9–3 in light of the probability assessments in the first three columns of Table 9–2 provides a very useful broad-stroke sensitivity analysis to complement the detailed threshold analyses.

Sensitivity to Utilities.   Another kind of sensitivity analysis involves altering the utilities assigned to different outcomes to see to what extent the result changes. In both studies this sort of sensitivity analysis is done by considering several sets of preference characteristics (the four types in study A and the active and sedentary types in study B). In the latter study the parameter of interest is the proportional rate of trade-off between years of life and relief from angina, that is, the number P, which represents the proportion of life years one would give up to obtain relief from severe angina. For the active patient, P was taken to be 0.3; for the sedentary patient, P was assumed to be 0.2. A full sensitivity analysis would allow P to vary from 0.0 (for one who values life years only and does not value pain relief) to 1.0 (for one who values only life years without anginal pain). In study B a change in the value of P from 0.2 (for the sedentary patient) to 0.0 (for the patient who is not concerned with pain) does not change any decisions. However, there are differences in decisions between the active and sedentary patients ($P = 0.3$ versus $P = 0.2$).

Intended Uses of the Published Analysis

The two studies differ somewhat with respect to their intended uses. Study A appears to be intended mainly as an aid to decision making for the individual physician, whereas study B is oriented more toward societal cost-effectiveness implications. As a result, the presentations of the analyses differ.

Because of the intention that study A be used by clinical decision makers, great emphasis is placed on the adaptation of the study for actual use by the individual physician. Ideally, physicians could enter their own assessments of probabilities and utilities and generate an analysis specifically for their own beliefs and preferences. However, the full analysis, while relatively straightforward, is still too complex for a busy practitioner (cardiologist or cardiac surgeon) to carry out. Therefore, the author of the analysis provides a simplified version that can realistically be used by the physician. The simplified version requires only ten probability and ten utility assessments, and a run through the analysis can be done easily on a standard calculator (i.e., the expected utilities are calculated as the sums of utilities multiplied by the corresponding probabilities). The complicated five-year outcomes are replaced by simple outcome descriptions similar to those shown in Figure 9–3. The easy method of calculation is illustrated by three hypothetical cases in the article, and it is realistic to suppose that the procedure could be replicated by a physician who is far less skilled at decision analysis than one who has read this book. It should be added that the author of study A conducted the utility assessments by actually "debriefing" the patients in question in a manner analogous to the hypothetical scenario in Chapter Seven. Since only ten assessments are required in the simplified version, this procedure can be replicated quickly and easily by the clinician.

The analysis in study B is not, however, so easily adapted for bedside use, nor is it intended to be. Rather, it is designed primarily as a guide to policy making and to the allocation of resources. The study presents estimates of the cost-effectiveness of CABG surgery in terms of dollar cost per year of increased quality-adjusted life expectancy. While such considerations might not be relevant for the individual physician caring for an individual patient, they would be most relevant at the levels of decision making at which limited resources must be allocated among health practices. The cost-effectiveness estimates — from less than $2,000 per quality-adjusted life year for the active 40-year-old patient with severe angina and a strong heart to more than $25,000 per quality-adjusted life year for most of the other patient types considered — provide a guide to the setting of priorities among candidates for CABG surgery as well as between CABG surgery and other uses of medical resources.

CLINICAL SERIES, CLINICAL TRIALS, AND CLINICAL DECISION ANALYSIS

As we have mentioned earlier, clinical decision analysis is not a substitute for empirical data obtained from clinical trials, nor is the reverse true. Rather, they complement each other. The evidence from clinical trials can provide the basis for certain probability assessments and structural assumptions in the decision tree, and the decision-analytic framework itself can raise key questions that a clinical trial or clinical data base might help to answer. Ultimately, the decision should be guided by the synthesis of evidence and value judgments that a clinical decision analysis can provide; this synthesis is done informally by every good clinician and is made explicit by decision analysis.

The first pieces of quantitative evidence on coronary artery bypass graft surgery derived from several patient series in hospitals in which the procedure was being performed. In a study at the Cleveland Clinics,[229] for example, a group of 997 surgical patients were observed, and their outcomes were compared with those in a group of 469 medically managed patients who had been candidates for a CABG but had not undergone surgery. Many of these "control" patients were presumably on the waiting list for the operation. The surgical group experienced a 4 per cent operative mortality, but only a 2.5 per cent subsequent annual mortality compared with a 9.3 per cent annual mortality in the control patients. Relief of symptoms was said to be excellent in 85 per cent of the surgical patients. In a Texas study,[103] operative mortality was 6.6 per cent, but subsequent mortality was only 2.3 per cent per year. Symptoms were relieved in 94 per cent of patients and disappeared completely in 62 per cent. In a Stanford study,[25] operative mortality was 6.5 per cent, but subsequent deaths averaged less than 1 per cent per year. Pain relief occurred in 79 per cent of patients. Thus, when viewed in isolation, these data suggest that CABG surgery involves a trade-off: a risk of early death in exchange for a high probability of at least short-term pain relief and a possibility of reduced later mortality among survivors.

An observational (nonrandomized) study at Duke University[159] is especially interesting because it compares outcomes for all surgically and medically treated patients who were regarded as potential CABG candidates. The analysis suggests that with respect to nearly all important physical and personal characteristics (e.g., with respect to severity of disease, heart function, and symptoms), the two groups were comparable. The results were as follows. Pain relief was realized in 69 per cent of the surgical cohort at six months and in 53 per cent at 24 months compared with 23 per cent of the medical cohort at six months and 26 per cent at 24 months. Mortality in the surgical cohort was high at six months (more than 10 per cent) owing to the surgery, but the rate then leveled off such that the two-year mortality was just 15 per cent. In the medical group, the two-year mortality was 13 per cent. Thus, the survival curves for medically and surgically treated patients cross at just about two years, as shown in Figure 9–6. The early operative mortality is gradually compensated for by a reduced number of deaths in the ensuing years. However, the expected number of years lost of the first two following treatment is smaller in the medical group than in the surgical group because the surgical deaths tend to occur earlier. Results for mortality and pain relief are also provided for 12 patient types defined by the number of arteries occluded and by heart function.

It is noteworthy that none of these published studies present data beyond a three-year horizon. If the trend in survival continues as shown by the dotted lines in Figure 9–6, then surgery will yield a greater life expectancy despite the early mortality. The evidence on this subject is not yet available as this book goes to press.

Thus, to summarize what can be learned from the observational series, we find that early mortality appears greater following surgery than following medical management, but later mortality is lower, and the survival curves intersect within a few years. The studies also suggest that pain relief is achieved in a high percentage of surgical patients, at least in the short term. The remaining questions concern (1) long-term mortality and pain relief, (2) the significance of these data and the trade-offs that they suggest in the context of clinical decision

Figure 9–6 *Results of the Duke University CABG study.*[159] *The solid curved line denotes the surgical group; the dashed curved line denotes the medical group; and the dotted curved line denotes the survival rate as extrapolated from data on the groups.*

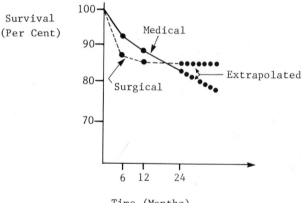

making, and (3) the validity of these observational studies in comparing surgical and medical therapies in patient groups assigned to treatments by choice rather than at random.

The latter concern, at least, can be alleviated by a randomized clinical trial. In 1977 the three-year mortality results from the Veterans Administration randomized trial of CABG surgery were published.[178] Qualitatively, these confirmed the indications of the observational studies: that surgery involves the risk of early death but offers a subsequent reduction in annual mortality relative to medical management. The probabilities of survival derived from this study are shown in Figure 9–7.

It must be stressed that these data alone are not sufficient to guide decision making. First, the survival curves to three years do not give enough information to determine even whether surgery or medical management results in a greater life expectancy. If the curves in Figure 9–7 extend together along the same trajectory, then life expectancy with medical management would be greater because of the lower rate of survival with surgery in the first two years. If, however, the curves, having crossed, continue to diverge, with the death rate following surgery less than that following medical management, then life expectancy with surgery would be greater. Given the limited available objective evidence, one can only assess subjectively what extrapolation is appropriate.

A second gap between the clinical trial and decision making lies in the fact that the trial gives no information relevant to pain relief, let alone the value judgments involved in trading off pain relief against longevity. Probabilities of pain relief over time must be assessed from other evidence, such as the non-experimental clinical series, and the utility assessments that describe patients' attitudes toward longevity and pain relief are an individual matter that cannot be revealed by a clinical trial of this kind.

Finally, there is the question of the adaptability of the results of the Veterans Administration trial in different settings. Indeed, the study revealed substantial variation in operative mortality among participating institutions. A physician would be ill-advised simply to apply the overall findings of the study in actual practice. Operative mortality may be lower or higher, and the graft patency rate may be different. Therefore, data from such a trial may provide qualitative evidence of efficacy and some quantitative guidance in estimating probabilities, but the decision analysis must incorporate assessments appropriate to the

Figure 9–7 Results of the Veterans Administration randomized trial of CABG. (Modified from Murphy et al.[178])

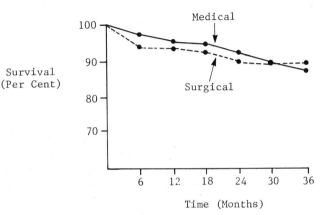

individual setting. Indeed, one value of the decision-analytic framework is that it permits one to apply any probabilities and utilities one chooses and to perform sensitivity analysis. The value of a well-conducted clinical trial is that it provides an objective basis for some probability assessments that are needed for decision making.

One last point concerning the relation between clinical trials and clinical decision analysis should be noted. Just as clinical trials contribute to a full decision analysis, so too can decision analysis improve the formulation of clinical trials. If analysis indicates that the decision depends critically on a certain probability (e.g., the ten-year survival rate or the five-year pain relief rate), then this suggests a priority for clinical trials. Often, in fact, a clinical decision analysis — or even just the process of structuring the decision tree — can raise central questions that might not otherwise have been apparent.

9.4 THE COMPUTER AS AN AID TO CLINICAL DECISION MAKING

Computers are being used to aid clinical decision making in a variety of ways, ranging from automated record storage and retrieval to automated clinical algorithms, programs that use Bayes' formula to aid in the diagnosis of illnesses, and artificial intelligence approaches to complex clinical problems. Several volumes[50, 195] and literally thousands of articles attest to the vigor and diversity of efforts to harness computer technology in the service of medical decision makers. In this section we will not attempt to review, even superficially, the variety of uses of computers in medical decision making. Rather, our purpose is to illustrate how the computer can enhance the decision-analytic approach to the diagnosis and treatment of medical problems.

THE LEEDS (ENGLAND) STUDY OF COMPUTER-AIDED DIAGNOSIS OF ACUTE ABDOMINAL PAIN

This example relates to our familiar diagnostic problem of acute abdominal pain. Specifically, we will discuss the research conducted by F. T. deDombal and his colleagues in Leeds, England.[49] This research, begun in 1971, initially involved 552 consecutive patients admitted to the emergency ward with the chief complaint of abdominal pain. Selected findings from each patient's history and physical examination were recorded on special forms and then entered into a computer. Using Bayes' formula and conditional probabilities derived from 700 previous patients, the computer generated the probabilities of alternative possible diagnoses (appendicitis, diverticulitis, perforated duodenal ulcer, cholecystitis, small bowel obstruction, pancreatitis, and nonspecific abdominal pain). The computer's predictions were then compared with the diagnostic guesses of attending physicians, and, in the first phase of the experiment at least, there followed discussion between the researchers and clinicians about discrepancies in the guesses.

The proportion of correct diagnoses for various physician groups ranged from 42 to 81 per cent. The computer system was correct in 91 per cent of cases. Even more striking was the improvement noted in patient management decisions after the computer-aided system was introduced: The rate of perforation of appendices fell from between 36 and 40 per cent to 6 per cent, and the rate of nondiseased appendices removed at laparotomy fell from between 20 and 25 per cent to 7 per cent. Most interestingly, the frequency of erroneous decisions rose after computer feedback was discontinued.

The effects of computer feedback and of its cessation were confirmed in a second trial. Not only did the performance of physicians revert toward the "base line" after feedback was discontinued, but the computer's performance also declined, implying that physicians may have been recording less "accurate" data in the absence of feedback. Indeed, one of the principal advantages of the computer system may have been that it imposed the discipline of precise observation and notation of clinical signs and symptoms.

DeDombal stresses the importance of orienting the computer system to the clinicians' needs and of adequate preparation and instruction (in, for example, precise definitions of physical signs). His colleagues have discussed the practical problems of implementing systems in other geographic areas[112]; this particular computer-aided system was successful in only 65 per cent of cases during a trial in Copenhagen.[17] Still, this work is an outstanding example of the potential for computer assistance in everyday clinical management problems.

PROGRAMMABLE CALCULATORS

The advent of hand-held calculators that can be programmed raises the prospect of the bedside computation of diagnostic probabilities and even of patient utilities and expected values. One article recently reported the use of a pocket calculator program for computing Bayesian probabilities for up to 9 diseases with 16 symptoms.[166,230] The major limitation of present calculators is the capacity of register storage, and a secondary problem is the slow speed of computation. But these problems are sure to be reduced over time, and better programs are certain to be developed. The doctor's black bag of the future may be as likely to contain a programmed calculator as an ophthalmoscope.

ARTIFICIAL INTELLIGENCE APPROACHES

Artificial intelligence computer programs use flexible programming languages to model complicated real-world decision situations typified by inexact reasoning and an incomplete prior specification of the situation.[191] These programs typically make use of the available information to reach the "best" decision, that is, the decision that best accords with informal judgmental knowledge acquired from experts. Artificial intelligence approaches thus can avoid explicit decision trees and statistical analyses, in effect attempting to respond to clinical questions according to a set of decision rules based on the behavior of experts. They can be highly interactive with physician users and, in some programs, provide explanations that are readily understood by clinical users. The more elaborate systems are expensive, but the approach holds promise as an aid to clinical decision making.

9.5 SUMMARY OF CHAPTER NINE

Clinical decision analysis has many potential uses in medical decision making, and this chapter has presented a few illustrative applications.

An analysis of the results of exercise stress testing was able to reconcile apparently divergent results from earlier investigations. Different degrees of association between test results and disease status in earlier studies were attributable to differences in the prior probabilities of disease among the patients studied. This analysis also demonstrates that the predictive value of ST-segment depression depends on the degree of depression and that the simple dichotomy into positive and negative results obscures available diagnostic information.

Two decision-analytic approaches to the question of coronary artery bypass graft surgery were examined in some detail. The comparison is instructive for the methodological issues it raises. One lesson from this comparison is that the specification of a clinical situation in greater detail increases the potential for patient-specific conclusions but also increases the number or probabilities and utilities to be assessed. In addition, changing the time horizon in an analysis can greatly alter apparent differences in life expectancy among various alternatives. Finally, clinical trials are complementary to clinical decision analysis in that they provide an objective basis for probability assessment.

The computer has been used extensively as an aid to clinical decision making. Researchers in Leeds, England, applied probabilistic analysis and Bayes' formula to the diagnosis of acute abdominal pain and found the diagnoses generated by the computer system to be more accurate than those offered by the attending physicians, even though the computer's diagnoses were based on data supplied by the physicians. Future applications of computer technology to clinical decision making may involve the bedside use of pocket calculators that can be programmed. Finally, an artifical intelligence approach using computers may become an increasingly useful aid to medical decision making in the future.

≡≡≡≡≡≡≡≡

EXERCISES FOR CHAPTER NINE

EXERCISES FOR SECTION 9.2

1. *Choice of a Positivity Criterion for Exercise Stress Testing*
Refer to Figure 9–1. Assume that you can select as a single positivity criterion any level of ST-depression from between 1.00 and 1.49 mm to between 2.00 and 2.49 mm. Which level would give you the most sensitive test, and which would be the most specific?

*2. *ROC Curves for Exercise Stress Testing*
Explain the relation of the curve in Figure 9–2 to the receiver-operating characteristic (ROC) curve as presented in Chapter Four.

---

*This exercise relates to an optional section of Chapter Four and should be attempted only by readers who have studied that section.

Chapter Ten

Advantages, Shortcomings, and Ethical Implications

10.1 ROADS ONCE TAKEN

Set into the wall of one of the buildings in the medical center where this book was conceived is, appropriately enough, a stone tablet on which is carved one version of the first aphorism of Hippocrates:

> Life is short
> And the art long
> The occasion instant
> Experiment perilous
> Decision difficult.

We have not studied the impact of this primitive visual aid on our students, but in writing this book we have responded to our perception of the Hippocratic challenge. Recognizing the risks in paraphrasing Hippocrates, we might nevertheless transform this aphorism into the language of this book:

> Nature is probabilistic
> And information incomplete
> Outcomes are valued
> Resources limited
> Decisions unavoidable.

Given the fact that decisions must and will be made, our basic stance is that the interests of the patient are best served if the process of decision making is as explicit as possible. Decision analysis provides a model for thinking explicitly about a patient's clinical problem. It is a model that stresses rational choice based on understanding of the clinical situation, probabilistic events, and personal preferences. As a map is not the territory, so the model of decision analysis is not itself the clinical reality.

The question is whether such a formal model can sufficiently reflect clinical reality to be a useful aid to decision making. While there are a few instances in which formal modeling has proved demonstrably superior to unaided clinical intuition, such as the work by deDombal and others cited in Chapter Nine, empirical validations of such formal analytic methods are rare. Some may be convinced by the logic of decision analysis that enables them to utilize rationally whatever clinical information is available. Others charge that important aspects of most, if not all, clinical decisions cannot possibly be dealt with by such a formal analytic approach.[67,207]

Throughout this book we have purposely minimized the difficulties, disadvantages, and limitations of the decision-analytic method in the setting of individual clinical decisions. We pleaded the didactic imperatives of an introductory text, and now we attempt to balance the record, or at least to qualify our evident enthusiasm. We begin by describing some of the difficulties encountered in the application of decision analysis to the clinical encounter. Next, we summarize the salient advantages of the method as developed in previous chapters. Finally, we discuss some ethical aspects of cost-effectiveness analysis as these arise in the care of individual patients.

10.2 DISADVANTAGES OF CLINICAL DECISION ANALYSIS

The major shortcomings of clinical decision analysis derive from three sources: (1) the complexity and other characteristics of the clinical encounter, (2) the technical features of the analytic method itself, and (3) the behavioral qualities of the clinical decision makers.

CHARACTERISTICS OF THE CLINICAL ENCOUNTER

Among the major obstacles to modeling the clinical situation in a decision-analytic framework are multiple medical problems in a single patient, a complex array of alternative actions and events, and urgency in the need to make decisions.

Many patients, particularly the elderly who so commonly need medical care, have more than one health problem. Potential interactions among the decisions involved in diagnosis and management increase very rapidly as the number of medical problems rises. This creates simultaneously a greater need for the help that systematic analysis supplies and an unwieldy arborization of a decision tree that may be used to structure the set of problems. Even a single problem, when fully elaborated, may be so complex as to yield a cumbersome decision tree unless simplifying assumptions are made.

Independent of the physician's attitudes toward decision analysis, the most useful strategy under these circumstances is to disaggregate the problems while bearing in mind those interactions of potential importance, to address them separately, and then to reassess possible interactions in the light of tentative decisions reached for the individual problems. Implementation of this strategy may isolate individual components of the overall problem in a form that permits the application of more formal analysis. Intrinsic complexity in the clinical presentation, we might add, is at least as burdensome to the intuitive decision maker as it is to the analytic practitioner.

A more serious concern has its origin in the urgency frequently associated with the clinical encounter. The problem often brings the patient and physician together for the first time and under circumstances of anxiety, discomfort, or altered mental status. Formal analysis is both demanding and time-consuming, which are characteristics that are not well served by the "occasion instant" of the Hippocratic challenge. Further, the conditions are not supportive of the compassionate and leisurely exploration of the patient's personal utilities, and this, as we have seen, is a precondition of appropriately individualized decision making. An additional complication results from the instability of personal preferences over time. Only rarely are a patient's utilities exhaustively discussed previous to the occurrence of the medical problem, a discussion that, if held at all, usually centers around the prolongation of life by various life-support devices. In the event that such devices are necessary, however, physicians surely are left to wonder whether the preferences then so clearly expressed by the patient are the same as those the patient is unable to express now.

TECHNICAL PROBLEMS IN USING THE METHOD

The validity of the results of an analysis may be compromised by difficulties in obtaining a patient's utilities and their instability over time, as noted in the previous section. A proper utility assessment also often requires satisfying certain technical assumptions, such as constant proportional trade-offs, which were discussed in Chapter Seven.

Beyond utility, the quality of an analysis depends upon the correctness of the structure devised for the clinical situation and on the appropriate use of probabilistic information. Medical science is a dynamic enterprise that is continuously yielding new understanding and new possible diagnostic tests and therapies. A particular analysis remains valid only so long as its structural and quantitative components are current. It is one thing for a study to provide objective evidence for a particular probability assessment; the new estimate can be readily incorporated in an updated analysis. More serious for the analysis is the discovery of an altogether new therapeutic alternative or other development requring major structural change. Elaborate analysis may be futile in areas in which clinical understanding and opportunities are rapidly evolving.

Data based upon multiple diagnostic tests, physical signs, and the patient's history are normally gathered to revise the estimated probability of disease in a patient. The simplifying assumption of independence among the tests is sometimes made in formal analyses, although it need not be, as we have shown in Chapter Five. To the extent that tests are conditionally dependent, the assumption of independence distorts estimates of the likelihood of disease. The difficulty in practice arises from the fact that the degree of departure from independence among the relevant clinical tests is usually unknown. Of course, such uncertainties about the independence of clinical tests pose equal problems for informal and decision-analytic approaches to medical choice.

PROBLEMS INTRODUCED BY THE USER OF
CLINICAL DECISION ANALYSIS

Not all of the difficulties encountered in applying decision analysis to medical problems stem from the nature of the clinical encounter or the requirements of the method. Clinicians may bring to the application a variety of attitudes that, although they are also deleterious in the setting of informal decision making, are more apparent in the context of formal decision analysis.

Traditional medical education, which is preoccupied with deterministic explanations of disease, has not emphasized the probabilistic character of much of the information on which clinical decisions are based. As a consequence, physicians may have difficulty manipulating probabilities, constructing coherent sets of probabilities, or quantifying their degree of belief. We believe that these skills are learned rather than innate and think that instruction and practice in using probabilities would be a useful adjunct to the training of most clinicians.

Those of us in medical practice find the responsibility of clinical decisions a heavy load and welcome maxims, heuristics, or authoritative pronouncements that lighten the burden of rigorous thinking. How else can we explain our recollections of professorial dicta or the conclusions of medical reports shorn of their original qualifications and warnings? The results of formal analyses of clinical problems are similarly susceptible to this process of reification, in which they acquire a life of their own. It is both easy and convenient to forget that an analysis may simply be wrong or, if it were right at one time, that new alternatives have emerged, that the original probabilities have been superseded by better values, or that a particular patient's utilities are different from those in the published example. In our view, formal analysis, whether it is published or personal, is a guide to clinical judgment and not a substitute for it. Although the efforts of others are often instructive, they cannot in the nature of the clinical encounter replace the thoughtful accumulation of information about the individual patient and its critical analysis in the light of personal as well as recorded experience.

The decision-analytic approach is both normative and action oriented and thus differs from a traditional approach to decision making in which the selection and accumulation of information as well as the details of inference and application are left entirely to the individual physician. As the decision-analytic method develops and published applications become more common, uncritical acceptance and use may raise questions as to who is responsible for the particular medical decisions. Clearly that responsibility must continue to rest with the practitioner caring for the patient. By writing this book we hope to encourage in practitioners not only the development of their own analytic skills but also the capacity to critically evaluate the analyses of others.

Finally, while we believe decision analysis to be useful in dealing with acknowledged or suspected disease, we recognize that it does not address the reason many patients seek medical attention: the desire to be cared for and about. Although decision analysis will not create wise and compassionate physicians, we believe that it will powerfully assist those who are.*

10.3 SOME ADVANTAGES OF THE DECISION-ANALYTIC METHOD

In the course of our discussion of the components of decision analysis in earlier chapters, occasional note was made of features that seemed to us partic-

---

*For further response to objections raised against clinical decision analysis, see Schwartz.[224]

ularly advantageous in the clinical setting. In this section we will bring together in summary form what we believe to be the principal benefits of the method.

HELPING PHYSICIANS DO WHAT THEY DO BETTER

Structuring the Decision Problem

The decision-analytic method encourages the breaking of complex problems into simpler components: choices, probabilistic events, and alternative outcomes. Breaking down the problem enables the physician to focus on the separate parts without losing sight of the whole. In addition, because a decision tree incorporates the dimension of time, it encourages the logical sequencing of tests and interventions.

Assessing Probabilities

The search for explicit estimates of probability promotes a proper quantitative interpretation of clinical tests. This result, along with improvements in test sequencing, may reduce the likelihood of ordering redundant tests and hence promote the more efficient use of medical resources.

Assessing Utilities

Because the method focuses attention on the values placed on different outcomes, it encourages concern about the source of the utilities to be considered in decisions. We believe that the predominant source of the utilities should be the patient rather than the physician. In addition to providing an opportunity for the patient's preferences to be incorporated into the decision, the description of the utility structure serves to focus on any ethical issues concerning the choices to be made.

HELPING PHYSICIANS COMMUNICATE WITH EACH OTHER

The Value of Vocabulary

Formal analysis of clinical decisions requires a vocabulary for assessing clinical tests and weighing individual preferences. This vocabulary provides a basis for meaningful communication among physicians regarding strategy for patient care. Medical students devote a good deal of time to mastering the vocabulary of anatomy, physiology, and pathology; understanding and meaningfully discussing strategies for clinical care are no less important.

Structuring Medical Controversies

The decision-analytic approach can clarify the nature of disagreements among clinicians. Do they see the structure of the problem differently, that is, conceive different alternative tests or treatments or perceive different risks? Do they disagree over the probabilities or over the utilities? If probabilities are in question, perhaps further inquiry can produce better estimates. Failure to find better information identifies a potential area for clinical research.

THE SPECIAL VALUE OF SENSITIVITY ANALYSIS

Decision analysis specifies each of the structural and quantitative assumptions that go into a particular clinical decision. Given a structured problem, it is a straightforward matter to hold all but one parameter fixed and to let that one vary over a plausible range of values to see what effect, if any, this has on the preferred clinical strategy. This sensitivity testing can reassure the physician about the conclusions of the analysis. It also directs the user to uncertainties whose effect on the result justifies the effort required to obtain more reliable estimates.

THE CLOSE CALL

Individuals who are learning to apply decision analysis to clinical problems may be disturbed by the small quantitative difference between the expected values of alternative choices. Intuitively aware of the vagaries of probability estimation and appropriately burdened by a sense of their responsibility to the patient, they are reluctant to launch themselves on a course of action based on apparently trivial differences in the expected value of alternative strategies. Often the closeness in the expected value of different strategies reflects the fact that the balance between the advantages and disadvantages for one strategy may be very similar to that for another strategy. In any close call it is worthwhile to think harder about what considerations may have been omitted from the analysis: Would they tend to strengthen or weaken the currently preferred choice? If the former is the case, well and good; if the latter is so, the analysis at least provides a base line for contemplating the additional considerations.

Unfortunately, the reality of clinical decision making is often not clear-cut whether one's approach is earnest but informal or decision analytic. In any case, physicians are obliged to seek the best strategies available to their patients, even if the choice is only slightly better than that dictated by the flip of a coin. Decision analysis does not guarantee that an overwhelmingly dominant strategy exists, nor does it convert a genuinely close call into a clear-cut choice. On appropriate application, decision analysis claims only to help physicians and patients identify the best choice available given their beliefs and preferences.

10.4   DOLLARS AND LIVES: SOME ISSUES IN COST-EFFECTIVENESS ANALYSIS

Contemporary physicians enjoy an unparalleled capacity to intervene effectively in the disease processes of their patients. In addition, in a secular society they continue to enjoy a public esteem that approaches reverence. Given the level of public regard and the opportunities for professional satisfaction, why do practitioners manifest so many signs of discomfort in their vocation? Surely one contributing factor is the conflict inherent in the dual role assumed by physicians as agents for individual patients and for society as a whole.

Traditionally, physicians act as advocates for their individual patients. The advocacy relationship is expressed in the allocation of medical resources, including the time and the personal concern of the physician, to do whatever is possible to assist the "preservation of life capacities for the realization of a reasonable, realistic life plan."[76] On the average, medical encounters have become increasingly expensive, and the resources allocated for health care come increasingly from the public sector. The practitioner has become burdened with an additional responsibility to society for the efficient use of these resources.

Medical interventions themselves are designed to affect the quality of life or to prolong it or both. In the former case, and sometimes in the latter, we lack the methods or information to document the extent of benefit. The physician thus is left with a perceived obligation to intervene vigorously in the problems of individual patients, often without compelling evidence to administrators and policy makers that the intervention is a cost-effective use of public resources.

To compound the problem, there is an emerging consensus that the total resources allocated to health care will not be permitted to expand without limit. It is not a question of whether present levels of expenditure are appropriate; what matters is that at some point a limit will be set. At that time we shall have to choose among medical services, and the question is, What ought to be the practitioner's role in those choices? In the remainder of this chapter we will express briefly our views of the contemporary physician's role as it relates to the use of cost-effectiveness criteria in judging medical care.

THE PRACTITIONER AND COST-EFFECTIVENESS ANALYSIS

The concept of cost-effectiveness, which was developed in Chapter Eight, is an important and useful way of describing the consequences of medical interventions. The description combines two general kinds of information, and it is instructive to ask again who has what stake in its components. For the individual medical encounter, the bulk of medical costs are borne both collectively and remotely in time from the intervention itself. As a result, the differential in cost between alternative strategies of management is unlikely to have much influence on the patient's preferred choice. To the extent, however, that these costs are met out of public resources — that is, collectively — their magnitude is a matter of intense concern to society. The effectiveness of the medical intervention, on the other hand, is a matter of very great interest to the patient, who hopes that it will lead to a beneficial change. Society's interest in the effectiveness of an intervention is generally expressed with respect to groups of patients rather than individuals.

The decision of whether to intervene — that is, to allocate medical resources to the care of an individual — rests under ordinary circumstances with the physician. The practitioner, we have noted earlier, properly stands as an advocate for the well-being of the patient, and this responsibility is expressed in efforts to promote the patient's "reasonable, realistic life plan." The physician's decisions should thus reflect the patient's utilities, which are influenced and constrained by the physician's knowledge of the patient.

Although the patient's utilities are of the greatest importance, in an appropriately personal and humane relation they cannot always prevail over those of the physician, who is also an ethical being. The open, rational, and prepared patient, for example, who is suffering from an incurable, advanced malignancy and asks for a large amount of morphine with the clear intent to shorten life, is expressing a personal and perhaps coherent utility structure. The compact between patient and physician, part of which is to honor and promote the patient's values, does not require the physician to violate a closely held personal utility, which in this case is a scruple about abetting suicide.

We would argue, however, that the physician's utilities should not generally override those of the patient; the physician's attitudes toward life style, social worth, and reproductive behavior, for example, are irrelevant in the exploration of the patient's values. Indeed, as we have pointed out on several occasions, one of the major advantages of the analytic requirement for explicit utilities is its reminder to ask, Whose utilities?

If the values with which the physician deals are generally those of the patient, of what use is the concept of cost-effectiveness to the practitioner? We identify five reasons for the practitioner as the primary decision maker to be familiar with cost-effectiveness analysis.

First, to the extent that individual patients are responsible for their own medical bills, physicians acting purely as advocates for the well-being of the patient should consider the cost-effectiveness of care. Individual patients responsible for paying part or all of their own bills might rationally decide to spend varying amounts on health care. Different people face different family and health circumstances, and outlays for medical care must compete with other expenditures.

Second, if the physician, who is an advocate primarily for the patient, places any value whatsoever on preserving society's resources, then given two ways of achieving the same expected value for the patient, the physician will choose the less costly. Exposure to cost-effectiveness analysis should help physicians think clearly about what constitutes societal resource costs.

Third, the physician must understand cost-effectiveness analysis in order to be a responsible critic and a resourceful advocate for the patient's well-being, a point to which we will return shortly.

Fourth, the physician is in a unique situation to collect the information regarding outcomes and the use of resources on which societal cost-effectiveness analyses may be based. Compelling evidence of efficacy is lacking for many common medical interventions, and lack of information about costs is the rule rather than the exception. For these reasons we believe that the physician has an obligation to accumulate medical experience in an ordered form that is both credible and usable by societal decision makers, who are charged with the responsibility for allocating resources to groups of people rather than to individuals. The physician, in short, should be prepared to serve as a technical expert and an advisor to secondary decision makers. The content of that advice is more useful in the form of statements about cost-effectiveness.

Finally, physicians will practice increasingly in situations in which resources are limited. Physicians are already forced to allocate certain resources that are limited, such as beds for intensive care and their own time. The principles of cost-effectiveness analysis apply as well to the efficient allocation of such constrained resources as to society's resources generally. Moreover, a growing number of physicians in the United States practice in prepaid group settings in which resources that are generally available for health care are explicitly limited. The importance to the physician of understanding cost-effectiveness analysis increases as limits on available resources become more and more tangible.

SOCIETAL VALUES AND COST-EFFECTIVENESS ANALYSIS

While the physician operates as the primary decision maker in the allocation of medical resources, the size and composition of the pool from which the resources are disbursed will increasingly be determined by secondary decision makers, including administrators, government policy makers, regulators, fiscal intermediaries, and the like, who are concerned with the medical care of populations. As expectations of medical service increase in relation to the available resources, the admissibility of claims on the resource pool seems likely to be determined by more explicit and specific criteria than is currently the case.

Rights, Interests, and Utilities

Decisions as to who gets what, as distinct from who pays, are likely to be based on two types of principles: rights and interests. With respect to medical resources, rights are claims of all members of the society that take precedence over allocational priorities based on criteria such as cost-effectiveness or a particular subset of diseases or patient groups. In the political sphere, an appropriate example would be the right to vote; the evolution of rights in the arena of health care, however, is less advanced in the United States, but a right to personal medical care may become analogous to the right to a grade school education.

The existence of a right with respect to medical care will never become a blanket entitlement to all of the resources that might conceivably be applied to the problem of an individual patient. Societal decision makers are responsible for delimiting individual rights to medical care and establishing a set of social priorities. These priorities would order the expression of further interests in medical care on the basis of such criteria as cost-effectiveness. It is on these interests in medical care, which are above and beyond what society deems to be the individual's due by right, that the impact of limited resources will fall.

Is it possible that societal decision makers could elicit a consensus that fairly and accurately reflects all individual priorities and that could then be used as a hierarchy of social utilities? For both theoretical and practical reasons, the prospect is remote. In practice, physicians can expect to operate within a schedule of social priorities devised by secondary decision makers, the rankings of which will be in conflict with the utilities of individual patients to some extent.

The Role of the Physician in a World of Limited Resources

Where does this leave the physician? In the role of advocate for the patient, the physician inevitably will make decisions that invade areas in which resource constraints are being defined or are already established by secondary decision makers. In our view, it would compromise the physician's advocacy role to anticipate the limits of available resources in situations not yet clearly defined by secondary decision makers or to impose a personal judgment less generous than socially defined contemporary levels for the particular problem at hand. If society entitles every patient to payment for renal dialysis, it is not the physician's role to deny that treatment to any patient who might benefit. In situations in which the constraints are ambiguous or undefined, we believe that physicians are obliged to seek any resources that might benefit their patients. When resource limits are clearly defined, the physician is obliged to accept compromises in the care of some patients in order to use available resources to gain greater benefits for these or other patients.

The expectation that the physician should serve both the patient and some conception of social welfare is not a new phenomenon. Long before limitations on total medical resources were the focus of public concern, physicians in the armed forces and industry, for example, were being asked to care for the patient in the traditional sense and simultaneously to make judgments as agents under a societal charge. In the usual circumstances of the medical encounter, assumption of this dual responsibility invites anxiety on the part of the patient and uncertainty on the part of the physician. The burdens of the therapeutic role are heavy enough without the additional weight of allegiance to societal values that are unlikely to be congruent with those of the patient. For this reason, physicians must make clear to the public at large and to its secondary decision makers that in the role of providers of care, physicians serve individual patients, not social priorities. Two mandates are one too many. On the other hand, society, operating through its secondary decision makers, has the obligation to articulate a clear set of criteria that translate into limits on resource allocation. These, in turn, set the currently legitimate boundaries for the physician's decisions regarding the individual patient. An understanding of cost-effectiveness analysis by the practitioner is useful not simply to serve some specific social utility but to judge more capably the validity and appropriateness of priorities for patient care within socially imposed resource constraints.

TOWARD A RESOLUTION OF THE DOCTOR'S DILEMMA

A physician makes a pledge to care for the patient. Two central characteristics of this pledge are candor and faithfulness, expressed in part by the physician's willingness to be truthful with and an advocate for the patient. Neither attribute can long survive the mismatch of expectations created when the physician is simultaneously the agent for a set of social priorities of which the patient may be unaware. Both parties to the therapeutic contract deserve and should insist upon a fair, clear, and widely accepted set of social values that define the limits of resource allocation in the particular case. The physician stands in the role only of expert advisor in the process of establishing this hierarchy of values; given an appropriately developed set, the physician may then serve with candor and faithfulness as the patient's advocate.

Social priorities, expressed in the form of decisions about resource allocation, will be influenced by information regarding the costs and effectiveness of possible medical interventions. Without compromising the role of advocate for the patient, the physician should provide systematic information for the determination of cost-effectiveness, serve as an informed critic of such analyses, and use the results to promote the welfare of patients as efficiently as possible.

10.5 SUMMARY OF CHAPTER TEN

Decision analysis offers a prescriptive model for clinical decision making. It is an aid, not a substitute, for clinical reasoning.

Important limitations in the application of clinical decision analysis derive from the complexity of and the urgency in clinical problems and from technical advances or other developments that alter the structure of a clinical situation. Other problems include difficulty in ascertaining the patient's utilities and their instability over time or through changing circumstances. In addition, physicians may be reluctant to think probabilistically and may naturally prefer generally applicable clinical maxims and clear-cut choices.

Despite its shortcomings, decision analysis can help physicians structure and work through a clinical decision problem, improve their interpretation of quantitative test results, and prompt their attention to patient preferences. Decision analysis provides a vocabulary to describe clinical strategies and can thereby improve communication among physicians, clarify controversy, and provide reassurance that decisions are rational and consistent with the beliefs and preferences of physicians and patients.

As public investment in health care grows, physicians become increasingly responsible for allocating society's health resources. Limited resources may force doctors to compromise their primary role as advocates for the individual patient, but only within total resource constraints set by societal decision makers. Methods for efficient resource allocation, such as cost-effectiveness analysis, are important for physicians to understand so that they themselves may make intelligent decisions within resource limits and act as informed technical advisors and responsible critics in the process of setting society's health-care priorities.

Bibliography

The bibliography contains a selection of publications in the English language related to medical decision analysis. Entries are numbered and listed alphabetically by author. Each reference also has been classified, where appropriate, into one or more of the following categories:

1. Acton JP: Evaluating public programs to save lives: The case of heart attacks, Report R–950–RC. Santa Monica, Calif, The Rand Corp, 1973 [B7, C1, D7].
2. Aitchison J: Decision-making in clinical medicine. J R Coll Physicians Lond *4*:195–202, 1970 [D2].
3. Albert DA: Decision theory in medicine: A review and critique. Milbank Mem Fund Q *56*:362–401, 1978 [A3, B3].
4. Alpérovitch A, LeMinor M, Lellouch J: The determination of sequential strategies of diagnostic tests: Comparison of different methods by simulation. Methods Inf Med *18*:75–79, 1979 [B3, B6, C4, D6].
5. American Heart Association: Coronary Risk Handbook: Estimating Risk of Coronary Heart Disease in Daily Practice. New York, American Heart Association, 1973 [B5, C1].
6. Anderson G, Llerena C, Davidson D, et al.: Practical application of computer-assisted decision-making in an antenatal clinic — a feasibility study. Methods Inf Med *15*:224–229, 1976 [C9, D6].
7. Anderson JA, Boyle JA: Computer diagnosis: Statistical aspects. Br Med Bull *24*:230–235, 1968 [D6].
8. Archer PG: The predictive value of clinical laboratory test results. Am J Clin Pathol *69*:32–35, 1978 [B2, C2].
9. Barnoon S, Wolfe H: Measuring the Effectiveness of Medical Decisions: An Operations Research Approach. Springfield, Ill, Charles C Thomas, Publisher, 1972 [A2, A3, B3, B4, D6, E].
10. Bay KS, Flatham D, Nestman L: The worth of

a screening program: An application of a statistical decision model for the benefit evaluation of screening projects. Am J Public Health 66:145-150, 1976 [D5].

11. Bayes T: An essay towards solving a problem in the doctrine of chances. Philos Trans R Soc Lond 53:370-375, 1763 [B3].

12. Beach BH: Expert judgment about uncertainty: Bayesian decision making in realistic settings. Organizational Behavior and Human Performance 14:10-59, 1975 [B5].

13. Bendixen HH: The cost of intensive care, in Bunker JP, Barnes BA, Mosteller F (eds): Costs, Risks, and Benefits of Surgery. New York, Oxford University Press, 1977, pp 372-384 [A1, B7, C7].

14. Benson ES, Rubin M (eds): Logic and Economics of Clinical Laboratory Use. New York, Elsevier North-Holland Publishing Co, 1978 [C2, E].

15. Berry RE Jr: Estimating the economic costs of alcohol abuse. N Engl J Med 295:620-621, 1976 [B7, C13].

16. Betaque NE, Gorry GA: Automating judgmental decision making for a serious medical problem. Management Science 17B:421-434, 1971 [D2].

17. Bjerregaard B, Brynitz S, Holst-Christensen J, et al.: Computer aided diagnosis of the acute abdomen: A system from Leeds used on Copenhagen patients, in de Dombal FT, Grémy F (eds): Decision Making and Medical Care: Can Information Science Help? New York, American Elsevier Publishing Co, 1976, pp 165-171 [B3, B5, C4, C17, D6].

18. Bleich HL: Computerized clinical diagnosis. Fed Proc 33:2317-2319, 1974 [D6].

19. Blumberg MS: Evaluating health screening procedures. Operations Research 5:351-360, 1957 [B2, D5].

20. Bunch WH, Andrews GM: Use of decision theory in treatment selection. Clin Orthop 80:39-53, 1971 [D2].

21. Bunker JP, Barnes BA, Mosteller F (eds): Costs, Risks, and Benefits of Surgery. New York, Oxford University Press, 1977 [A3, B1, B7, C17, E].

22. Bunker JP, McPherson K, Henneman PL: Elective hysterectomy, in Bunker JP, Barnes BA, Mosteller F (eds): Costs, Risks, and Benefits of Surgery. New York, Oxford University Press, 1977, pp 262-276 [B2, C9, C10].

23. Bush JW, Chen MM, Patrick DL: Health status index in cost-effectiveness: Analysis of PKU program, in Berg RL (ed): Health Status Indexes. Chicago, Hospital Research and Educational Trust, 1973, pp 172-209 [B6, C5, D5].

24. Bush JW, Fanshel S, Chen MM: Analysis of a tuberculin testing program using a health status index. Socio-Econ Planning Sci 6:49-68, 1972 [B6, C6, D5].

25. Cannom DS, Miller DC, Shumway NE, et al.: The long-term follow-up of patients undergoing saphenous vein bypass surgery. Circulation 49:77-85, 1974.

26. Card WI: Choice of diagnostic tests. J R Coll Physicians Lond 9:264-268, 1975 [D2].

27. Card WI: Mathematical method in diagnosis. J R Coll Physicians Lond 9:193-196, 1975 [D2].

28. Card WI, Good IJ: The estimation of the implicit utilities of medical consultants. Math Biosci 6:45-54, 1970 [B6].

29. Card WI, Rusinkiewicz M, Phillips CI: Utility estimation of a set of states of health. Methods Inf Med 16:168-175, 1977 [B6, C11].

30. Carrera GF, Gerson DE, Schnur J, et al.: Computerized tomography of the brain in patients with headache or temporal lobe epilepsy: Findings and cost-effectiveness. J CAT 1:200-203, 1977 [B7, C8, C15].

31. Casscells W, Schoenberger A, Graboys TB: Interpretation by physicians of clinical laboratory results. N Engl J Med 299:999-1000, 1978 [B2, B5].

32. Cattaneo AD, Lucchelli PE, Rocca E: Decision theory and surgical risk. Methods Inf Med 13:238-241, 1974 [C17, D2].

33. Centerwall BS, Criqui MH: Prevention of the Wernicke-Korsakoff syndrome: A cost-benefit analysis. N Engl J Med 299:285-289, 1978 [B7, C8].

34. Cochrane AL: Effectiveness and Efficiency: Random Reflections on Health Services. London, Nuffield Provincial Hospital Trust, 1972 [B5, D8, E].

35. Cochrane AL, Holland WW: Validation of screening procedures. Br Med Bull 27:3-8, 1971 [D5].

36. Collen MF, Feldman R, Siegelaub AB, et al.: Dollar cost per positive test for automated multiphasic screening. N Engl J Med 283:459-463, 1970 [B7, C2, D5].

37. Cooper BS, Brody W: 1972 Lifetime Earnings by Age, Sex, Race and Educational Level: Research and Statistical Note, US Dept of Health, Education, and Welfare Publication (SSA) 75-11701. Washington, DC, Government Printing Office, 1975, pp 1-12 [B6].

38. Cooper BS, Rice DP: The economic cost of illness revisited. Soc Secur Bull, 39:21-36, 1976 [B7].

39. Coppleson LW, Brown B: Estimation of the screening error rate from the observed detection rates in repeated cervical cytology. Am J Obstet Gynecol 119:953-958, 1974 [B2, C9, C10].

40. Cornfield J: Bayes Theorem: Proceedings of the Sixth IBM Medical Symposium. New York, International Business Machines Corp, 1964, pp 163-196 [B3].

41. Cornfield J: The Bayesian outlook and its application. Biometrics 25:617-657, 1969 [B1, B3].

42. Cox AG: Choosing an operation for duodenal ulcer. Ann R Coll Surg Engl 55:124-128, 1974 [A1, C4, C17].

43. Cretin S: Cost/benefit analysis of treatment and prevention of myocardial infarction. Health Serv Res *12*:174–189, 1977 [B7, C1].

44. Croft DJ: Is computerized diagnosis possible? Comput Biomed Res *5*:351–367, 1972 [D6].

45. Croft DJ, Machol RE: Mathematical methods in medical diagnosis. Ann Biomed Eng *2*:69–89, 1974 [D2].

46. Cutler P: Problem Solving in Clinical Medicine: From Data to Diagnosis. Baltimore, The Williams & Wilkins Company, 1979 [B1, E].

47. Dalkey NC: The Delphi Method: An Experimental Study of Group Opinion, Research Memorandum RM-58888-PR. Santa Monica, Calif, The Rand Corp, 1969 [B5].

48. de Dombal FT: Surgical diagnosis assisted by a computer. Proc R Soc Lond (Biol) *184*:433–440, 1973 [B3, B5, C4, C17, D6].

49. de Dombal FT: Computer aided diagnosis: A practical proposition?, in de Dombal FT, Grémy F (eds): Decision Making and Medical Care: Can Information Science Help? New York, American Elsevier Publishing Co, 1976, pp 153–157 [B3, B5, C4, C17, D6].

50. de Dombal FT, Grémy F (eds): Decision Making and Medical Care: Can Information Science Help? New York, American Elsevier Publishing Co, 1976 [B2, B3, B4, B5, D2, D6, E].

51. de Dombal FT, Horrocks JC: Use of receiver operating characteristic (ROC) curves to evaluate computer confidence threshold and clinical performance in the diagnosis of appendicitis. Methods Inf Med *17*:157–161, 1978 [B4, C17].

52. de Dombal FT, Horrocks JC, Staniland JR: The computer as an aid to gastroenterological decision making. Scand J Gastroenterol *10*:225–227, 1975 [B3, B5, C4, C17, D6].

53. de Dombal FT, Horrocks JC, Staniland JR, et al.: Pattern-recognition: A comparison of the performance of clinicians and non-clinicians with a note on the performance of a computer-based system. Methods Inf Med *11*:32–37, 1972 [D2, D6].

54. de Dombal FT, Horrocks JC, Walmsley G, et al.: Computer-aided diagnosis and decision-making in the acute abdomen. J R Coll Physicians Lond *9*:211–218, 1975 [A1, A2, B3, B5, C4, C17, D6].

55. de Dombal FT, Leaper DJ, Horrocks JC, et al.: Human and computer aided diagnosis of abdominal pain: Further report with emphasis on performance of clinicians. Br Med J *1*:376–380, 1974 [A1, A2, B3, B5, C4, C17, D6].

56. de Dombal FT, Leaper DJ, Staniland JR, et al.: Computer-aided diagnosis of acute abdominal pain. Br Med J *2*:9–13, 1972 [B3, B5, C4, C17, D6].

57. de Zeeuw G, Vlek CAJ, Wagenaar WA (eds): Subjective Probability: Theory, Experiments, Applications: Proceedings of a research conference on subjective probability, Amsterdam Acta Psychol *34*:129–397, 1970 [B5].

58. Diamond GA, Forrester JS: Analysis of probability as an aid in the clinical diagnosis of coronary artery disease. N Engl J Med *300*:1350–1358, 1979 [B3, C1].

59. Drum DE: Optimizing the clinical value of hepatic scintiphotography. Semin Nucl Med *8*:346–357, 1978 [B2, C4, C15, D2].

60. Elstein AS: Clinical judgment: Psychological research and medical practice. Science *194*:696–700, 1976 [D1].

61. Elstein AS, Shulman LS, Sprafka SA: Medical Problem Solving: An Analysis of Clinical Reasoning. Cambridge, Mass, Harvard University Press, 1978 [D1, D2, E].

62. Emerson PA: Decision theory in the prevention of thrombo-embolism after myocardial infarction. J R Coll Physicians Lond *9*:238–251, 1975 [C1, D2].

63. Emerson PA, Teather D, Handley AJ: The application of decision theory to the prevention of deep vein thrombosis following myocardial infarction. Q J Med *43*:389–398, 1974 [C1, D2].

64. Fagan TJ: Nomogram for Bayes's theorem. N Engl J Med *293*:257, 1975 [B3].

65. Feduska NJ, Dent TL, Lindenauer SM: Results of palliative operations for carcinoma of the pancreas. Arch Surg *103*:330–333, 1971.

66. Feinstein AR: Clinical Biostatistics. St Louis, The C. V. Mosby Co, 1977 [B2, E].

67. Feinstein AR: Clinical biostatistics: XXXIX. The haze of Bayes, the aerial palaces of decision analysis, and the computerized Ouija board. Clin Pharmacol Ther *21*:482–496, 1977 [B3, D2].

68. Feinstein AR: Clinical Judgment. Huntington, NY, Robert E. Krieger Publishing Co, Inc, 1974 [B2, D2, E].

69. Fineberg HV: Clinical chemistries: The high cost of low-cost diagnostic tests, in Altman SH, Blendon R (eds): Medical Technology: The Culprit Behind Health Care Costs? US Dept of Health, Education, and Welfare Publication (PHS) 79-3216. Washington, DC, Government Printing Office, 1979, pp 144–165 [B7, C2].

70. Fineberg HV, Bauman R, Sosman M: Computerized cranial tomography: Effect on diagnostic and therapeutic plans. JAMA *238*:224–227, 1977 [B5].

71. Fishburn PC: Utility Theory for Decision Making. Huntington, NY, Robert E. Krieger Publishing Co, Inc, 1979 [B6, E].

72. Fitzpatrick G, Neutra R, Gilbert JP: Cost-computer program for diagnosis of thyroid disease. Am J Roentgenol *97*:901–905, 1966 [B2, C3, C15, D6].

73. Fitzpatrick G, Neutra R, Gilbert JP: Cost-effectiveness of cholecystectomy for silent gallstones, in Bunker JP, Barnes BA, Mosteller F (eds): Costs, Risks, and Benefits of Surgery. New York, Oxford University Press, 1977, pp 246–262 [B7, C4, C17].

74. Fox SH, Moskowitz M, Saenger EL, et al.:

Benefit/risk analysis of aggressive mammographic screening. Radiology *128*:359-365, 1978 [B2, C15].

75. Fraser PM, Franklin DA: Mathematical models for the diagnosis of liver disease: Problems arising in the use of conditional probability theory. Q J Med *43*:73-88, 1974 [B2, C4].

76. Fried C: Medical Experimentation: Personal Integrity and Social Policy. New York, American Elsevier Publishing Co, 1974 [D3, E].

77. Fried C: Rights and health care — beyond equity and efficiency. N Engl J Med *293*:241-245, 1975 [D3].

78. Friedman GD: Medical usage and abusage: "Prevalence" and "incidence." Ann Intern Med *84*:502-504, 1976 [B2].

79. Friedman M, Savage LJ: The utility analysis of choices involving risk. J Polit Econ *56*:279-304, 1948 [B6].

80. Fryback DG, Thornbury JR: Evaluation of a computerized Bayesian model for diagnosis of renal cyst vs. tumor vs. normal variant from excretory urogram information. Invest Radiol *11*:102-111, 1976 [B3, B5, C15, C16, D6].

81. Fryback DG, Thornbury JR: Informal use of decision theory to improve radiological patient management. Radiology *129*:385-388, 1978 [B5, C16, C16].

82. Galen RS, Gambino SR: Beyond Normality: The Predictive Value and Efficiency of Medical Diagnoses. New York, John Wiley & Sons, Inc, 1975 [B2, B3, B4, C2, E].

83. Gardiner PE, Edwards W: Public values: Multiattribute utility measurement for social decision making, in Kaplan MF, Schwartz S (eds): Human Judgment and Decision Processes. New York, Academic Press, 1975, pp 2-37 [B6].

84. Gardner JW, Lyon JL: Efficacy of cervical cytologic screening in the control of cervical cancer. Prev Med *6*:487-499, 1977 [C9, C10, D5].

85. Garland H: Studies on the accuracy of diagnostic procedures. Am J Roentgenol *82*:25-38, 1959 [B2].

86. Gill PW, Leaper DJ, Guillou PJ, et al.: Observer variation in clinical diagnosis — a computer-aided assessment of its magnitude and importance in 552 patients with abdominal pain. Methods Inf Med *12*:108-113, 1973 [B5, C4, C17, D6].

87. Ginsberg AS: The diagnostic process viewed as a decision problem, in Jacquez JA (ed): Computer Diagnosis and Diagnostic Methods. Springfield, Ill, Charles C Thomas, Publisher, 1972, pp 203-240 [B1, B3, B5, B6, C14].

88. Ginsberg AS, Offensend FL: An application of decision theory to a medical diagnosis-treatment problem. IEEE Trans Systems Sci Cybernetics *SSC-4*:355-362, 1968 [B3, B5].

89. Glass N: The cumulative cost of death. Lancet *1*:1341-1342, 1975 [B7].

90. Goldberg MF, Oakley GP Jr: Interpreting elevated amniotic fluid alpha-fetoprotein levels in clinical practice: Use of the predictive value

positive concept. Am J Obstet Gynecol *133*:126-131, 1979 [B2, C9, D5].

91. Good IJ, Card WI: The diagnostic process with special reference to errors. Methods Inf Med *10*:176-188, 1971 [B2, D2].

92. Gorry GA, Barnett GO: Sequential diagnosis by computer. JAMA *205*:849-854, 1968 [D6].

93. Gorry GA, Kassirer JP, Essig A, et al.: Decision analysis as the basis for computer-aided management of acute renal failure. Am J Med *55*:473-484, 1973 [B3, C16, D6].

94. Gorry GA, Pauker SG, Schwartz WB: The diagnostic importance of the normal finding. N Engl J Med *298*:486-489, 1978 [A2, B3].

95. Greibe J, Bugge P, Gjørup T, et al.: Long-term prognosis of duodenal ulcer: Follow-up study and survey of doctors' estimates. Br Med J *2*:1572-1574, 1977 [B5, C4].

96. Grim CE, Luft FC, Weinberger MH, et al.: Sensitivity and specificity of screening tests for renal vascular hypertension. Ann Intern Med *91*:617-622, 1979 [B2, C1, C15, C16, D5].

97. Grosse RN: Cost-benefit analysis of health service. Ann Am Acad Polit Soc Sci *399*:89-99, 1972 [B7].

98. Gustafson DH, Kestly JJ, Greist JH, et al.: An initial evaluation of a subjective Bayesian diagnostic system. Health Serv Res *6*:204-213, 1971 [B5].

99. Habbema JDF, Hilden J, Bjerregaard B: The measurement of performance in probabilistic diagnosis: I. The problem, descriptive tools, and measures based on classification matrices. Methods Inf Med *17*:217-227, 1978 [B2, B5, C17, D6].

100. Hagard S, Carter FA: Preventing the birth of infants with Down's syndrome: A cost-benefit analysis. Br Med J *1*:753-756, 1976 [B7, C5].

101. Hagard S, Carter F, Milne RG: Screening for spina bifida cystica: A cost-benefit analysis. Br J Prev Soc Med *30*:40-53, 1976 [B7, C5].

102. Hall GH: The clinical application of Bayes' theorem. Lancet *2*:555-557, 1967 [B3].

103. Hall RJ, Dawson JT, Cooley DA, et al.: Coronary artery bypass. Circulation *48* (suppl III):146-150, 1973.

104. Hamilton GW, Trobaugh GB, Ritchie JL, et al.: Myocardial imaging with [201]Thallium: An analysis of clinical usefulness based on Bayes' theorem. Semin Nucl Med *8*:358-364, 1978 [B3, C1, C15].

105. Henschke UK, Flehinger BJ: Decision theory in cancer therapy. Cancer *20*:1819-1826, 1967 [B3, C10].

106. Hershey JC: Consequence evaluation in decision analytic models of medical screening, diagnosis, and treatment. Methods Inf Med *13*:197-203, 1974 [B3, B6].

107. Hiatt HH: Protecting the medical commons: Who is responsible? N Engl J Med *293*:235-241, 1975 [D3].

108. Hilden J, Habbema JDF, Bjerregaard B: The

measurement of performance in probabilistic diagnosis: II. Trustworthiness of the exact values of the diagnostic probabilities. Methods Inf Med 17:227–237, 1978 [B2, B5, C17, D6].

109. Hilden J, Habbema JDF, Bjerregaard B: The mesurement of performance in probabilistic diagnosis: III. Methods based on continuous functions of the diagnostic probabilities. Methods Inf Med 17:238–246, 1978 [B2, B5, C17, D6].

110. Hockstra DJ, Miller SD: Sequential games and medical diagnosis. Comput Biomed Res 9:205–215, 1976 [B2].

111. Holland WW, Whitehead TP: Value of new laboratory tests in diagnosis and treatment. Lancet 2:391–394, 1974 [C2].

112. Horrocks JC, McAdam WAF, Devroede G, et al.: Some practical problems in transferring computer-aided diagnostic systems from one geographical area to another, in de Dombal FT, Grémy F (eds): Decision Making and Medical Care: Can Information Science Help? New York, American Elsevier Publishing Co, 1976, pp 159–164 [C4, C17, D6].

113. Horvath WJ: The effect of physician bias in medical diagnosis. Behav Sci 9:334–340, 1964 [D1].

114. Howard R: The foundations of decision analysis. IEEE Trans Systems Sci Cybernetics SSC-4: 211–219, 1968 [B1].

115. Howie JG: Death from appendicitis and appendectomy: An epidemiological survey. Lancet 2:1334–1337, 1966.

116. Jacquez JA (ed): Computer Diagnosis and Diagnostic Methods: Proceedings of a Conference on the Diagnostic Process, University of Michigan. Springfield, Ill, Charles C Thomas, Publisher, 1972 [B1, B2, B3, B4, B5, B6, D6, E].

117. Kahneman D, Tversky A: On the psychology of prediction. Psychol Rev 80:237–251, 1973 [B5, D1].

118. Kaplan RM, Bush JW, Berry CC: Health status index: Category rating versus magnitude estimation for measuring levels of well-being. Med Care 17:501–525, 1979 [B6].

119. Kaplan RM, Bush JW, Berry CC: Health status: Types of validity and the index of well-being. Health Serv Res 11:478–507, 1976 [B6].

120. Kassirer JP: The principles of clinical decision making: An introduction to decision analysis. Yale J Biol Med 49:149–164, 1976 [B1, B3].

121. Kassirer JP, Gorry GA: Clinical problem solving: A behavioral analysis. Ann Intern Med 89:245–255, 1978 [D2].

122. Kassirer JP, Pauker SG: Should diagnostic testing be regulated? N Engl J Med 299:947–949, 1978 [A3, D2].

123. Katz MA: A probability graph describing the predictive value of a highly sensitive diagnostic test. N Engl J Med 291:1115–1116, 1974 [B3].

124. Keeney RL, Raiffa H: Decisions with multiple objectives: Preferences and value tradeoffs. New York, John Wiley & Sons, Inc, 1976 [B1, B6, E].

125. King DJ, Manegold RF: The consistency of cardiologists' prognostic judgments in cases of myocardial infarction. Am J Cardiol 15:27–32, 1965 [B5, C1].

126. Klarman HE: Socioeconomic impact of heart disease, in Andrus EC, Maxwell CH (ed): The Heart and Circulation: Second National Conference on Cardiovascular Disease, Vol. II. Bethesda, Md, Federation of American Societies for Experimental Biology, 1965, Vol. II, pp 693–707 [B7, C1].

127. Klarman HE: Syphilis control programs, in Dorfman R (ed): Measuring Benefits of Governmental Investments. Washington, DC, The Brookings Institution, 1965, pp 367–414 [B7, C6].

128. Klarman HE, Francis JO, Rosenthal GD: Cost-effectiveness analysis applied to the treatment of chronic renal disease. Med Care 6:48–54, 1968 [B7, C16].

129. Klarman HE: Application of cost-benefit analysis to the health services and the special case of technologic innovation. Int J Health Serv 4:325–352, 1974 [B7].

130. Klarman HE: Application of cost-benefit analysis to health systems technology. J Occup Med 16:172–186, 1974 [B7].

131. Knill-Jones RP: The diagnosis of jaundice by the computation of probabilities. J R Coll Physicians Lond 9:205–210, 1975 [B3, B5, C4, D6].

132. Knill-Jones RP, Stern RB, Girmes DH, et al.: Use of sequential Bayesian model in diagnosis of jaundice by computer. Br Med J 1:530–533, 1973 [B3, B5, C4, D6].

133. Kodlin D: A note on the cost-benefit problem in screening for breast cancer. Methods Inf Med 11:242–247, 1972 [B7, C10].

134. Koplan JP, Schoenbaum SC, Weinstein MC, et al: Pertussis vaccine — an analysis of benefits, risks, and costs. N Engl J Med 301:906–911, 1979 [B7, C6].

135. Koran LM: Increasing the reliability of clinical data and judgments. Ann Clin Res 8:69–73, 1976 [B5, D1].

136. Koran LM: The reliability of clinical methods, data and judgments (first of two parts). N Engl J Med 293:642–646, 1975 [A3, B5, D1].

137. Koran LM: The reliability of clinical methods, data and judgments (second of two parts). N Engl J Med 293:695–701, 1975 [A3, B5, D1].

138. Kraus J: Use of Bayes theorem in clinical decision: Suicidal risk, differential diagnosis, response to treatment. Br J Psychiatry 120:561–567, 1972 [B3, C13].

139. Krause RD, Anand VD, Gruemer HD, et al.: The impact of laboratory error on the normal range: A Bayesian model. Clin Chem 21:321–324, 1975 [B3, C2].

140. Krischer JP: An annotated bibliography of decision analytic applications to health care. Operations Research 28:97–113, 1980 [A4].

141. Kyburg HE, Smokler HE (eds): Studies in Subjective Probability. New York, John Wiley & Sons, Inc, 1964 [B5, E].

142. Leaper DJ, Horrocks JC, Staniland JR, et al.: Computer-assisted diagnosis of abdominal pain using "estimates" provided by clinicians. Br Med J 4:350–354, 1972 [B5, C4, C17, D6].

143. Ledley RS, Lusted LB: Reasoning foundations of medical diagnosis. Science 130:9–21, 1959 [D2].

144. Levi S, Grant JR, Westphal MC, et al.: Development of a decision guide—optimal discriminators for meningitis as determined by statistical analysis. Methods Inf Med 15:87–90, 1976 [C6, C8, D4].

145. Lilienfeld AM: Some limitations and problems of screening for cancer. Cancer 33:1720–1724, 1974 [C10, D5].

146. Lindberg DAB, Watson FR: Imprecision of laboratory determinations and diagnostic accuracy: Theoretical considerations. Methods Inf Med 13:151–158, 1974 [B2, C2].

147. Lindley DV: The role of utility in decision-making. J R Coll Physicians Lond 9:225–230, 1975 [B6].

148. Lindsay PH, Norman DA: Human Information Processing: An Introduction to Psychology. New York, Academic Press, 1977 [D1, E].

149. Lodwick GS: A probabilistic approach to the diagnosis of bone tumors. Radiol Clin North Am 3:487–497, 1965 [B3, C10, C12].

150. Longmore DB, Rehahn M: The cumulative cost of death. Lancet 1:1023–1025, 1975 [B7].

151. Lusted LB: Introduction to Medical Decision Making. Springfield, Ill, Charles C Thomas, Publisher, 1968 [A3, B3, B4, D2, D6, E].

152. Lusted LB: Decision-making studies in patient management. N Engl J Med 284:416–424, 1971 [B3, B4].

153. Lusted LB: Signal detectability and medical decision-making. Science 171:1217–1219, 1971 [B4, C15].

154. Lusted LB: Observer error, signal detectability and medical decision-making, in Jacquez JA (ed): Computer Diagnosis and Diagnostic Methods. Springfield, Ill, Charles C Thomas, Publisher, 1972, pp 29–44 [B4, C15].

155. Lusted LB: General problems in medical decision making with comments on ROC analysis. Semin Nucl Med 8:299–306, 1978 [B3, B4, C15].

156. Mark RK, Stuart-Alexander DE: Disasters as a necessary part of benefit-cost analyses. Science 197:1160–1162, 1977 [B7].

157. McDonald CJ: Protocol-based computer reminders, the quality of care and the non-perfectability of man. N Engl J Med 295:1351–1355, 1976 [D6].

158. McDonald CJ: Use of a computer to detect and respond to clinical events: Its effect on clinician behavior. Ann Intern Med 84:162–167, 1976 [D6].

159. McNeer JR, Starmer CF, Bartel AG, et al.: The nature of treatment selection in coronary disease: Experience with medical and surgical treatment of a chronic disease. Circulation 49:606–614, 1974.

160. McNeil BJ: Rationale for the use of bone scans in selected metastatic and primary bone tumors. Semin Nucl Med 8:336–345, 1978 [C10, C12, C15].

161. McNeil BJ, Adelstein SJ: Measures of clinical efficacy: II. The value of case finding in hypertensive renovascular disease. N Engl J Med 293:221–226, 1975 [B7, C1, C15, C16].

162. McNeil BJ, Adelstein SJ: Determining the value of diagnostic and screening tests. J Nucl Med 17:439–448, 1976 [B3, B4, D5].

163. McNeil BJ, Collins JJ, Adelstein SJ: Rationale for seeking occult metastases in patients with bronchogenic carcinoma. Surg Gynecol Obstet 144:389–393, 1977 [C10, C14].

164. McNeil BJ, Hessel SJ, Branch WT, et al.: Measures of clinical efficacy: III. The value of the lung scan in the evaluation of young patients with pleuritic chest pain. J Nucl Med 17:163–169, 1976 [B3, B4, C14, C15].

165. McNeil BJ, Keeler E, Adelstein SJ: Primer on certain elements of medical decision making. N Engl J Med 293:211–215, 1975 [A2, B3, B4].

166. McNeil BJ, Sherman H: Bayesian calculations for the determination of the etiology of pleuritic chest pain in young adults in a teaching hospital. Comput Biomed Res 11:187–194, 1978 [B3, D6].

167. McNeil BJ, Varady PD, Burrows BA, et al.: Measures of clinical efficacy: I. Cost-effectiveness calculations in the diagnosis and treatment of hypertensive renovascular disease. N Engl J Med 293:216–221, 1975 [B7, C15, C16].

168. McNeil BJ, Weber E, Harrison D, et al.: Use of signal detection theory in examining the results of a contrast examination: A case study using the lymphangiogram. Radiology 123:613–617, 1977 [B4].

169. McNeil BJ, Weichselbaum R, Pauker SG: Fallacy of the five-year survival in lung cancer. N Engl J Med 299:1397–1401, 1978 [B6, C10, C14].

170. McPeek B, Gilbert JP, Mosteller F: The end result: Quality of life, in Bunker FP, Barnes BA, Mosteller F (eds): Costs, Risks, and Benefits of Surgery. New York, Oxford University Press, 1977, pp 170–175 [B6, C17].

171. Metz CE: Basic principles of ROC analysis. Semin Nucl Med 8:283–298, 1978 [A2, B4].

172. Meyer RF, Pratt JW: The consistent assessment and fairing of preference functions. IEEE Trans Systems Sci Cybernetics SCC-4:270–278, 1968 [B6].

173. Milholland AV, Wheeler SG, Heieck JJ: Medical

assessment by a Delphi group opinion technic. N Engl J Med *288*:1272–1275, 1973 [B5].

174. Mosteller F: Assessing unknown numbers: Order of magnitude estimation, in Fairley WB, Mosteller F (eds): Statistics and Public Policy. Reading, Mass, Addison-Wesley Publishing Co, Inc, 1977, pp 163–184 [B5].

175. Mosteller F, Rourke REK, Thomas GB Jr: Probability With Statistical Applications. Reading, Mass, Addison-Wesley Publishing Co, Inc, 1961, [B2, E].

176. Murphy EA: The Logic of Medicine. Baltimore, Johns Hopkins University Press, 1976 [B2, E].

177. Murphy EA, Mutalik GS: The application of Bayesian methods in genetic counseling. Hum Hered *19*:126–151, 1969 [B3, C5].

178. Murphy ML, Hultgren HN, Detre K, et al.: Treatment of chronic stable angina: A preliminary report of survival data of the randomized Veterans Administration cooperative study. N Engl J Med *297*:621–627, 1977.

179. Neuhauser D: Elective inguinal herniorrhaphy versus truss in the elderly, in Bunker JP, Barnes BA, Mosteller F (eds): Costs, Risks, and Benefits of Surgery. New York, Oxford University Press, 1977, pp 223–239 [A1, B7, C17].

180. Neuhauser D, Lewicki AM: What do we gain from the sixth stool guaiac? N Engl J Med *293*:226–228, 1975 [A2, B7, C4, C10].

181. Neutra R: Indications for the surgical treatment of suspected acute appendicitis: A cost-effectiveness approach, in Bunker JP, Barnes BA, Mosteller F (eds): Costs, Risks, and Benefits of Surgery. New York, Oxford University Press, 1977, pp 277–307 [A1, A2, B3, B7, C4, C17].

182. Neutra R, Neff R: Fetal death in eclampsia: II. The effect of non-therapeutic factors. Br J Obstet Gynaecol *82*:390–396, 1975 [C9].

183. Newhouse JP: The Economics of Medical Care: A Policy Perspective. Reading, Mass, Addison-Wesley Publishing Co, Inc, 1978 [B7, E].

184. Nugent CA, Warner HR, Dunn JT, et al.: Probability theory in the diagnosis of Cushing's syndrome. J Clin Endocrinol Metab *24*:621–627, 1964 [B3, C3].

185. Office of Technology Assessment, Congress of the United States: Assessing the Efficacy and Safety of Medical Technologies, Office of Technology Assessment Publication OTA-H-75. Washington, DC, Government Printing Office, 1978 [B7].

186. Overall JE, Williams CM: Conditional probability program for diagnosis of thyroid function. JAMA *183*:307–313, 1963 [B3, C3].

187. Patrick DL, Bush JW, Chen MM: Methods for measuring levels of well-being for a health status index. Health Serv Res *8*:228–245, 1973 [B6].

188. Patrick EA: Decision Analysis in Medicine: Methods and Applications. Boca Raton, Florida, CRC Press, Inc, 1979 [B1, E].

189. Patton DD: Introduction to clinical decision making. Semin Nucl Med *8*:273–282, 1978 [A3, B2, B3].

190. Pauker SG: Coronary artery surgery: The use of decision analysis. Ann Intern Med *85*:8–18, 1976 [A1, B1, B3, B6, C1, C17].

191. Pauker SG, Gorry GA, Kassirer JP, et al.: Towards the simulation of clinical cognition: Taking a present illness by computer. Am J Med *60*:981–996, 1976 [D2, D6].

192. Pauker SG, Kassirer JP: Therapeutic decision making: A cost-benefit analysis. N Engl J Med *293*:229–234, 1975 [B7].

193. Pauker SG, Kassirer JP: Clinical applications of decision analysis: A detailed illustration. Semin Nucl Med *8*:324–335, 1978 [B1, B3, B6, C14, C15].

194. Pauker SP, Pauker SG: Prenatal diagnosis: A directive approach to genetic counseling using decision analysis. Yale J Biol Med *50*:275–289, 1977 [B3, C5].

195. Perkins WJ: Biomedical Computing. Baltimore, University Park Press, 1977 [D6, E].

196. Peters RJ: Zero order and nonzero order decision rules in medical diagnosis. IBM J Res Develop *21*:449–460, 1977 [B2].

197. Pliskin JS, Beck CH Jr: Decision analysis in individual clinical decision making: A real-world application in treatment of renal disease. Methods Inf Med *15*:43–46, 1976 [B1, B6, C16].

198. Pliskin JS, Beck CH Jr: A health index for patient selection: A value function approach with application to chronic renal failure patients. Management Science *22*:1009–1021, 1976 [B6, C16].

199. Pliskin JS, Shepard DS, Weinstein MC: Utility functions for life years and health status: Theory, assessment, application. Operations Research *28*:206–224, 1980 [B6].

200. Pliskin N, Taylor AK: General principles: Cost-benefit and decision analysis, in Bunker JP, Barnes BA, Mosteller F (eds): Costs, Risks, and Benefits of Surgery. New York, Oxford University Press, 1977, pp 5–27 [A2, B1, B6, B7].

201. Polissar J: Transfusion hepatitis: Use of statistical decision theory. Transfusion *9*:15–22, 1969 [B3, C6].

202. Prewitt JMS: Experiments with statistical and quasi-statistical methods in diagnosis, in Jacquez JA (ed): Computer Diagnosis and Diagnostic Methods. Springfield, Ill, Charles C Thomas, Publisher, 1972, pp 294–354 [B2, D4].

203. Pryor TA, Warner HR: Some approaches to computerized medical diagnosis, in Jacquez JA (ed): Computer Diagnosis and Diagnostic Methods. Springfield, Ill, Charles C Thomas, Publisher, 1972, pp 241–254 [B3, D6].

204. Raiffa H: Decision Analysis: Introductory Lectures on Choices Under Uncertainty. Reading, Mass, Addison-Wesley Publishing Co, Inc, 1968 [A2, B1, E].

205. Raiffa H, Schwartz WB, Weinstein MC: Evaluating health effects of societal decisions and

programs, in Decision Making in the Environmental Protection Agency. Washington, DC, National Academy of Sciences, 1977 [B1, B3, B6].

206. Raiffa H, Thompson LT: Analysis for Decision Making: An Audiographic, Self-Instructional Course. Chicago, Encyclopaedia Britannica Educational Corp, 1974 [A2, B1, E].

207. Ransohoff DF, Feinstein AR: Is decision analysis useful in clinical medicine? Yale J Biol Med 49:165-168, 1976 [D2].

208. Rawls J: A Theory of Justice. Cambridge, Mass, Harvard University Press, 1971 [D3].

209. Reich T, Robins LN, Woodruff RA, et al: Computer-assisted derivation of a screening interview for alcoholism. Arch Gen Psychiatry 32:847-852, 1975 [C13, D6].

210. Rice D: Estimating the cost of illness. Am J Public Health 57:424-440, 1967 [B7].

211. Rifkin RO, Hood WB Jr: Bayesian analysis of electrocardiographic exercise stress testing. N Engl J Med 297:681-686, 1977 [A1, B3].

212. Robin ED: Overdiagnosis and overtreatment of pulmonary embolism: The emperor may have no clothes. Ann Intern Med 87:775-781, 1977 [B3, C14].

213. Ross P: Computers in medical diagnosis. CRC Crit Rev Radiol Sci 3:197-243, 1972 [D6].

214. Sackett DL: Clinical diagnosis and the clinical laboratory. Clin Invest Med 1:37-43, 1978 [A2, B2, C2].

215. Sackett DL, Chambers LW, MacPherson AS, et al.: The development and application of indices of health: General methods and a summary of results. Am J Public Health 67:423-428, 1977 [B6].

216. Safran C, Desforges JF, Tsichlis PN, et al.: Decision analysis to evaluate lymphangiography in the management of patients with Hodgkin's disease. N Engl J Med 296:1088-1092, 1977 [B3, C10, C15].

217. Safran C, Tsichlis PN, Bluming AZ, et al.: Diagnostic planning using computer assisted decision-making for patients with Hodgkin's disease. Cancer 39:2426-2434, 1977 [C10, D6].

218. Salamon R, Bernadet M, Samson M, et al.: Bayesian method applied to decision making in neurology — methodological considerations. Methods Inf Med 15:174-179, 1976 [B3, C8].

219. Scheff TJ: Decision rules, types of error and their consequences in medical diagnosis. Behav Sci 8:97-107, 1963 [D2].

220. Schelling TC: The life you save may be your own, in Chase SB (ed): Problems in Public Expenditure Analysis. Washington, DC, The Brookings Institution, 1968, pp 127-176 [B7].

221. Schmidt WM: Health and welfare of colonial American children. Am J Dis Child 130:694-701, 1976.

222. Schoenbaum SC, Hyde JN, Bartoshesky LB, et al.: Benefit-cost analysis of rubella vaccination policy. N Engl J Med 294:306-310, 1976 [B7, C6, D7].

223. Schoenbaum SC, McNeil BJ, Kavet J: The swine influenza decision. N Engl J Med 295:759-765, 1976 [A1, B1, B5, B7, C6, D7].

224. Schwartz WB: Decision analysis: A look at the chief complaints. N Engl J Med 300:556-559, 1979 [A3, B1].

225. Schwartz WB, Gorry GA, Kassirer JP, et al.: Decision analysis and clinical judgment. Am J Med 55:459-472, 1973 [A2, B1, B3, B6, C16].

226. Selvidge J: A three-step procedure for assigning probabilities to rare events, in Wendt D, Vlek C (eds): Utility, Probability, and Human Decision Making. Boston, Reidel Publishing Co, 1975, pp 199-216 [B5].

227. Shapiro AR: The evaluation of clinical predictions: A method and initial application. N Engl J Med 296:1509-1514, 1977 [B5].

228. Sheiner LB, Halkin H, Peck C, et al.: Improved computer-assisted digoxin therapy: A method using feedback of measured serum digoxin concentrations. Ann Intern Med 82:619-627, 1975 [C1, D6].

229. Sheldon WC, Rincon G, Effler DB, et al.: Vein graft surgery for coronary artery disease: Survival and angiographic results in 1,000 patients. Circulation 48(suppl III):184-189, 1973.

230. Sherman H: A pocket diagnostic calculator program for computing Bayesian probabilities for nine diseases with sixteen symptoms: Part A. Comput Biomed Res 11:177-186, 1978 [B3, D6].

231. Shortliffe EH: Computer-Based Medical Consultations: MYCIN. New York, American Elsevier Publishing Co, 1976 [C6, D6].

232. Shulman LS, Elstein AS: Studies of problem solving, judgment and decision making: Implications for educational research, in Kerlinger FN (ed): Review of Research in Education. Itasca, Ill, FT Peacock Publishers, 1975, Vol 3, pp 3-42 [D1].

233. Sisson JC, Schoomaker EB, Ross JC: Clinical decision analysis: The hazard of using additional data. JAMA 236:1259-1263, 1976 [B1].

234. Siu TO, Hancock JR: Test sequences in screening for breast cancer. Health Serv Res 12:250-268, 1977 [B3, C10].

235. Slack WV, Peckham BM, Van Cura LJ, et al.: A computer-based physical examination system. JAMA 200:224-228, 1967 [D6].

236. Slovic P: Choice between equally valued alternatives. J Exp Psychol (Hum Percept) 1:280-287, 1975 [B6].

237. Slovic P, Fischhoff B, Lichtenstein S: Behavioral decision theory. Annu Rev Psychol 28:1-39, 1977 [B5, D1].

238. Smedslund J: The concept of correlation in adults. Scand J Psychol 4:165-173, 1963 [D1].

239. Smith WF: Cost-effectiveness and cost-benefit analyses for public health programs. Public Health Rep 83:899-906, 1968 [B7].

240. Sokal RR: Classification: Purposes, principles, progress, prospects. Science 185:1115–1123, 1974 [D4].

241. Staniland JR, Ditchburn J, de Dombal FT: Clinical presentation of acute abdomen: Study of 600 patients. Br Med J 3:393–398, 1972 [B3, C4, C17, D6].

242. Staquet M, Sylvester R: A decision theory approach to Phase II clinical trials. Biomedicine 26:262–266, 1977 [D8].

243. Stason WB, Weinstein MC: Allocation of resources to manage hypertension. N Engl J Med 296:732–739, 1977 [A1, B7, C1, D7].

244. Stern RS, Jennings M, Delbanco TL, et al.: Graduate education in primary care: An economic analysis. N Engl J Med 297:638–643, 1977 [B7].

245. Swets JA: Signal detection in medical diagnosis, in Jacquez JA (ed): Computer Diagnosis and Diagnostic Methods. Springfield, Ill, Charles C Thomas, Publisher, 1972, pp 8–28 [B4].

246. Swets JA: The relative operating characteristic in psychology. Science 182:990–1000, 1973 [B4].

247. Swets JA: ROC analysis applied to the evaluation of medical imaging techniques. J Invest Radiol 14:109–121, 1979 [A2, B4, C15].

248. Taylor TR: Clinical decision analysis. Methods Inf Med 15:216–224, 1976 [A3, B1].

249. Taylor TR, Aitchison J, McGirr EM: Doctors as decision-makers: A computer-assisted study of diagnosis as a cognitive skill. Br Med J 3:35–40, 1971 [D6].

250. Taylor TR, Shields S, Black R: Study of cost-conscious computer-assisted diagnosis in thyroid disease. Lancet 2:79–83, 1972 [C3, D6].

251. Teather D, Emerson PA, Handley AJ: Decision theory applied to the treatment of deep vein thrombosis. Methods Inf Med 13:92–97, 1974 [B3, C1].

252. Thompson M, Milunsky A: Policy analysis for prenatal genetic diagnosis. Public Policy 27:25–48, 1979 [B7, C5, C9].

253. Thornbury JR, Fryback DG, Edwards W: Likelihood ratios as a measure of the diagnostic usefulness of excretory urogram information. Radiology 114:561–565, 1975 [B3, B5, C15, C16].

254. Thrall RM, Cardus D: Benefit-cost and cost-effectiveness analyses in rehabilitation research programs. Methods Inf Med 13:147–151, 1974 [B7, C12].

255. Tompkins RK, Burnes DC, Cable WE: An analysis of the cost-effectiveness of pharyngitis management and acute rheumatic fever prevention. Ann Intern Med 86:481–492, 1977 [B3, B7, C1, C6].

256. Torrance GW, Sackett DL, Thomas WH: Utility maximization model for program evaluation: A demonstration application, in Berg RL (ed): Health Status Indexes. Chicago, Hospital Research and Educational Trust, 1973, pp 156–172 [B6].

257. Torrance GW, Thomas WH, Sackett DL: A utility maximization model for evaluation of health care programs. Health Serv Res 7:118–133, 1972 [B6].

258. Turner DA, Fordham EW, Pagano JV, et al.: Brain scanning with the Anger multiplane tomographic scanner as a second examination: Evaluation by the ROC method. Radiology 121:115–124, 1976 [B4, C8, C15].

259. Turner DA, Ramachandran PC, Ali AA, et al.: Brain scanning with the Anger multiplane tomographic scanner as a primary examination: Evaluation by the ROC method. Radiology 121:125–129, 1976 [B4, C8, C15].

260. Tversky A, Kahneman D: Judgment under uncertainty: Heuristics and biases. Science 185:1124–1131, 1974 [A3, B5, D1].

261. Vanderplas JM: A method for determining probabilities for correct use of Bayes' theorem in medical diagnosis. Comput Biomed Res 1:215–220, 1967 [B3, B5].

262. Vecchio TJ: Predictive value of a single diagnostic test in unselected populations. N Engl J Med 274:1171–1173, 1966 [A2, B3].

263. Wagner G, Tautu P, Wolber U: Problems of medical diagnosis — a bibliography. Methods Inf Med 17:55–74, 1978 [A4].

264. Warner HR, Rutherford BD, Houtchens B: A sequential Bayesian approach to history taking and diagnosis. Comput Biomed Res 5:256–262, 1972 [B3].

265. Warner HR, Toronto AF, Veasy LG: Experience with Bayes' theorem for computer diagnosis of congenital heart disease. Ann NY Acad Sci 115:558–567, 1964 [B3, C1, C5, D6].

266. Warner HR, Toronto AF, Veasy LG, et al.: A mathematical approach to medical diagnosis: Application to congenital heart disease. JAMA 177:177–183, 1961 [B3, C1, C5, D6].

267. Weinstein MC: Allocation of subjects in medical experiments. N Engl J Med 291:1278–1286, 1974 [D8].

268. Weinstein MC: Economic evaluation of medical procedures and technologies: Progress, problems and prospects, in Wagner JL (ed): Medical Technology, US Department of Health, Education, and Welfare Publication (PHS)79-3254. Washington, DC, Government Printing Office, 1979, pp 52–68 [B7].

269. Weinstein MC, Fineberg HV: Cost-effectiveness analysis for medical practices: Appropriate laboratory utilization, in Benson ES, Rubin M (eds): Logic and Economics of Clinical Laboratory Use. New York, Elsevier North-Holland Publishing Co, 1978, pp 3–32 [B7, C2].

270. Weinstein MC, Shepard DS, Pliskin JS: The economic value of changing mortality probabilities: A decision-theoretic approach. Q J Econ 95:373–396, 1980 [B6].

271. Weinstein MC, Pliskin JS, Stason WB: Coronary artery bypass surgery: Decision and policy

analysis, in Bunker JP, Barnes BA, Mosteller F (eds): Costs, Risks, and Benefits of Surgery. New York, Oxford University Press, 1977, pp 342–371 [A1, B1, B3, B6, B7, C1, C17].

272. Weinstein MC, Stason WB: Hypertension: A Policy Perspective. Cambridge, Mass, Harvard University Press, 1976 [B7, D5, D7, C1, E].

273. Weinstein MC, Stason WB: Foundations of cost-effectiveness analysis for health and medical practices. N Engl J Med 296:716–721, 1977 [A2, B7].

274. Williams A: The cost-benefit approach. Br Med Bull 30:252–256, 1974 [B7].

275. Winkler RL: The quantification of judgment: Some methodological suggestions. J Amer Stat Assoc 62:1105–1120, 1967 [B2, B5].

276. Woodbury MA: Inapplicabilities of Bayes' theorem to diagnosis, in Bostem FH (ed): Medical Electronics: Digest of the Fifth International Conference in Medical Electronics, Liège, Belgium. Springfield, Ill, Charles C Thomas, Publisher, 1963, pp 860–868 [B3].

277. Wulff HR: Rational Diagnosis and Treatment. London, Blackwell Scientific Publications, 1976 [A3, B2, D2, E].

278. Zeckhauser R: Procedures for valuing lives. Public Policy 23:419–464, 1975 [B6].

279. Zelen M, Feinleib M: On the theory of screening for chronic diseases. Biometrika 56:601–614, 1969 [D5].

280. Zieve L: Misinterpretation and abuse of laboratory tests by clinicians. Ann NY Acad Sci 134:563–572, 1966 [B2, C2].

Solutions to Exercises

SOLUTIONS TO EXERCISES FOR CHAPTER TWO

1. A possible decision tree for this problem may be found in Chapter Seven, Figure 7–1, p. 187.
2. a. A possible structure for the portion of the decision tree following "wait six hours" is shown in Figure S–1.
   b. If waiting is of any value at all, it must be that the best possible outcome (much better) will result in no operation. Similarly, the worst possible outcome (much worse) must result in an operation if waiting six hours makes any sense. The "pruning" suggested by these considerations has already been incorporated into Figure S–1.
   c. A possible decision tree is shown in Figure S–2.
3. A possible decision tree for this problem is shown in Figure S–3. Note that following "arteriography +" and "operable" the only option shown is "operate". This is because it makes no sense to perform arteriography if you are going to elect "medical Rx" regardless of the result. Note also that the decision tree indicates that it is possible to do arteriography without a prior intravenous pyelogram (IVP); this is theoretically possible but rarely, if ever, done in practice.
4. A possible decision tree for this problem is shown in Figure S–4. Note that, if a culture is taken, the decision whether to prescribe penicillin is determined: Treat if the culture is positive, and do not treat if the culture is negative.
5. a. Possible strategies are the following:
      i. Do an IVP. Perform an arteriogram if the IVP result is positive; treat medically if the IVP result is negative. If the result of the arteriogram is positive and the renovascular disease (RVD) is operable, then operate; if the result of the arteriogram is negative or the RVD is not operable, then treat medically.
      ii. Do not do an IVP. Do an arteriogram. If the result of the arteriogram is positive and the RVD is operable, operate; if the result of the arteriogram is negative or the RVD is not operable, then treat medically. (This would rarely, if ever, be done in practice.)
      iii. Do not perform an IVP. Treat medically.
   b. Unless the decision whether to do an arteriogram depends on the results of the IVP ("Do an IVP. Perform an arteriogram if the IVP result is positive"), you would not bother doing an IVP. This is an example of a test that has no value because no subsequent decision depends on its result.

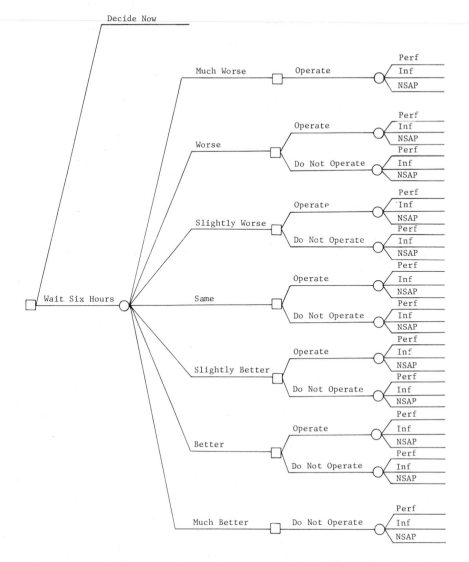

Figure S–1 *A solution to Exercise 2a, Chapter Two. (The "Decide Now" branch is the same as in Figure 2–8.)*

SOLUTIONS TO EXERCISES FOR CHAPTER THREE

1. a. $P[\text{IVP}^+ \text{ and } \text{RG}^+] = 0.69.$

   b. $P[\text{IVP}^+|\text{RG}^+] = \dfrac{P[\text{IVP}^+, \text{RG}^+]}{P[\text{RG}^+]}$

   $\qquad\qquad\quad = \dfrac{0.69}{0.85}$

   $\qquad\qquad\quad = 0.81.$

   c. $P[\text{RG}^+|\text{IVP}^+] = \dfrac{P[\text{IVP}^+, \text{RG}^+]}{P[\text{IVP}^+]}$

   $\qquad\qquad\quad = \dfrac{0.69}{0.78}$

   $\qquad\qquad\quad = 0.88.$

2. a. $P[\text{Test}_1 \text{ Abn}] = P[\text{Test}_2 \text{ Abn}] = \ldots = P[\text{Test}_6 \text{ Abn}] = 0.05.$
By independence,
$P[\text{Test}_1 \text{ Abn and Test}_2 \text{ Abn and} \ldots \text{and Test}_6 \text{ Abn}] =$
$P[\text{Test}_1 \text{ Abn}] \cdot P[\text{Test}_2 \text{ Abn}] \cdot \ldots \cdot P[\text{Test}_6 \text{ Abn}] \quad = (0.05)^6$
$= 1.56 \times 10^{-8},$

or a little more than one in a hundred million!

b. The probability that all six test results will be *normal* is

$$P[\text{Test}_1 \text{ Nor}] \circ P[\text{Test}_2 \text{ Nor}] \circ \ldots \circ P[\text{Test}_6 \text{ Nor}] = (0.95)^6 = 0.735.$$

By the summation principle, the probability that at least one test result will be *abnormal* is

$$1.000 - 0.735 = 0.265,$$

or 26.5 per cent.

Figure S–2 A solution to Exercise 2c, Chapter Two.

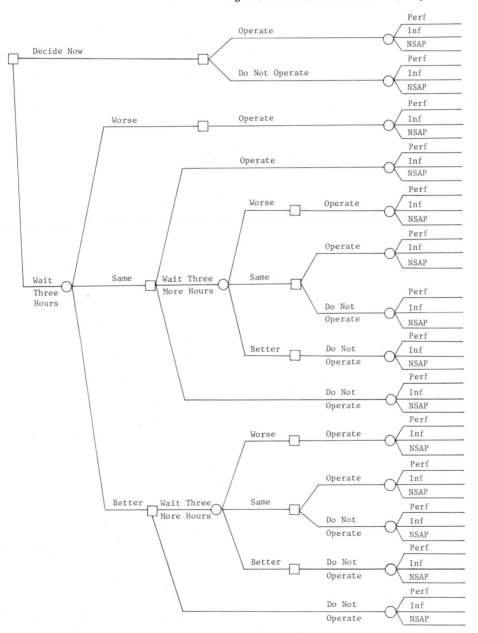

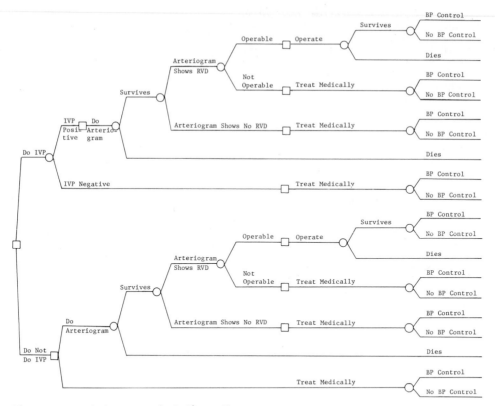

Figure S–3 *A solution to Exercise 3, Chapter Two.*

3. This is a problem in averaging out and can be solved either algebraically or with the aid of a probability tree.

Algebraically, let IVP⁺ stand for a positive IVP result and let RVD stand for renovascular disease. Then,

$$P[\text{IVP}^+] = P[\text{IVP}^+ \text{ and RVD}] + P[\text{IVP}^+ \text{ and No RVD}]$$

by the summation principle for joint probabilities, since a patient either has RVD or does not. Then,

$$P[\text{IVP}^+] = P[\text{IVP}^+ | \text{RVD}] \circ P[\text{RVD}] + P[\text{IVP}^+ | \text{No RVD}] \circ P[\text{No RVD}]$$
$$= (0.78)(0.10) + (0.11)(1.00 - 0.10)$$
$$= 0.078 + 0.099$$
$$= 0.177.$$

About 17.7 per cent of IVP results will be positive.

A probability tree for this simple problem is shown in Figure S–5.

4. The solution to this problem is given by the decision tree in Figure S–6. The best strategy is to administer radiotherapy, which gives the patient a 0.8 chance of survival compared with a 0.75 chance with the exploratory procedure.

5. a. You would not operate because the death rate with surgery would be 10 per cent compared with 8 per cent without surgery. Figure S–7 shows the analysis of this problem.

 b. The test would have to detect at least 50 per cent of cases. If a positive AT test result indicates acute tarkism with a probability of 0.5, then the mortality without surgery is

$$(0.5)(0.2) = 0.1,$$

which is the same as with surgery. Any proportion above 50 per cent would lead to a higher mortality without surgery.

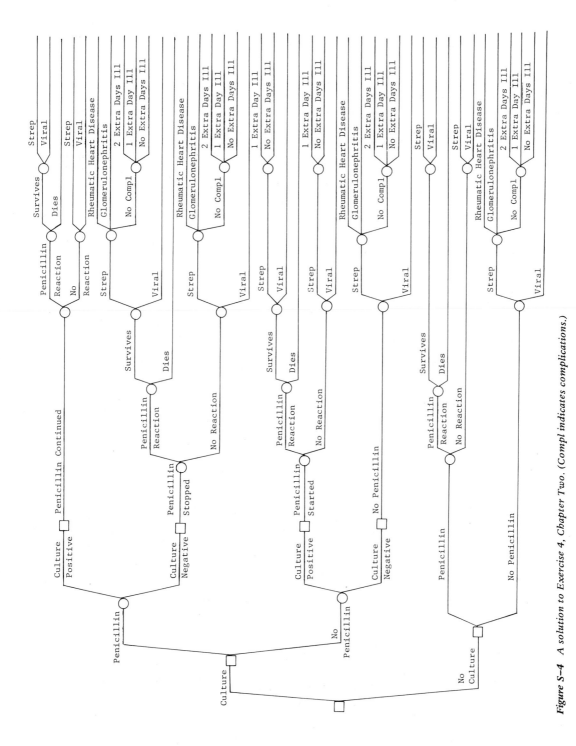

Figure S–4 A solution to Exercise 4, Chapter Two. (Compl indicates complications.)

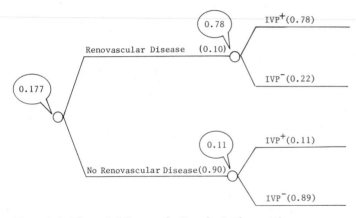

Figure S–5 *The probability tree for Exercise 3, Chapter Three.*

6. A decision tree for the evaluation of patients with possible *Pneumocystis* is shown in Figure S–8.
   a. The decision whether to administer pentamidine in the absence of biopsy information occurs at node 4 . The averaged-out six-month survival rate following the "pentamidine" branch is

$$(0.2)\ (0.50) + (0.8)\ (0.63) = 0.604.$$

Figure S–6 *A solution to Exercise 4, Chapter Three. (Rates shown are survival probabilities.)*

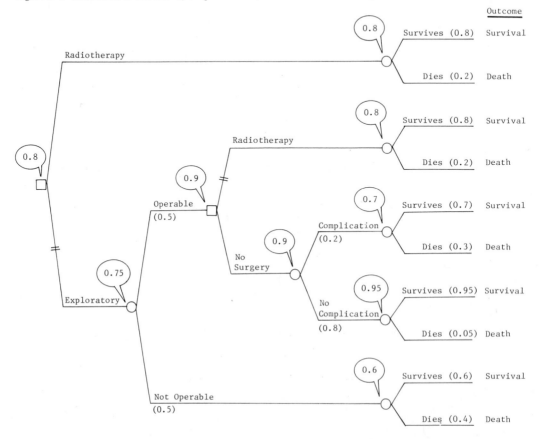

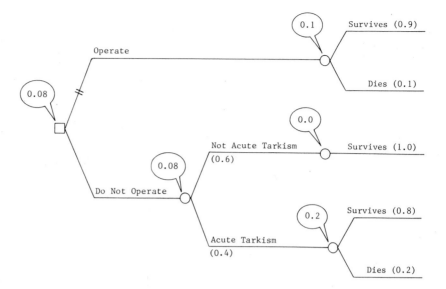

Figure S-7 *A solution to Exercise 5, Chapter Three. (Rates shown are mortality probabilities.)*

The six-month survival rate following the "no pentamidine" branch is

$$(0.2)\,(0.10) + (0.8)\,(0.65) = 0.540.$$

Hence, the preferred strategy in the absence of biopsy information (the choice with the highest survival probability) is the administration of pentamidine.

b. To compute the survival probability of the "biopsy" branch, we first average out at chance node Ⓑ :

$$(0.2)\,(0.50) + (0.8)\,(0.65) = 0.62.$$

Figure S-8 *A solution to Exercise 6, Chapter three.*

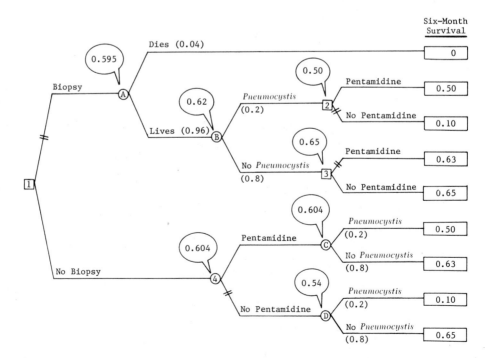

Hence, the expected value of perfect information is

$$0.62 - 0.604 = 0.016.$$

However, the survival probability when the risk of the biopsy is taken into account, which is shown at chance node $\textcircled{A}$, equals

$$(0.96) (0.62) + (0.04) (0) = 0.595.$$

Since this is *less* than the expected value of simply treating everyone with pentamidine, it is better *not* to do the biopsy. The net expected value (additional six-month survival) of seeking biopsy information is negative:

$$0.595 - 0.604 = -0.009.$$

    c. At the point of indifference between the "biopsy" and "no biopsy" strategies, the averaged-out values of both branches at decision node $\boxed{1}$ would be equal. If M represents the mortality from the biopsy itself, then at the point of indifference

$$(1 - M) [(0.2) (0.50) + (0.8) (0.65)] = 0.604,$$

or

$$(1 - M) (0.62) = 0.604.$$

Solving for M yields

$$M = 1 - \frac{0.604}{0.620} = 0.0258.$$

This means that if the expected mortality from open-lung biopsy were less than 2.58 per cent, then performing the biopsy would be preferable to treating without the biopsy.

    d. A possible decision tree for this refinement is shown in Figure S–9.

7. Algebraic proof that the point of indifference between treatment with steroids and without steroids occurs when the probability of cirrhosis equals 0.9 is as follows:

    i. Let P represent the probability of cirrhosis.

    ii. The survival rate when all patients are treated with steroids would be

$$(P) (0.48) + (1 - P) (0.85).$$

    iii. The survival rate when all patients are treated without steroids would be

$$(P) (0.50) + (1 - P) (0.67).$$

    iv. The point of indifference between treatment with steroids and without steroids occurs when the quantity in part ii equals that in part iii, or when

$$(P) (0.48) + (1 - P) (0.85) = (P) (0.50) + (1 - P) (0.67).$$

    v. The preceding equality reduces algebraically to P equals 0.9.

SOLUTIONS TO EXERCISES FOR CHAPTER FOUR

1. The complete probability table is as follows:

Sign	Appendicitis	NSAP	Row Totals
Rovsing's	0.000016	0	0.000016
No Rovsing's	0.159984	0.84	0.999984
Column totals	0.16	0.84	1.00

    a. $P[\text{Rovsing's}|\text{App}] = 0.0001$, by assumption.
    b. $P[\text{Rovsing's}|\text{NSAP}] = 0$, by assumption.

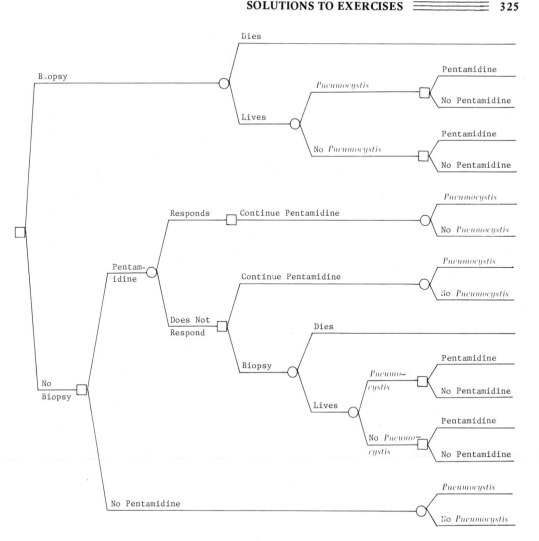

Figure S-9 A possible solution to Exercise 6d, Chapter Three.

c. $P[\text{App} \mid \text{Rovsing's}] = \dfrac{P[\text{App, Rovsing's}]}{P[\text{Rovsing's}]}$

   $= \dfrac{0.000016}{0.000016 + 0}$

   $= 1.0.$

d. $P[\text{App} \mid \text{No Rovsing's}] = \dfrac{P[\text{App, No Rovsing's}]}{P[\text{No Rovsing's}]}$

   $= \dfrac{0.159984}{0.999984}$

   $= 0.159987.$

   Compare this with the prior probability of 16 per cent.
2. The complete probability table is as follows:

Test Result	Cancer	No Cancer	Row Totals
Positive	0.002	0.00997	0.01197
Negative	0.001	0.98703	0.98803
Column totals	0.003	0.997	1.000

a. —

b. i. $P[\text{No Ca}|\text{Neg}] = \dfrac{P[\text{No Ca, Neg}]}{P[\text{Neg}]}$

$$= \dfrac{0.987}{0.988}$$

$$= 0.999$$

$$= 99.9\%.$$

ii. $P[\text{Ca}|\text{Pos}] = \dfrac{P[\text{Ca, Pos}]}{P[\text{Pos}]}$

$$= \dfrac{0.002}{0.012}$$

$$= 0.167$$

$$= 16.7\%.$$

Most people will have guessed higher in part a than the calculation shows here.

3. a. $P[\text{Rovsing's}|\text{App}] = 0.0001.$
    b. $P[\text{Rovsing's}|\text{No App}] = 0.$

c. $P[\text{App}|\text{Rovsing's}] = \dfrac{P[\text{Rovsing's}|\text{App}] \cdot P[\text{App}]}{\begin{array}{l} P[\text{Rovsing's}|\text{App}] \cdot P[\text{App}] + \\ P[\text{Rovsing's}|\text{No App}] \cdot P[\text{No App}] \end{array}}$

$$= \dfrac{(0.0001)\,(0.16)}{(0.0001)\,(0.16) + (0)\,(0.84)}$$

$$= 1.0.$$

d. $P[\text{App}|\text{No Rovsing's}] = \dfrac{P[\text{No Rovsing's}|\text{App}] \cdot P[\text{App}]}{\begin{array}{l} P[\text{No Rovsing's}|\text{App}] \circ P[\text{App}] + \\ P[\text{No Rovsing's}|\text{No App}] \cdot P[\text{No App}] \end{array}}$

$$= \dfrac{(0.9999)\,(0.16)}{(0.9999)\,(0.16) + (1)\,(0.84)}$$

$$= 0.159987.$$

4. a. —

b. i. $P[\text{No Ca}|\text{Neg}] = \dfrac{P[\text{Neg}|\text{No Ca}] \cdot P[\text{No Ca}]}{P[\text{Neg}|\text{No Ca}] \cdot P[\text{No Ca}] + P[\text{Neg}|\text{Ca}] \cdot P[\text{Ca}]}$

$$= \dfrac{(0.99)\,(0.997)}{(0.99)\,(0.997) + (0.33)\,(0.003)}$$

$$= 0.999.$$

ii. $P[\text{Ca}|\text{Pos}] = \dfrac{P[\text{Pos}|\text{Ca}] \circ P[\text{Ca}]}{P[\text{Pos}|\text{Ca}] \cdot P[\text{Ca}] + P[\text{Pos}|\text{No Ca}] \cdot P[\text{No Ca}]}$

$$= \dfrac{(0.67)\,(0.003)}{(0.67)\,(0.003) + (0.01)\,(0.997)}$$

$$= 0.167.$$

5. Of 10 million patients with acute abdominal pain, about 10 will have appendicitis, and of these 8 will also have "the symptoms." Of these 10 million patients, almost all will not have appendicitis, and of these about 100,000 will have "the symptoms." So just over 100,000 patients have "the symptoms," but only 8 of these have appendicitis. Hence, "other abdominal pain" is by far the more likely explanation for these symptoms.

6. a. $P[\text{RVD}|\text{IVP}^+] = \dfrac{P[\text{IVP}^+|\text{RVD}] \cdot P[\text{RVD}]}{P[\text{IVP}^+|\text{RVD}] \cdot P[\text{RVD}] + P[\text{IVP}^+|\text{No RVD}] \cdot P[\text{No RVD}]}$

$$= \dfrac{(0.78)\,(0.1)}{(0.78)\,(0.1) + (0.11)\,(0.9)}$$

$$= 0.441$$

$$= 44.1\%.$$

b. $P[\text{RVD}|\text{IVP}^-] = \dfrac{P[\text{IVP}^-|\text{RVD}] \cdot P[\text{RVD}]}{P[\text{IVP}^-|\text{RVD}] \circ P[\text{RVD}] + P[\text{IVP}^-|\text{No RVD}] \circ P[\text{No RVD}]}$

$= \dfrac{(0.22)\,(0.1)}{(0.22)\,(0.1) + (0.89)\,(0.9)}$

$= \dfrac{0.022}{0.022 + 0.801}$

$= 0.027$

$= 2.7\%.$

7. $P[\text{Abused}|\text{T}^+] = \dfrac{P[\text{T}^+|\text{Abused}] \cdot P[\text{Abused}]}{P[\text{T}^+|\text{Abused}] \cdot P[\text{Abused}] + P[\text{T}^+|\text{Not Abused}] \cdot P[\text{Not Abused}]}$

$= \dfrac{(0.95)\,(X)}{(0.95)\,(X) + (0.1)\,(1-X)},$

where X is the prevalence of abuse.

  a. When $X = 0.03$, $P[\text{Abused}|\text{T}^+] = 23\%$.
  b. When $X = 0.003$, $P[\text{Abused}|\text{T}^+] = 2.8\%$.
  c. When $X = 0.0003$, $P[\text{Abused}|\text{T}^+] = 0.28\%$.

8. Here we use the method of tree inversion. The original probability tree is shown in the text in Figure 4–11. This time we invert the tree so that the "factor X present" and "factor X absent" node precedes the "D" and "D̄" node. The inverted tree is shown in Figure S–10; branches whose probability is 0 have been omitted. We see that the revised probability that the patient has factor X is 4/9.

9. a. $P[\text{Perf}] = P[\text{Perf}|\text{App}] \circ P[\text{App}]$

$= (0.1875)\,(0.16)$

$= 0.03.$

  b. $P[\text{Perf}] = P[\text{Perf}|\text{App}] \circ P[\text{App}]$

$= (0.24)\,(0.16)$

$\cong 0.038.$

Figure S–10   *A solution to Exercise 8, Chapter Four.*

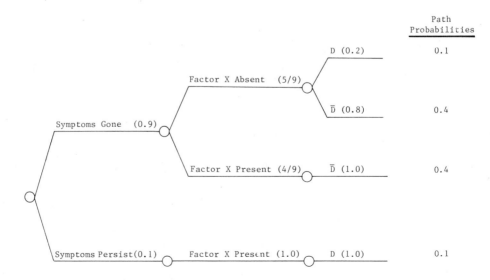

c. We use a 3 × 3 contingency table and fix the column totals according to the result from part b and the given probability of appendicitis of 0.16:

Patient's Condition	Appendix Perforated	Appendix Inflamed	NSAP	Row Totals
Worse	0.032	0.098	0	0.13
Same	0.006	0.024	0.33	0.36
Better	0	0	0.51	0.51
Column totals	0.038	0.122	0.84	1.00

The row totals indicate that
  i. $P[\text{Worse}] = 0.13$;
  ii. $P[\text{Same}] = 0.36$;
  iii. $P[\text{Better}] = 0.51$.

d. i. $P[\text{Perf}|\text{Worse}] = \dfrac{P[\text{Perf and Worse}]}{P[\text{Worse}]}$

$$= \frac{0.032}{0.13}$$

$$= 0.25.$$

  ii. $P[\text{Perf}|\text{Same}] = \dfrac{P[\text{Perf and Same}]}{P[\text{Same}]}$

$$= \frac{0.006}{0.36}$$

$$= 0.017.$$

  iii. $P[\text{Perf}|\text{Better}] = \dfrac{P[\text{Perf and Better}]}{P[\text{Better}]}$

$$= 0.$$

e. i. $P[\text{Inf}|\text{Worse}] = \dfrac{P[\text{Inf and Worse}]}{P[\text{Worse}]}$

$$= \frac{0.098}{0.13}$$

$$= 0.75.$$

  ii. $P[\text{Inf}|\text{Same}] = \dfrac{P[\text{Inf and Same}]}{P[\text{Same}]}$

$$= \frac{0.024}{0.36}$$

$$= 0.066.$$

  iii. $P[\text{Inf}|\text{Better}] = \dfrac{P[\text{Inf and Better}]}{P[\text{Better}]}$

$$= 0.$$

10. a. i. The prior probability, or prevalence, of appendicitis among patients with abdominal pain is *lower* for older persons than for younger persons.
    ii. The ratio,

$$\frac{CTN - CFP}{CTP - CFN},$$

is larger for older than for younger patients. To demonstrate this, we note that

$$CFP \text{ (old)} = 4.0; \; CTN \text{ (old)} = 0; \; CFN \text{ (old)} = 67.3; \; CTP \text{ (old)} = 5.7;$$

and that

$$CFP \text{ (young)} = 0.7; \; CTN \text{ (young)} = 0; \; CFN \text{ (young)} = 13.8; \; CTP \text{ (young)} = 0.9.$$

Hence,

$$\frac{CTN - CFP}{CTP - CFN}(\text{old}) = \frac{0 - 4.0}{5.7 - 67.3}$$

$$= 0.065;$$

and

$$\frac{CTN - CFP}{CTP - CFN}(\text{young}) = \frac{0 - 0.7}{0.9 - 13.8}$$

$$= 0.054.$$

    iii. In older patients with appendicitis the distribution of the separator variable based on symptoms and signs *overlaps more* with the corresponding distribution for patients with NSAP than is the case in younger patients.

b. i. The lower prevalence raises the prior odds against disease in Equation 4–21. This shifts the optimal likelihood ratio to a larger value, which corresponds to more severe symptoms. As the prevalence of appendicitis approaches 0, you should require more and more florid symptoms to warrant surgery.

    ii. The ratio,

$$\frac{CTN - CFP}{CTP - CFN},$$

is larger in older persons. The implication is that the penalty for the removal of a nondiseased appendix is even worse relative to the penalty for perforation in older persons than is the case in younger persons. This tends to make one even more anxious to avoid unnecessary surgery in older as compared with younger patients. Thus, we ought to become more cautious and willing to forgo operations on older patients with milder symptoms.

    iii. By shifting the appendicitis distribution to the left in older persons (Figure S–11), the likelihood ratio for appendicitis has become greater for milder symptoms. In order to reduce the likelihood ratio to its initial level, the cut-off point would tend to shift to the left (milder symptoms) as well. Thus, of the three factors, the first two tend to lead to a more stringent criterion for surgery in older persons, and the last tends to lead to a less stringent criterion.

c. Additional data that would be helpful include the following:

    i. The prevalence of appendicitis in older patients with acute abdominal pain;

    ii. The conditional probabilities of signs, symptoms, and laboratory tests in each diagnostic category, so that a separator variable can be developed.

11. The plot of *TPR* versus *TNR* would be a right-left mirror image of the conventional ROC curve, as shown in Figure S–12. An economist might see this relation as resembling a "production possibility frontier" showing the possible combinations of true-positive and true-negative rates that might be attained. The line with a slope equal to the product of the prior odds and the net consequence ratio in this plot would then be analogous to the economist's "indifference" curve and would run from upper left to lower right in this plot. The point of tangency between this line and the curve would correspond to the optimal operating point on the ROC curve.

Figure S–11 A solution to Exercise 10, Chapter Four. To preserve the likelihood ratio, a/b, the cutoff point must move to the left.

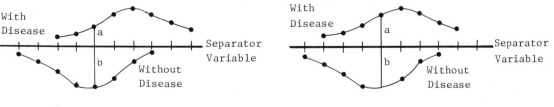

Younger Persons   Older Persons

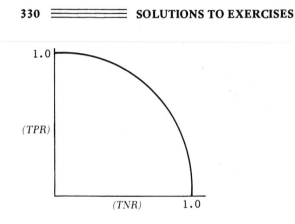

Figure S–12 *A solution to Exercise 11, Chapter Four.*

SOLUTIONS TO EXERCISES FOR CHAPTER FIVE

1. The answers are contained in Figure 5–10. Using Bayes' formula,

$$P[\text{Hep}|\text{Indicates Hep}] = \frac{P[\text{Indicates Hep}|\text{Hep}] \cdot P[\text{Hep}]}{P[\text{Indicates Hep}|\text{Hep}] \cdot P[\text{Hep}] + P[\text{Indicates Hep}|\text{Cirr}] \cdot P[\text{Cirr}]}$$

$$= \frac{(0.9)(0.6)}{(0.9)(0.6) + (0.05)(0.4)}$$

$$= 0.96;$$

$$P[\text{Hep}|\text{Indicates Cirr}] = \frac{P[\text{Indicates Cirr}|\text{Hep}] \cdot P[\text{Hep}]}{P[\text{Indicates Cirr}|\text{Hep}] \cdot P[\text{Hep}] + P[\text{Indicates Cirr}|\text{Cirr}] \cdot P[\text{Cirr}]}$$

$$= \frac{(0.1)(0.6)}{(0.1)(0.6) + (0.95)(0.4)}$$

$$= 0.14.$$

2. a. The decision tree is shown in Figure S–13. To derive the probabilities at chance nodes Ⓐ, Ⓑ, Ⓒ, Ⓓ, and Ⓔ, we use Bayes' formula:

$P[Pneumo|\text{Indicates } Pneumo]$

$$= \frac{P[\text{Indicates } Pneumo|Pneumo] \cdot P[Pneumo]}{P[\text{Indicates } Pneumo|Pneumo] \cdot P[Pneumo] + P[\text{Indicates } Pneumo|\text{No } Pneumo] \cdot P[\text{No } Pneumo]}$$

$$= \frac{(1)(0.2)}{(1)(0.2) + (0.1)(0.8)}$$

$$= 0.71;$$

$P[Pneumo|\text{Indicates No } Pneumo] = 0.$

The averaging out at Ⓑ and Ⓒ indicates that pentamidine is indicated if the biopsy indicates *Pneumocystis*, but the averaging out at Ⓓ and Ⓔ demonstrates that pentamidine is not indicated if the biopsy does not indicate *Pneumocystis*. After folding back and averaging out to Ⓐ, we find a six-month survival rate of 0.619 with the biopsy. This is compared with 0.604 without the biopsy, for an EVCI of

$$0.619 - 0.604 = 0.015,$$

or a 1.5 per cent survival rate.

b. Let the mortality from the biopsy be r. Then $(r)(0.619)$ is the reduction in survival, owing to the biopsy. For the EVCI to exceed the risk, we must have

$$0.015 > (r)(0.619).$$

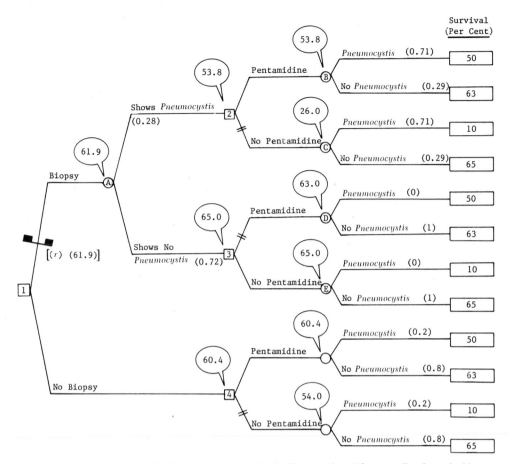

Figure S–13 *A decision tree for Exercise 2, Chapter Five. (The mortality from the biopsy is indicated by r.)*

Hence, if the mortality is less than 2.4 per cent, the biopsy is indicated.

c. In this case we find that

$$P[Pneumocystis | \text{Biopsy Indicates No } Pneumocystis] = 0.05,$$

$$P[\text{No } Pneumocystis | \text{Biopsy Indicates No } Pneumocystis] = 0.95.$$

Hence, the expected value at Ⓓ is 0.624, and at Ⓔ it is 0.623. At decision node ③ following a negative finding from the biopsy, pentamidine is still preferred, if ever so slightly. Without averaging out and folding back the rest of the tree, we are safe in concluding that the EVCI of the biopsy is 0, because the decision regarding pentamidine is unaffected by the result.

3. a. By Bayes' formula,

$$P[X | A^+, B^+] = \frac{P[A^+, B^+ | X] \cdot P[X]}{P[A^+, B^+ | X] \cdot P[X] + P[A^+, B^+ | \overline{X}] \cdot P[\overline{X}]}.$$

By conditional independence,

$$P[X | A^+, B^+] = \frac{P[A^+ | X] \cdot P[B^+ | X] \cdot P[X]}{P[A^+ | X] \cdot P[B^+ | X] \cdot P[X] + P[A^+ | \overline{X}] \cdot P[B^+ | \overline{X}] \cdot P[\overline{X}]}$$

$$= \frac{(0.8)(0.7)(0.01)}{(0.9)(0.7)(0.01) + (0.1)(0.1)(0.99)}$$

$$= 0.36,$$

or 36 per cent.

b. $P[A^+, B^+|\overline{X}]$ is at *most* 0.1 (if *all* patients without disease who have positive results on test A also have positive results on test B). $P[A^+, B^+|X]$ is at *least* 0.5 (if, among patients with disease, *all* patients with a negative result on test A have a positive result on test B, and *all* patients with a negative result on test B have a positive result on test A).

Therefore,

$$P[X|A^+, B^+] > \frac{(0.5)\,(0.01)}{(0.5)\,(0.01) + (0.1)\,(0.99)}$$

$$= 0.048.$$

The revised probability of disease could be as low as 4.8 per cent.

4. a. 25.0 per cent.
   b. 47.1 per cent.
   c. i.   72.7 per cent.
      ii.   17.4 per cent.
     iii.   40.9 per cent.
      iv.   5.2 per cent.
   d. i.   87.0 per cent.
      ii.   0.0 per cent.
     iii.   19.8 per cent.
      iv.   7.2 per cent.
   e. Given that conditional independence no longer holds, when both test results are negative we can be less confident in ruling out the disease, but when both test results are positive we can be more confident in ruling in the disease.

SOLUTIONS TO EXERCISES FOR CHAPTER SEVEN

1. The expected dollar costs of the alternative strategies are computed in the same way as the expected mortality using the decision tree in Figure 3–10.

For the "decide now" branch, the expected cost would be

$$(0.03)\,(\$3,000) + (0.13)\,(\$1,500) + (0.84)\,(\$1,500) = \$1,545.$$

The expected cost for the "wait six hours" branch would be

$$(0.13)\,[(0.25)\,(\$3,060) + (0.75)\,(\$1,560)]$$

$$+ (0.36)\,[(0.017)\,(\$3,060) + (0.066)\,(\$1,560) + (0.917)\,(\$1,560)]$$

$$+ (0.51)\,[(1.0)\,(\$60)]$$

$$= \$251.55 + \$570.78 + \$30.60$$

$$= \$852.93.$$

Hence, the expected dollar *savings* following the "wait six hours" strategy would be

$$\$1,545 - \$853 = \$692.$$

The alert reader may have realized that if all we cared about were dollar savings, the cheapest strategy of all would have been simply to send every patient home without surgery (assuming that no one would come back later for more care). Of course, that is both undesirable and unrealistic. On the other hand, effect on mortality is usually not the only outcome we care about. Dealing with both cost and clinical outcome in a clinical situation is the subject of Chapter Eight.

2. The probability of surviving exactly n years is the difference between the survival rate to $n - 1$ years and the survival rate to n years. For example, the probability of living exactly five years is 0.56 minus 0.49, or 0.07.

Life expectancy is the expected value of length of survival. It is equal to

$$(0.20)\,(1) + (0.08)\,(2) + (0.08)\,(3) + (0.08)\,(4) + \ldots + (0.01)\,(23),$$

or

6.46 years.

An easy way to compute life expectancy is simply to *add* the survival probabilities in Table 7-2. In this way the 0.2 mortality in year 1 is counted once, the 0.08 mortality in year 2 is counted twice, and so forth up to the 0.01 mortality in year 23, which is counted 23 times. Hence, the result agrees with the formula for expected value, as given previously.

3. a. Let b stand for $u(B)$. Then the expected utility with surgery is

$$(0.99)\,(b),$$

and the expected utility with delay is

$$(0.7)\,(1) + (0.3)\,[(0.9)\,(0.95) + (0.1)\,(0)]$$
$$= 0.957.$$

Delaying surgery is preferred if

$$0.957 > (0.99)\,(b),$$

or

$$b < 0.966.$$

Hence, delay is preferred if the outcome of amputation below the knee is less desirable than a gamble consisting of a 96.6 per cent chance of total cure and a 3.4 per cent chance of death.

b. Let a stand for $u(A)$. Then the expected utility with surgery is

$$(0.99)\,(0.99) = 0.98,$$

and the expected utility with delay is

$$(0.7)\,(1) + (0.3)\,[(0.9)\,(a) + (0.1)\,(0)]$$
$$= 0.7 + (0.27)\,(a).$$

Delaying surgery is preferred if

$$0.7 + (0.27)\,(a) > 0.98,$$

or

$$0.27a > 0.28,$$

or

$$a > 0.28/0.27 = 1.04.$$

Now, the utility of A cannot be greater than 1 if cure is better than the loss of limb. Hence, if $u(B)$ equals 0.99, then surgery is preferable regardless of the utility assigned to the outcome of amputation above the knee.

c. The question is whether the gamble

$$<(0.75,\ C);\ (0.25,\ A)>$$

is better or worse than B for certain. In terms of expected utilities, is

$$(0.75)\,u(C) + (0.25)\,u(A) > u(B)?$$

Substituting the utilities given, we have for the left-hand side of the inequality

$$(0.75)\,(1.0) + (0.25)\,(0.95) = 0.9875,$$

which is less than 0.99. Hence, this patient would prefer amputation below the knee.

4. a. The three possible outcomes are survival without recurrence (S, $\overline{R}$), survival with recurrence (S, R), and death ($\overline{S}$). The decision maker must first determine the best and worst outcomes, which are obviously (S, $\overline{R}$) and $\overline{S}$, respectively. Assign values of 1.0 and 0.0 to these outcomes. To get the values for the intermediate outcome, get an assessment of the probability, p, such that the patient or physician is indifferent between (S, R) for sure and a gamble giving a chance of p at (S, $\overline{R}$) and a chance of $1 - p$ at $\overline{S}$.

In the following dialogue, A represents the decision analyst and P represents the patient or physician. The conversation might proceed as follows:

A: Imagine that you have previously had a gastrectomy but that your ulcer has recurred. If there were an operation that could absolutely guarantee elimination of the ulcer with no further recurrence but it had a 70 per cent chance of mortality, would you elect to undergo this surgery?

P: Definitely not at that high risk of death!

A: What if the operation had a mortality of only 1 per cent?

P: Well, then I'd take it.

A: What if the operation had a mortality of 10 per cent?

P: I don't think I would risk that. I guess I place a high value on avoiding death, particularly if it's my own. (Here is an insight!)

A: Well, then, what about a risk of 5 per cent to alleviate your present suffering?

P: That starts to get tough, but I still prefer no surgery. I think I see what you're driving at.

A: It seems that somewhere between 1 per cent and 5 per cent there must be a point where you'd be just as willing to undergo surgery as to remain as you are.

P: I guess so. I think it would be around 3 per cent.

They have just determined that p is equal to 0.97, which equals $u(S, R)$.

b. Suppose that your utilities are

$$u(S, \overline{R}) = 1.00,$$

$$u(S, R) = 0.97,$$

and

$$u(\overline{S}) = 0.00.$$

If we substitute these utilities into the decision tree of Figure 7–2, we derive Figure S-14. The expected utilities are as follows:

$$\text{Expected } u(\text{Gastrectomy}) = 0.959,$$

$$\text{Expected } u(\text{Vagotomy}) = 0.987,$$

$$\text{Expected } u(\text{No Surgery}) = 0.976.$$

Hence, if the preceding are your utilities, your preferred course of action is vagotomy.

c. If we average out the decision tree, we have, in general,

$$\text{Expected } u(\text{Gastrectomy}) = (0.96)(0.98) + (0.96)(0.02) \, u(S, R)$$

$$= 0.9408 + 0.0192 \, u(S, R);$$

$$\text{Expected } u(\text{Vagotomy}) = (0.99)(0.90) + (0.99)(0.10) \, u(S, R)$$

$$= 0.891 + 0.099 \, u(S, R);$$

$$\text{Expected } u(\text{No Surgery}) = (0.2) + (0.8) \, u(S, R).$$

If gastrectomy were optimal, then it would have a higher expected utility than vagotomy:

$$0.941 + 0.019 \, u(S, R) > 0.891 + 0.099 \, u(S, R),$$

or

$$0.05 > 0.08 \, u(S, R),$$

or

$$u(S, R) < 0.625.$$

Hence, the utility of recurrence must be less than 0.625, so that survival with recurrence would be *less* desirable than a lottery giving a 5/8 chance of survival without recurrence but a 3/8 chance of death.

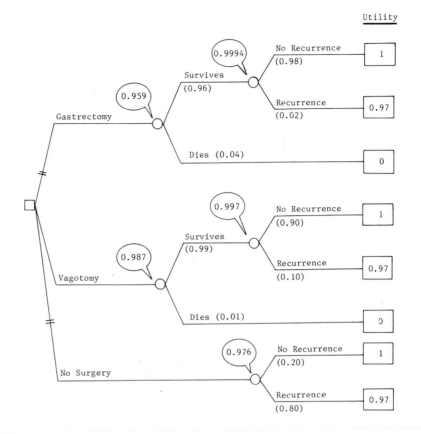

Figure S–14 A solution to Exercise 4b, Chapter Seven.

Also, the expected utility for gastrectomy would have to exceed that for no surgery. Hence,

$$0.941 + 0.019 \, u(S, R) > 0.2 + 0.8 \, u(S, R),$$

or

$$0.741 > 0.781 \, u(S, R),$$

or

$$u(S, R) < 0.95,$$

which is superfluous given that $u(S, R)$ must be less than 0.625. Thus, for gastrectomy to be optimal the utility of (S, R) must be less than 0.625:

$$u(S, R) < 0.625:$$

d. For no surgery to be optimal, it must have a higher expected utility than vagotomy. Hence,

$$0.2 + 0.8 \, u(S, R) > 0.891 + 0.099 \, u(S, R),$$

or

$$0.701 \, u(S, R) > 0.691,$$

or

$$u(S, R) > 0.986.$$

Thus, in order that no surgery be optimal, survival with recurrence would have to be preferable as an outcome to a lottery giving a 98.6 per cent chance of survival without recurrence and a 1.4 per cent chance of death.

5. a. One possible formulation is shown in Figure S–15. We assume that repeated surgery (if there is no change in symptoms) is not possible, but the reader, as an additional exercise, may wish to modify the tree to allow for repeated surgery.

b. The four possible outcomes are relief (R), no change in symptoms (S), above-knee amputation (A), and death (D). Assign the following utilities: $u(R)$ equals 1; $u(S)$ equals u_S; $u(A)$ equals u_A; and $u(D)$ equals 0.
Surgery is preferred if

$$0.80 + 0.12\, u_S + (0.06)\,(0.96)\, u_A > u_S,$$

or

$$0.80 + 0.0576 u_A > 0.88 u_S. \qquad \text{(S–1)}$$

Suppose that for your patient u_S equals 0.95 and u_A equals 0.9. Then the inequality reads

$$0.80 + (0.0576)\,(0.9) > (0.88)\,(0.95),$$

or

$$0.80 + 0.052 > 0.836,$$

which is true. Hence, surgery is indicated.

c. Surgery would not be preferred if the utility of continued symptoms relative to amputation were high enough. If, for example, the golfer assesses a utility of 0.99 for continued symptoms (u_S) and a utility of 0.9 for amputation (u_A), then it would be best not to operate on this patient.

d. Inequality S–1 gives us the combinations of utilities for which surgery is indicated. Note that relatively higher values of u_A and lower values of u_S favor surgery, as would be expected. We can portray this graphically, as in Figure S–16. Surgery is preferred if the utilities fall within the shaded area.

Figure S–15 *A solution to Exercise 5, Chapter Seven.*

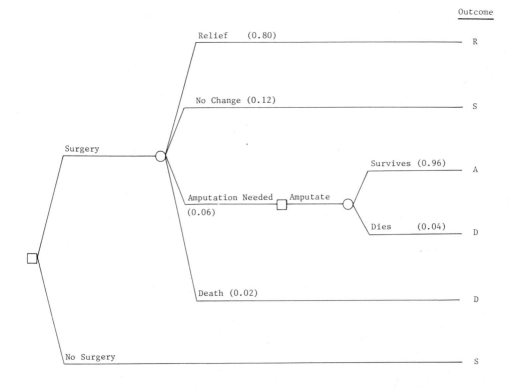

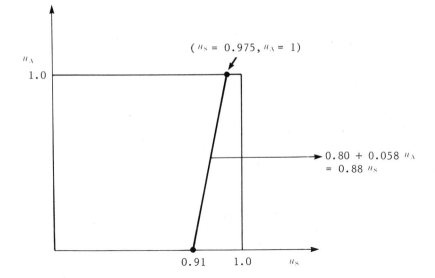

Figure S–16 *A solution to Exercise 5d, Chapter Seven.*

6. Quality weights for T_1, T_2, D_1, and D_2 are derived from i through iii as follows:

$$u(T_1) = 1.0;$$
$$u(T_2) = 0.6 \text{ (from i)};$$
$$u(D_1) = 0.8 \text{ (from iii)};$$
$$u(D_2) = 0.4 \text{ (from ii and iii)}.$$

The problem is made tractable by a decision tree such as that in Figure S–17.

a. Quality-adjusted life expectancy with dialysis equals

$$(0.5) (10) u(D_1) + (0.5) (10) u(D_2)$$
$$= 4.0 + 2.0$$
$$= 6.0 \text{ years}.$$

b. Quality-adjusted life expectancy for a patient who survives a transplant operation and accepts the kidney equals

$$(0.6) (12.5) u(T_1) + (0.4) (12.5) u(T_2)$$
$$= 7.5 + 3.0$$
$$= 10.5 \text{ years}.$$

c. Quality-adjusted life expectancy for a patient who survives the transplant operation equals

$$P[\text{Accept}] \ (10.5) + P[\text{Reject}] \ (6.0)$$
$$= (0.6) (10.5) + (0.4) (6.0)$$
$$= 6.3 + 2.4$$
$$= 8.7 \text{ years}.$$

d. Quality-adjusted life expectancy with transplantation equals

$$P[\text{Survive}] \ (8.7)$$
$$= (0.8) (8.7)$$
$$= 6.96 \text{ years}.$$

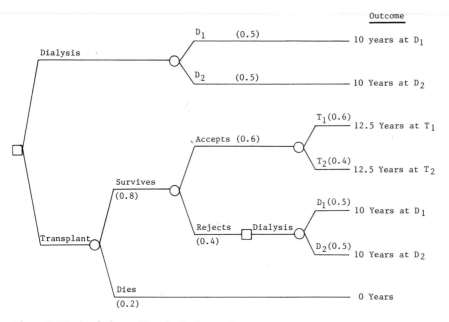

Outcome

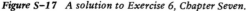

Figure S-17 A solution to Exercise 6, Chapter Seven.

e. Transplantation yields a greater quality adjusted life expectancy than dialysis, 6.96 years versus 6.00 years, given the assumptions made about preferences and probabilities.

f. Let $u(D_1)$ equal y. Then $u(D_2)$ would equal $(0.5)y$.
Quality-adjusted life expectancy with dialysis equals

$$(0.5)(10)(y) + (0.5)(10)(0.5)(y)$$
$$= (5.0)y + (2.5)y$$
$$= (7.5)y.$$

Quality-adjusted life expectancy for a patient who survives a transplant operation equals

$$P[\text{Accept}](10.5) + P[\text{Reject}](7.5)(y)$$
$$= (0.6)(10.5) + (0.4)(7.5)(y)$$
$$= 6.3 + (3.0)y.$$

Quality-adjusted life expectancy with transplantation, therefore, equals

$$(0.8)(6.3 + 3.0y)$$
$$= 5.04 + (2.4)y.$$

Dialysis is preferred to transplantation if

$$(7.5)y > 5.04 + (2.4)y,$$

or

$$(5.1)y > 5.04,$$

or

$$y > 0.988.$$

For dialysis to be preferred, therefore, the patient would have to prefer ten years with state D_1 (successful dialysis) to 9.88 years with state T_1 (successful transplant). In other words, the patient would have to be unwilling to give up 1.2 per cent of life expectancy to avoid being on dialysis.

SOLUTIONS TO EXERCISES FOR CHAPTER EIGHT

1. Surgery and no surgery would have the same quality-adjusted survival time when the following equation holds:

$$(0.5)\,(x) = (0.58)\,(0) + (0.42)\,(134),$$

or

$$x = 112.6 \text{ days}.$$

Note that this is just twice the number of days calculated in Section 8.3. Since each day of survival without surgery is worth half as much here as it is in the example in the text, survival time must be at least twice as long before surgery becomes the inferior choice.

2. a. We may use Bayes' formula to calculate the probability that a patient with a positive result on the screening test actually has the disease:

$$P[D|T^+] = \frac{P[T^+|D] \circ P[D]}{P[T^+|D] \circ P[D] + P[T^+|\overline{D}] \circ P[\overline{D}]}$$

$$= \frac{(0.95)\,(0.00001)}{(0.95)\,(0.00001) + (0.01)\,(0.99999)}$$

$$= \frac{0.0000095}{0.0000095 + 0.0099999}$$

$$\cong 0.00095.$$

With surgery the mortality is 0.001. Without surgery the mortality is 50 per cent for those who have the disease, or

$$(0.5)\,(0.00095) = 0.000475$$

among all patients with positive test results. Since performing surgery leads to a higher mortality than doing nothing among those with positive test results, surgery is not indicated under the assumptions given.

b. With the higher prevalence, the predictive value of a positive result on a screening test increases to

$$P[D|T^+] \cong 0.0095,$$

and the probability of death without surgery is

$$(0.5)\,(0.0095) = 0.00475.$$

This is higher than the 0.001 mortality with surgery. Hence, surgery is indicated for those with positive test results if the prevalence is 10^{-4}.

The net benefit of surgery for patients with positive test results is a difference in the mortality probability of

$$0.00475 - 0.001 = 0.00375.$$

That is, of every 100,000 patients with positive test results, surgery will save 375 lives.

c. Consider the decision tree in Figure S–18. Notice that all outcomes have two attributes: the percentage who survive and resource cost. Costs represent simply the sums of the costs of screening or surgery or both along each path. Probabilities on the tree are calculated from the data given using Bayes' formula. For example,

$$P[D|T^-] = \frac{P[T^-|D] \cdot P[D]}{P[T^-|D] \cdot P[D] + P[T^-|\overline{D}] \cdot P[\overline{D}]}$$

$$= \frac{(0.05)\,(0.0001)}{(0.05)\,(0.0001) + (0.99)\,(0.9999)}$$

$$= \frac{0.000005}{0.000005 + 0.989901}$$

$$\cong 0.00000505.$$

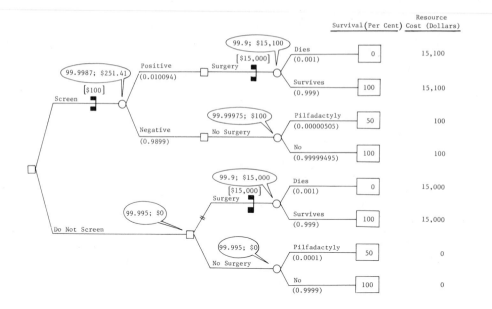

Figure S-18   A solution to Exercise 2, Chapter Eight.

Next we average out both costs and survival as a percentage and indicate the averaged-out values in the "balloon" at each node. Folding back to the initial choice, we find that screening yields an expected net benefit of survival of

$$99.9987 - 99.995 = 0.0037$$

per cent at an expected net cost of

$$\$251.41 - \$0.00 = \$251.41.$$

The cost per life saved is, therefore,

$$\$251.41/(0.0037)\,(0.01) \cong \$6,800,000.$$

d. The result calculated is an extraordinarily high cost per life saved. It seems very likely that more cost-effective ways could be found to spend these resources in health care. Notice, however, that the result is particularly sensitive to the prevalence of disease; for example, the cost per life saved if the prevalence were as high as 10^{-3} (1/1,000) would be approximately \$570,000, less than one tenth of the amount calculated at the lower prevalence. If the surgery were free, however, at the original prevalence the cost per life saved by the screening test would still be

$$\$100/(0.0037)\,(0.01) \cong \$2,700,000.$$

Hence, the result does not depend so much on the induced costs of surgery as on the cost of screening itself and on the prevalence of disease.

3. a. Present-value costs are computed according to the formula

$$P = S_0 + \frac{S_1}{(1 + r)^1} + \frac{S_2}{(1 + r)^2} + \frac{S_3}{(1 + r)^3} + \frac{S_4}{(1 + r)^4},$$

as given in Section 8.4 (p. 249). For example, for program B at a discount rate of 5 per cent,

$$P = \$40,000 + \frac{\$30,000}{(1.05)^1} + \frac{\$10,000}{(1.05)^2} + \frac{\$10,000}{(1.05)^3} + \frac{\$10,000}{(1.05)^4} \cong \$94,500.$$

The rest of the results are given in Table S-1.

According to these results, program C is less expensive than either A or B at discount rates of 5 per cent and 10 per cent. This reflects the reduced weights assigned to costs borne in later years. Generally, a program that is least costly at one discount rate need not be the least costly at every discount rate.

b. To calculate the amortized cost, C, we use the formula given in Section 8.4 (p. 243), which can be rewritten as

$$C = \frac{Pr (1 + r)^{N-1}}{(1 + r)^{N} - 1},$$

TABLE S–1 SOLUTION TO EXERCISE 3a, CHAPTER EIGHT

DISCOUNT RATE	PRESENT-VALUE RESOURCE COST INVESTMENT*		
	Program A	Program B	Program C
0%	$100,000	$100,000	$100,000
5%	90,900	94,500	87,400
10%	83,400	89,900	77,100

*The present-value resource cost is rounded to the nearest hundred dollars.

where the discount rate r equals $i/100$. In this example, N equals four years; r equals 0, 0.05, or 0.1; and P is the present-value resource cost shown in Table S–1. For example, for program B at 5 per cent,

$$C \cong \frac{(\$94{,}500)\,(0.05)\,(1.05)^{4}}{(1.05)^{5} - 1}$$

$$\cong 20{,}800.$$

The rest of the results are given in Table S–2. Notice that at a discount rate of 0 the amortized cost of each project is simply its average annual cost. Note also that the amortized cost of program A is $20,000, regardless of the discount rate, because the costs of program A already accrue at a constant annual rate.

TABLE S–2 SOLUTION TO EXERCISE 3b, CHAPTER EIGHT

DISCOUNT RATE	AMORTIZED RESOURCE COST*		
	Program A	Program B	Program C
0%	$20,000	$20,000	$20,000
5%	20,000	20,800	19,200
10%	20,000	21,600	18,500

*The amortized resource cost is rounded to the nearest hundred dollars.

4. In a problem as complicated as this, it is usually worthwhile to begin by structuring the problem in the form of a decision tree. Such a tree is shown in Figure S–19. Note that the problem includes three kinds of outcomes: life expectancy, quality of life, and resource costs.

a. One could proceed to average out the expected number of years of life and the expected resource costs for each strategy. First, we want to compute the present value of benefits and costs for each possible outcome. These calculations are shown in Table S–3 for the seven possible outcomes corresponding to the seven paths in the decision tree. For the five possibilities following surgery, the path probabilities are given in parentheses. The life expectancy and expected cost for surgery are the averaged-out values across the five possibilities.

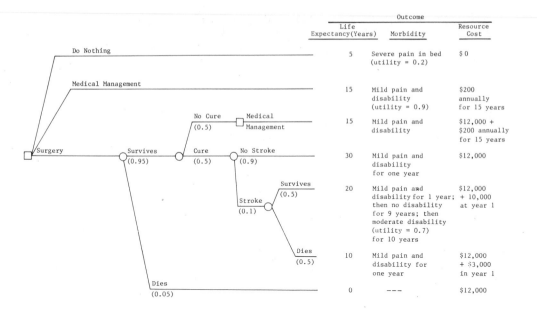

Figure S–19 *A possible decision tree for Exercise 4, Chapter Eight.*

TABLE S–3   SOLUTION (PART 1) TO EXERCISE 4a, CHAPTER EIGHT

STRATEGY OUTCOME (PROBABILITY)	LIFE EXPECTANCY*	EXPECTED COST*
Do nothing ...	4.55	$ 0
Medical management ...	10.90	2,180
Surgery	12.58	13,225
Survive, no cure (0.475)	10.90	14,180
Survive, cure, no stroke (0.4275)	16.14	12,000
Survive, cure, nonfatal stroke (0.02375)	13.09	18,139
Survive, cure, fatal stroke (0.02375)	8.11	13,842
Die (0.05)	0	12,000

*The present value is calculated at a 5 per cent annual discount rate.

    Next, we construct a table showing the incremental benefit and cost for each intervention (Table S–4). Medical management provides an additional year of life expectancy at a much lower cost than surgery, but surgery still would be the preferred strategy, so long as the cutoff point for dollars per year of life exceeds $6,574.40. If, for example, the next best use of resources could provide an additional year of life expectancy for $10,000, we would save more years of life by performing surgery on these patients. If, on the other hand, other interventions could save a year of life for less than $6,574.40 (but not less than $343.31), then surgery would be cost-ineffective and medical management would be the preferred use of resources.

b. First, we revise Table S–3 by "quality adjusting" the life expectancies. For example, in the "do nothing" strategy, the discounted life expectancy of 4.55 years is multiplied by 0.2 (the utility value for severe pain for a bedridden patient) to yield a quality-adjusted life expectancy of 0.91 years. These revised calculations are shown in Table S–5. The most complicated of these calculations is that for the outcome following surgery of "survive, cure, nonfatal stroke." We compute discounted quality-adjusted life expectancy for this outcome as follows. The first year, with mild pain and disability, is multiplied by 0.9. The next nine years have a present value equal to the difference between the present values of the first ten years (from data in the table provided in the problem) and the very first year, or

$$8.11 - 1.00 = 7.11.$$

This number is multiplied by 1.0, which is the utility of full health. The last ten years have a present value of

$$13.09 - 8.11 = 4.98,$$

and this quantity is multiplied by 0.7, the assumed utility for moderate disability from stroke. The total quality-adjusted life expectancy, then, is

$$(1) (0.9) + (7.11) (1) + (4.98) (0.7) = 11.50.$$

TABLE S–4   SOLUTION (PART 2) TO EXERCISE 4a, CHAPTER EIGHT

STRATEGY	ADDITIONAL YEARS OF LIFE EXPECTANCY*	INCREMENTAL RESOURCE COST*	INCREMENTAL COST PER ADDITIONAL YEAR OF LIFE EXPECTANCY*
Do nothing	...	...	...
Medical management	6.35	$ 2,180	$ 343.31
Surgery	1.68	11,045	6,574.40

*The present value is calculated at a 5 per cent annual discount rate.

TABLE S–5   SOLUTION (PART 1) TO EXERCISE 4b, CHAPTER EIGHT

STRATEGY	OUTCOME (PROBABILITY)	QUALITY-ADJUSTED LIFE EXPECTANCY*	EXPECTED COST*
Do nothing	...	0.91	$ 0
Medical management	...	9.81	2,180
Surgery		11.98	13,225
	Survive, no cure (0.475)	9.81	14,180
	Survive, cure, no stroke (0.4275)	16.04	12,000
	Survive, cure, nonfatal stroke (0.02375)	11.50	18,139
	Survive, cure, fatal stroke (0.02375)	8.01	13,842
	Die (0.05)	0	12,000

*The present value is calculated at a 5 per cent annual discount rate.

Next, we construct a table analogous to Table S–4 that shows the incremental benefit and cost for each intervention (Table S–6). In this example, considerations of the quality of life have not radically altered the comparative cost-effectiveness of the two alternatives, unless the cutoff point for the expenditure per QALY lies between $5,089.86 and $6,574.40. In that case, medical management would be preferred if considerations of the quality of life were ignored, but surgery would become the preferred choice if considerations of the quality of life were weighed in the decision.

TABLE S–6   SOLUTION (PART 2) TO EXERCISE 4b, CHAPTER EIGHT

STRATEGY	ADDITIONAL YEARS OF QUALITY-ADJUSTED LIFE EXPECTANCY*	INCREMENTAL RESOURCE COST*	INCREMENTAL COST PER ADDITIONAL YEAR OF QUALITY-ADJUSTED LIFE EXPECTANCY*
Do nothing	...	...	...
Medical management	8.90	$ 2,180	$ 244.94
Surgery	2.17	11,045	5,089.86

*The present value is calculated at a 5 per cent annual discount rate.

SOLUTIONS TO EXERCISES FOR CHAPTER NINE

1. A test is most sensitive when its results are most likely to be positive in patients who have the disease. This would occur at the most liberal possible test positivity criterion, or at a level between 1.00 and 1.49 mm. With this criterion, many patients would be classified as "positive," which would result in a large number of false positives but in very few false negatives. The most specific test positivity criterion would occur at the other extreme, at which only patients with a depression greater than 2.00 mm would be counted as "positive." Using this criterion would drastically reduce the number of false positives and concomitantly increase the number of false negatives.

2. The ROC curve plots the true-positive rate *(TPR)* against the false-positive rate *(FPR)* over the range of possible positivity criteria. As the criterion becomes progressively more restrictive, the curve arcs from upper right to lower left. Each point on the curve corresponds to a particular test likelihood ratio, namely, the ratio of the true-positive rate to the false-positive rate at the cutoff point. Thus, the entire curve of Figure 9–2 would be represented by a single point on the ROC curve. That point would have coordinates such that *TPR/FPR* equals 7.42 and would be obtained using a positivity criterion of an ST-segment depression greater than or equal to 1.0. The curve in Figure 9–2 is obtained by varying the prevalence of coronary artery disease from 0.0 to 1.0.

Index